To John for his sensitivity and existentialism

To Emmalea for her courage and creativity

To Joe for his humor and infinite patience

ACKNOWLEDGEMENTS

The truth is that although a book may be written by just one person, it is created by many. So, it is here that I hope to acknowledge everyone who participated in any way in creating this book. This book is the tangible product of many conversations, creative thoughts, different perspectives, and, of course, a lot of good old-fashioned hard work.

First, my husband and partner, Joe. We have been together since we were 17 years old. In many respects, this book started being written in 1976. He is the strength, the consistency, and where, appropriate, the humor, in this book. He is also the legal expert providing much input and critique into the content.

Emmalea, our daughter. Emmalea was the inspiration behind this book. Her stories provide many of the real life experiences that prove the recommendations I make to you are good and can produce effective results. In her short 21 years, she has already lived a life that many of us can only hope to aspire to – her experiences and her determination to figure it out and live the life she was meant to lead are part of that.

John, our son. John was the driving force for this book. His perspective on learning, by taking an interesting approach to everything, is embedded throughout the book. John's love of storytelling was the primary inspiration for my use of the stories of individuals to illustrate many of the points throughout the book.

Next, my mother, Helen Mamrak. My mother gave me so much positive feedback growing up that I have enough in the bank to last a lifetime. It took me almost 50 years to figure it out, but this positive feedback is the source of my ability to create and share with others, and endure the bad stuff that sometimes does happen. At the age of 70, she is also an inspiration to all of us as she keeps a trim figure, has excellent nutritional habits, and exercises at least 25 hours a week!

My father, Ed Mamrak. He was the computer geek and the entrepreneur who inspired and encouraged me to do my own thing. He continues to serve as an example of how to inject passion into your work. Having learned several new computer programs at the age of 70, he is also an inspiration to all of us for life-long learning.

My sister-in-law, Vera Reynolds. Vera is one of the "stars" of the book. She was gracious enough to allow her stories about how she successfully managed breast cancer. Vera's laugh, her love of life, her teaching, and her keen interest in other people were all part of the inspiration for this book.

Hank Franey, the CFO at the University of Maryland Medical Center has been a friend and a colleague for many years. On March 22, 2006, after a business meeting, Hank shared a few very touching stories with me about his two children, now young adults. What struck me the most was Hank's willingness to tell the stories with such emotion that his love for, and closeness with, his children was really reflected in every story. Hank's stories so affected me, that I changed my plans that night and went home to see my own children instead of heading for New York as planned. In some indirect way, I ended up the next morning with Emmalea during her first seizure, because of that conversation with Hank, for which I will always be grateful.

Charlie, Marti, and Kelly Mamrak, my brother and his family. They provided feedback, suggestions, direction, and a lot more editing than I am sure they planned on. Marti's input has been essential to the success of the book. Her editing, writing, marketing, and graphic artistry talents are responsible for how you see the finished product.

Ginger McQueen and David Moore, a dynamic duo that I have worked with for many years on many different ventures. Ginger has provided feedback, editing, and even encouragement that have all found their way into the book. David has taken the written word and spread it out into cyberspace so many more of us can benefit from this book. Other individuals who provided feedback, editing, design, or proofreading are: Kathleen Dunleavy, Esther Courtright, Lisa Horning, Ian Diener, Beth Sullivan, Mary Ann Haller, Maryann Marfia, Michelle Schafer, Cecilia Lucas, Jeff Russo, Valerie Reynolds, Steve Siegel, and Ruth Taswell.

Emmalea's doctors. Dr. Andrew Herzog at Harvard, and his groundbreaking research on the relationship between natural progesterone and seizures gave us a happy ending to the book (thanks!). Dr. Orrin Devinsky at NYU, and his proven techniques for assessing epilepsy have given us hope and stability when we thought there was none. And, Dr. Carl Bazil, at Columbia-Presbyterian in New York City, helped us to better understand the role of pharmaceuticals and epilepsy.

Lance Armstrong's writings about his own struggles have helped to make this book one that nearly everyone can relate to. Other "stars" in the book who shared their stories and helped make the book more interesting for everyone include: Christine and Jay Sostarecz, Maryann Marfia, John Russo, Kathy Gavin, Phoebe Moore, Lou Grujanac, Marsha Abraham and her daughters Wendy and Tammy, Dr. Kristen Jabbs, Dyanne and Rod Holt, Arnold Kauffman, and the 2,000 respondents to the Web-based survey on "positive experiences in healthcare" and the management team at Catholic Health Initiatives, Denver, Colorado and Lexington, Kentucky.

Sara, Michael, Kate and Todd Miller. Your story and your ability to embrace normalcy in the face of significant challenges has served as inspiration and your story is woven in between many lines of this book. Thank you for being an example of how proactive and positive we all can be.

Many physicians who have chosen to share their expertise by publishing books have contributed in some way to this book. They are: Ronald Hoffman, Andrew Weil, Jerome Groopman, Christiane Northrop, Mehmet Oz, Michael Roizen, and Joel Furhman.

Finally, all of my favorite authors in some way have made it into this book by the way they have shaped my view of the written word. They include: Steven Covey, Peter Senge, Napoleon Hill, Ken Blanchard, Jon Kabat-Zinn, Norman Cousins, Jim Collins, Jerry Porras, President Clinton, Jack Canfield, Peter Drucker, Kurt Eichenwald, Lois Frankel, Betty Rollins, Michael Porter, Marcus Buckingham, John Maxwell, Rick Warren, Jack Welch, John Grisham, Dale Carnegie, Norman Vincent Peale, Wayne Dyer, and Warren Bennis.

Thank you all.

7 Steps

to Your

Best Possible

Healthcare

Ruthann Russo
PhD, JD, MPH, RHIT

7 Steps to Your Best Possible Healthcare, by Ruthann Russo

Published by:
DJ Iber Publishing, Inc.
One Bethlehem Plaza, Suite 1010
Bethlehem, PA 18018
www.djiber.com

ISBN-13: 978-0-9799061-0-7
ISBN-10: 0-9799061-0-5

Manufactured in the United States of America
10 9 8 7 6 5 4 3 2 1

Library of Congress Control Number:

Editors: Marti Mamrak, Ginger McQueen, David Moore
Copyeditor: Mamrak and Associates, LLC
Proofreader: Cecilia Lucas
Cover and interior design: Concord Editorial and Design

Advice given is general. Neither the author nor the publisher is engaged in providing medical, health, or legal services. Readers should consult professional counsel for specific questions. The author and publisher expressly disclaim responsibility for any adverse effects arising from the use or application of the information contained in this book.

The author and editors have made every effort to verify the accuracy of all the resources, including Web sites, referred to in this book. However, organizations and Web sites mentioned may change or cease to operate after this book is published. Visit *www.ruthannruusso.com* and *www.djiber.com* for current resources.

TABLE OF CONTENTS

PREFACE

My son John and I had just completed our morning ritual, which included pulling him out from under our king-size bed, and scribbling cell phone numbers on a piece of paper folded up four times to fit neatly into his pocket. It was 1994. He was five. He did not have a cell phone, but those phone numbers provided him security to get through the long day in his kindergarten classroom, which was agonizing for him.

During the day, he would find security in the fact that my husband Joe, my mother, or I (the owners of the three phone numbers in his pocket) would be in the parking lot at the end of the day waiting for him. As we drove to school this one particular day, I explained to John that his dad would be picking him up at the end of the day. I had a class, I said, and would be home after dinner. He looked at me very intensely and asked, "Mommy, why do you go to school when you don't have to?"

One of the many things I have learned from John since that time is that everyone learns in different ways. Sometimes we do not even think of it as learning. In fact, it is when we are passionate about something and intensely engaged that we learn the best and usually don't even think of the process as work. This was the case with John.

A child with very high IQ scores, John initially was afraid of school and then grew quickly bored. He learned about the things he loved: filmmaking, music, baseball, computers, and other technology, on his own, outside of the system of traditional education. More importantly, through these pursuits he learned and exercised the skills he needed to succeed socially. A very popular teenager, John got there by practicing, albeit unconsciously, a specific set of skills. He supported others, shared what he had (including his brand new car, much to my husband's and my chagrin), and always contributed positively to conversations. I also learned from John that you can and you should make your own way in life. No one else will do that for you.

Lifelong learning, no matter how you achieve it, is a part of making your own way in life. No matter what your age, 9 or 109, or somewhere in between, it is my hope that this book can make a significant contribution to your lifelong learning and to your best possible health.

INTRODUCTION

It was a beautiful spring morning. My daughter Emmalea (pronounced like Emily) was enjoying her last day of spring break from Sarah Lawrence College. She had arrived home to Center Valley, Pennsylvania, the prior evening after 12 tiring hours of highway driving. We were talking casually about her recent trip to Atlanta. She was describing the blueberry-laden breakfast that her friend's father had prepared for them the day before: blueberry pancakes, blueberry waffles, blueberry grits. She kept losing her train of thought as she tried to finish a part of the story that had something to do with the syrup bottle. I teased her that she was becoming just like her father, unable to stay focused on the topic at hand.

I turned away for a second. When I turned back, Emmalea was face down on the floor, her body stiff and jerking in a hundred directions. The word seizure kept repeating in my mind and then the word made its way out of my mouth to the 911 operator. Emmalea would not remember those two minutes. I would relive them over and over.

At the hospital emergency room, the doctor's lips and mouth seemed to move in slow motion as the words *juvenile myoclonic epilepsy* poured out. So marked the beginning of our formal journey into healthcare consumerism.

Months later, Emmalea's statement to her father and me that her diagnosis of epilepsy was both a curse and a blessing became a primary inspiration for this book. She talked about how the epilepsy made her appreciate the good things in her life more than ever before, and she found herself focusing on living in the moment. There is an upside to health problems, even in the darkest of times.

The ultimate goal of this book is to increase your confidence in dealing with the healthcare system by educating you about the system in seven specific steps: create your own vision, own your story, build your relationships, assess quality, understand the people, know the places, and learn the language.

As a healthcare professional, I have been surrounded by hospitals and healthcare providers all of my working life. With the exception of the routine deliveries of my two children, I had never considered myself to be much of a healthcare consumer. Emmalea's experience changed that. We faced some significant challenges working our way through the system for the best possible healthcare solutions for Emmalea. I realized that if I had difficulty navigating the healthcare system as a consumer after spending 20 years working in healthcare, it must be much more difficult for the average healthcare consumer.

At some stage in life, each one of us is a healthcare consumer, whether directly or indirectly. Every healthcare consumer has a different story about how he or she was first thrust into the healthcare consumer maze. It may have been a personal experience with cancer or diabetes. A parent's stroke. A spouse's heart attack. A child's accident. The length and the intensity of the experience vary as well. A bump on the head and a few stitches to stop the bleeding can end your brief encounter as a healthcare consumer in the emergency room in just a few hours. For the lucky cancer survivor, whose tumor was caught through a needle biopsy the size of a pinhead, walking away from an acute phase of your role as a healthcare consumer may have occurred in a few months. For others, it can be months, years, and lifetimes of hospitals, doctors, and treatments.

For Emmalea, as the neurologist explained, there was good news and bad news. The good news is that *juvenile myoclonic epilepsy* (JME) is a form of epilepsy that is generally easy to control. The bad news is that JME is a lifetime disorder and may require treatment for the rest of Emmalea's life. Whatever the health situation, being informed about your options and confident in your decisions will help you navigate your way to the best possible healthcare.

HOW DO THE *7 STEPS* GET ME TO THE BEST POSSIBLE HEALTHCARE?

The topics in this book fall neatly into seven distinct areas, each essential for you, as a healthcare consumer, to understand. They address your vision, story, and relationships as well as the quality, people, places, and language of healthcare. You may be wondering, "If the goal is for me to get the best possible healthcare, how does this book get me there?" The simple answer is by increasing your knowledge, raising your sense of responsibility for your healthcare, and helping you make the best possible healthcare decisions.

The less obvious, but potentially more meaningful, answer is that if you read and follow the advice in this book, your confidence as a healthcare consumer is likely to grow. You can become more goal oriented and focused in your healthcare, saving time and money. By being more confident when interacting with your healthcare providers, you are more likely to increase their accountability to you. In the end, you will be the conductor of your own healthcare orchestra!

WHY THE HEALTHCARE CONSUMER?

I could have written this book with a focus on any number of groups. Learning how to better navigate the healthcare system provides benefits to many audiences: physicians, hospital administrators, students, and healthcare insurance companies. Physicians and other healthcare providers can benefit from learning about healthcare from the patient's perspective. They could also benefit from understanding how the consolidation of all health information on each patient into one location can help patients and the healthcare system overall. Hospital administrators could benefit from learning how better to respond to patients' needs to understand their health information and the healthcare system. Since administrators manage these processes, they have the ability and the resources to create this type of service for patients of their health systems. Medical students and other students in the healthcare provider professions also could benefit from an increased understanding of the importance of the health information that they document on every patient. Finally, health plans could implement a more holistic approach to the people they insure. Many health insurers have spent decades focusing on how to avoid payments to providers and how to force patients to comply with preventive health measures. Shifting their focus to patient education would likely empower patients, increase their responsibility and accountability, and potentially produce better healthcare results overall.

This book, however, is not specifically for any of these groups. This book is for you, the healthcare consumer, because you have the most challenges in the world of healthcare. You have the greatest degree of vulnerability and the greatest ability to do something about it. The power of each individual to obtain and act on knowledge about the healthcare system has the greatest potential to create change. We must use multiple strategies to improve healthcare delivery in this country. If we aren't engaged in what is going on, it is impossible to improve healthcare. This book shows how you can do your part to make the healthcare system work better for you.

The information in this book can empower you to get the best possible healthcare by increasing your knowledge of the healthcare system, its clinicians, and the information collected on you. If you and other healthcare consumers act on the information in this book, the healthcare system may serve everyone better.

WHY BUYING HEALTHCARE ISN'T LIKE BUYING ANYTHING ELSE

You find yourself in unfamiliar territory when buying treatment for a healthcare problem, yours or a family member's. No one prepares you for this role. Five factors make buying healthcare different from buying anything else: information, unpredictability, payment, emotion, and responsibility.

Information

There are two basic problems with medical information: complexity and excess. Most medical information is simply too technical for many patients to understand. The second problem is that the amount of medical information, available through the Internet, books, and other media, is overwhelming. You can begin to address these issues by learning basic medical terms and using only credible resources.

Unpredictability

You face two types of unpredictability in healthcare. The first is the unpredictability of the *results* you'll experience from the healthcare you receive. The second is the unpredictability of exactly *when* you will need healthcare intervention. You can take some actions to increase your control of unpredictability by engaging in preventive care, such as annual physicals, screening for certain conditions, eating healthy foods, and exercising.

Payment

Healthcare purchases are different from other purchases. If you are insured, you may pay for a small portion of the healthcare bill. For example, you may pay a $20 co-payment for a doctor visit. Because your insurer pays the majority of the bill, it changes your purchasing behavior in two ways. First, with someone else paying the bill, it relieves you of some responsibility. When you are not responsible for the payment, you may not be as responsible for your health. Second, in all other purchasing, you follow your own set of rules. When your insurance company is paying the bill, you must follow its rules, such as selecting in-network doctors. You can manage the payment process by being as familiar as possible with your health plan's policies.

Emotion

The emotional component of healthcare makes buying healthcare different from buying anything else. Your discomfort may be due to your lack of knowledge of healthcare information, systems, and processes. If so, you can manage the emotional component of healthcare by becoming more familiar with the healthcare systems.

Responsibility

Because of complex information, unpredictability, payment rules, and emotion, you may feel like a victim of the healthcare system. You can care more responsibly for yourself by focusing on how to improve your health. If you take responsibility for your healthcare and are engaged in understanding how your body works, you improve the chances of better health. As we all become more responsible for our healthcare and our health, a positive overall shift may occur in healthcare cost, quality, and processes.

HOW THIS BOOK IS ORGANIZED

As the title suggests, the book is organized into seven steps, summarized as follows:

- Step 1, *Create your vision,* helps you to create your healthcare values, vision, and mission statements. You develop a plan for your healthcare and health status using your own values, vision, and mission statements. These are dynamic and you can reference them for guidance and to reassess your priorities. In this section, I also discuss the process for ensuring you have the best possible primary care physician, medical mentors, and health insurance coverage.
- Step 2, *Own your story*, talks about how your medical records—or healthcare biography—are created. In this section, I also discuss why providers collect and maintain health information on you, as well as gaining, keeping, and limiting others' access to your health information. Health information is another term for medical record. Health information can also include x-ray films and other images that often are stored outside of the medical record. I use both terms throughout this book.
- Step 3, *Build your relationships,* describes your rights and responsibilities as a patient. I also discuss actions to improve communication between you and your physicians and other members of your healthcare team. I describe reasons why you may want a second opinion, how to obtain one, and what to do with the information once you have it.
- Step 4, *Assess quality,* helps you to define exactly what quality in healthcare means to you. I also describe how to use Internet-based tools to rate the quality of your healthcare providers and your health plan. In addition, in this chapter I explore the impact and

ethics of medical research. I also share my thoughts with you regarding what is referred to as the growing "medicalization" of life—a term referring to how more and more conditions previously thought of as normal are now being medically treated.

- Step 5, *Understand the people,* identifies different types of healthcare providers, how they are educated, and what they do. I specifically describe the education and training of physicians to help you better understand the rigor of their preparation and what drives and inspires them. I also explain complementary and alternative medicine options and the providers who practice in this area.
- Step 6, *Know the places,* acquaints you with the many different locations where you can receive healthcare, as well as the difference between teaching and non-teaching hospitals. I outline the steps you need to take to make sure your providers in various locations have access to your health information.
- Step 7, *Learn the language,* describes the most common medical terminology, phrases, and abbreviations. It also provides methods and resources to learn more on the topic. In addition, I talk how the documentation in your record is translated into coded data.

THE PATIENTS IN THIS BOOK

Many chapters in this book begin with a relevant, true healthcare story. You will read several stories from my daughter Emmalea (who has epilepsy) and my sister-in-law Vera (a cancer survivor). They have kindly agreed to share their stories with the hope of helping others to benefit from their experiences. I've included several stories of my own as well. In addition, you will read stories from many others. These stories are based upon the accounts from 2,000 respondents to a Web-based survey I conducted for this book. In the survey, I asked respondents to tell me three stories about positive experiences they had with the healthcare system. All respondents agreed to let me use their stories in this book without revealing their identities. To preserve anonymity, I have changed their names, and in some cases, modified some inconsequential facts, as well.

ONLINE ASSESSMENT

As you begin to read this book, you may be unsure how much you already know about the healthcare system and your own healthcare goals. If you are interested in finding out, you can complete my online assessment at *www.7stepshealth.com*. You may be surprised with the results.

A NOTE ON PRIVACY OF HEALTH INFORMATION

Chapter 4 discusses how you and your family may benefit from sharing your personal medical information. Federal law, known as the Health Insurance Portability and Accountability Act (HIPAA), protects all identified health information. Chapter 6 describes this law and other protections. Note that the law allows for you, as a healthcare consumer, to share your own healthcare information as desired.

A NOTE ON MEDICAL ADVICE

Although I use medical, surgical, and diagnostic terms throughout this book, they are for reference only and do not constitute medical advice. Nor do the examples I provide about patients' treatments. I have based descriptions, statements, and suggestions on personal experiences. They are for reference only and not intended as medical advice.

A NOTE ON LEGAL ADVICE

In different parts of the book, I describe legal rights about your health information, informed consent, and expected standards of care. Examples and statements I provide about violation of individuals' rights are based on personal experiences. These statements are for reference only and do not constitute legal advice.

STEP

1

CREATE YOUR VISION

CHAPTER

1

BECOMING A VISIONARY HEALTHCARE CONSUMER

The human body experiences a powerful gravitational pull in the direction of hope. That is why the patient's hopes are the physician's secret weapon. They are the hidden ingredients in any prescription. —Norman Cousins

VALUES, VISION, AND MISSION STATEMENTS: THEY APPLY TO HEALTHCARE, TOO

"I want to die at a hundred years old with an American flag on my back and the star of Texas on my helmet after screaming down an Alpine descent on a bicycle at 75 miles per hour." So begins famed cyclist and cancer survivor Lance Armstrong's book, *It's Not About the Bike: My Journey Back to Life*.[1] Whether you are currently healthy or facing an illness, Lance Armstrong's visionary perspective offers a valuable lesson. If you know what you want, you are more likely to get there, even if you have to take some detours in the process.

I have started (and sold) three companies. This may make me a serial entrepreneur. But, it has also made me someone who understands the necessity of articulating values, vision, and mission statements (VVMS). Without a clear understanding of where you want to go and how to get there, chances are slim that you will move along a satisfying and fulfilling path. And chances are even less that you will achieve your goals.

This chapter helps you develop a VVMS and a daily plan specifically for your healthcare and your health status goals. If you already have a personal VVMS, you can use the following exercises to complement it. If not, you can use what you develop here to help provide more focused direction to your life overall. You may find yourself repeating the exercises multiple times to revise and improve your initial VVMS. Your VVMS is a dynamic guide that will change as you do.

Your general life values are likely the same or similar to the values you identify to guide your healthcare. For example, my three most highly prized values, in general, are: growth, innovation and collaboration. These drive my personal and professional decisions. I am always looking to learn something new. I believe that being on the cutting edge can be the difference between an adequate and a phenomenal solution. Learning with one or more colleagues is the best way for me to learn. This process of learning (growth) something new or cutting edge (innovation) from colleagues (collaboration) embodies all three of my personal values.

In my healthcare planning, my values are the same. I look for care that is provided by a healthcare team, not just one individual. (I figure if two heads are better than one, then three heads must be better than two!) I am always looking for the most cutting-edge practices. Recently, for example, I converted to a raw vegetarian diet, upon the advice of several healthcare professionals and my own reading and research. A progressive nutritional philosophy, a raw vegetarian diet may not be for everyone, but it works for me. I am also always seeking to learn more about how I can improve my approach to healthcare as a consumer *and* benefit from new research. Then, I can better discuss specific topics with my healthcare team at my next visit.

Applying your core values to complex healthcare decisions can simplify a lot for you. For example, by applying my values, I realized that I want care provided by a healthcare team in a large academic medical center. These organizations conduct research and tend to be innovators in their field. In addition, they work as a team with physicians, residents (physicians in training), and mid-level practitioners, such as physician assistants. I feel comfortable, even invigorated, navigating my way through the complexities of a large academic medical center.

This approach, however, does not work for everyone. My husband Joe finds comfort in returning regularly to the same solo practitioner he has seen for the past decade. Joe is quite friendly with his physician. Having a physician who knows him well gives Joe confidence and a comfort level that leads to positive healthcare visits. By applying your own values to healthcare decision making, you are more likely to have positive and beneficial experiences wherever you seek care.

Values of a Cancer Survivor

When Lance Armstrong received his diagnosis of cancer, his first surgery took place less than 24 hours later. It is highly unlikely that he thought about his specific healthcare values, vision, and mission at all. However, his razor-sharp focus on values and vision, evident in his public life and his book, *It's Not About the Bike,* enabled him to make critical decisions quickly. Not everyone is so naturally driven. However, by thinking through and preparing a specific healthcare plan, ideally before a problem arises, each of us will be better able to achieve our healthcare goals. Here are some of the values Lance Armstrong identifies in his book:

- *Confidence in his healthcare team*: "I decided I had confidence in them, in their purposely laid-back styles, their lack of ego, and their refusal to be rattled by me . . . they wanted to alter my protocol to preserve my lungs . . . to get me back on the bike."
- *Positive attitude:* "To continue believing in yourself, the doctors, the treatment . . . was the most important thing."
- *Patience and focus:* "With this illness, I couldn't afford impatience or a lapse in concentration."

Values: What Do I Value in My Healthcare Providers and the Healthcare Process?

To identify the values that drive your healthcare planning and decision making, ask yourself: "What attributes am I looking for in healthcare providers and the healthcare process? What matters most to me?" Remember, you are the "customer." Without the patient, a healthcare provider has no business. If it seems like the balance of power in healthcare is not in your favor, reminding yourself who the customer is may help you to feel more empowered. To make a difference in your own healthcare, you need to be confident, knowledgeable, and in control. Creation of a VVMS is the starting point.

As you identify your values and the attributes of healthcare providers most important to you, think about previous positive healthcare experiences. Ask yourself: "What made my interaction with the physician good? Was she compassionate? Did she spend a lot of time with me? Was I able to trust her? Did she involve me in the decision-making process? Did she put my mind at ease immediately?" It is also useful to think about a healthcare interaction that did not go so well: "What made my interaction with the physician unsatisfactory? Did he really listen to my questions and concerns? Did he rush the appointment? Did I have to wait a long time to see the physician?" The importance you place on these questions will vary based on what you value most in your healthcare.

Below is a sample list of values. While not complete, this list provides suggestions to help you create your own list. As you read the sample list, think of other values that are important to you and add them to the list.

Sample List of Values

- Quality
- Cost
- Time and efficiency of care
- Comfort
- Collaboration (among healthcare team)
- Focus (one provider at all times, if possible)
- Location
- Innovation (treatment with new versus proven methods)
- Integrity and ethics
- Simplicity
- Complementary and alternative medicine (CAM)
- Trust and honesty
- Involvement
- Knowledge
- Freedom
- Responsibility and accountability
- Autonomy in decision making
- Friendliness
- Compassion and empathy
- Reliability and confidence
- Spirituality
- Communication
- Competence
- Dignity

Now, take some time and think about what you value. What matters to you?

DO IT NOW!

In the space below, list six to eight values that matter to you in seeking healthcare.

My Values

1. ______________________________

2. ______________________________

3. ______________________________

4. ______________________________

5. ______________________________

6. ______________________________

7. ______________________________

8. ______________________________

The most effective VVMS contains two or three core values, the values that are most important to you. Identify your three core values from the list you just created. Eliminate from the list—one by one, if necessary—those values that do not fall into your top three. Or, assign a number from 1 to 8, in order of importance, to each value. This exercise pulls you towards focusing and prioritizing your values. If you have competing priorities, it is difficult to make a decision. By identifying your top three values, your health planning and decision making will be easier and more reliable.

Will My Values Change?

For most people who have not experienced a life-transforming event, your top eight core values remain generally the same. Yet, you may re-prioritize your top three values as you grow older. Changes in your life may cause different values to become more important over time. In my 20s, my priorities in healthcare planning and decision making were *cost* and *location.* I was relatively healthy, but brought home a small paycheck each month, most of which went to pay the rent. My health insurance plan, a traditional HMO, did not have out-of-plan benefits. I had to pay for certain physicians or types of care myself. In addition, we lived in Washington, D.C. and did not have a car, so seeking care any place not serviced by public transportation was not an option.

In my 30s, *focus* and *time* were my most important values. I wanted the most efficient care in the least amount of time. And I needed doctors to fit my schedule. Luckily, my family and I remained in relatively good health, so my values coincided with my needs. I had two small children, was traveling a lot for business, and going to graduate school. Now, in my 40s, my top three values have changed again. As I mentioned previously, my top three values are growth, innovation, and collaboration.

Do It Now!

Now, it's time to make your choices and identify your top three values. In the space below, write your top three values and add comments about each value. Explain why the value is important, how you see using the value to make healthcare decisions, or what the value means to you.

Values can have different meanings for different people. For example, *you* may interpret collaboration as being involved in all aspects of the decision-making process along with your physician. I, however, view collaboration as teamwork among my healthcare providers, including a primary care physician, specialist, and nutritionist. It is important to be as clear as possible about your interpretations of your values. That way, when you re-evaluate or apply new information, you will not have to waste time redefining your values.

My Core Values and Why They are Important

1. ________________ -- ________________

2. ________________ -- ________________

3. ________________ -- ________________

HAPPY TIMES IN HEALTHCARE

As I gathered research for this book, I noticed almost every book on healthcare had a negative title and focused on problems with healthcare. This unfortunate trend undermines the positive experience we all seek and need. One of the lessons we learn from people such as Norman Vincent Peale (author of *The Power of Positive Thinking*), Louise L. Hay (author of *You Can Heal Your Life),* Norman Cousins (author of *Head First: The Biology of Hope and the Healing Power of the Human Spirit*), Mark Victor Hansen and Jack Canfield (authors of the *Chicken Soup for the Soul* series), and Wayne Dyer (author of *Change Your Thoughts—Change Your Life)* is that the power of focusing our energy on the positive dramatically influences our lives.

To create a healthcare vision statement, it is helpful to identify three positive healthcare experiences. Focusing on positive healthcare experiences sets a foundation for being a strong healthcare consumer, one who expects good outcomes and views future healthcare situations through an optimistic lens. Below, I have described three of my "happy times in healthcare" as an example.

Three Positive Healthcare Memories

1. **Birth of my children, Emmalea and John.** These were the best two days of my life. For most parents, having a child, whether biologically or through adoption, is a powerful, amazing occurrence. Many hospitals even play a lullaby throughout the hospital every time a baby is born. The music raises the spirits of patients, visitors, and employees alike.
2. **Finding and meeting with Dr. Herzog**. Dr. Herzog is the Harvard-based physician we found after months of searching for a credible alternative treatment of epilepsy for women likely to have a seizure related to their menstrual cycle. In addition to recommending a more natural treatment for Emmalea's epilepsy, his office environment was unassuming and welcoming. He listened intently to everything we said, taught us a lot, and demonstrated a clear expertise that made us feel confident that his was a reliable solution.
3. **A warm reception from a famed neurosurgeon at Johns Hopkins Hospital**. In 1997, my husband Joe and I worked on a project at Johns Hopkins Hospital interviewing members of the hospital's medical staff. The purpose of the project was to reduce the hospital's risk and make its processes more efficient. This is not a topic near and dear to most physicians. So, it was a relief to

> us that the physicians responded courteously. Still, the prospect of interviewing a famous neurosurgeon created much apprehension. Just thinking about what he did for a living, exploring and operating on people's brains, was intimidating. To our surprise, he welcomed us into his office and sat with us for quite some time. He was so soft-spoken, we had to move our chairs closer to his desk to hear every word. He answered all of our questions, providing more detail than we expected. He said he would do everything he could to help make the hospital a better place for patients. This neurosurgeon proved he was a gentleman who truly cared about his patients and showed it. He clearly was guided by a vision for happier, healthier patients. As I left his office (and for years after that), our encounter made me smile about doctors and the healthcare system.

Most memories about healthcare involve a key person or people. A hospital's welcoming lobby or imposing structure can make a good initial impression on you. However, the lasting impression that healthcare organizations make is through their people. It's not the hospital, the clinic, or the laboratory that typically stands out. The people who work there make the difference in the lives of patients.

In a Web-based survey I conducted for this book, I asked respondents to describe three "happy times in healthcare." The 2,000 respondents to the survey submitted almost 5,000 stories. Most stories did have a focus on an individual as well as several values, including compassion, caring, making the system easier, and healthcare providers' willingness to spend time with patients. Four of my favorite stories submitted by survey respondents follow.

Examples of Happy Times in Healthcare

When I had to have chemo treatments two years ago, my oncology nurse would sing to me as she was hooking my port up to the IV. I would hardly feel the big stick. **K.H., Oklahoma**

As a child I had many asthma attacks that inevitably led to many emergency room visits. I was always rushed right in for treatment and was medicated as soon as possible. I remember one time specifically after recovering from an asthma attack, I was hooked up to a machine and asked to blow in as hard a possible. After doing this a few times, the technicians (I think they were respiratory therapists), showed me how I did on a computer screen. They explained to me that even though I had asthma, my lungs were very strong. Of course, that cheered me right up and made me feel much better about myself and my condition. **P.V., Tennessee**

When I was pregnant and in labor, my nurse was a huge woman who held me so that my epidural would go well. She also took care of my husband when he passed out after seeing the epidural needle. **L.T., South Carolina**

My husband's brother died just days before I gave birth to my first child. When our son was born, the family used it as a way to focus on life after death. The staff in the hospital was so nice to us. They went out of their way to make us feel comfortable. The nurses allowed our family to order pizza into the room, have many and frequent guests, and to stay past normal visiting hours. They broke a lot of rules for us. They truly made a difficult time much easier to bear for my entire family, even though I was the only patient. **R.P., Pennsylvania**

The four patients in the previous stories were dealing with cancer, chronic asthma, pregnancy and death. In each case, the patient identified something pleasant in his or her healthcare experience. The pleasant interactions included healthcare providers who showed them sympathy and support, were comforting, and even pointed out the patient's strengths. These contacts had a positive impact on each of these individuals.

Betty Rollin, a journalist and cancer survivor, offers another example of the power of a positive attitude in healthcare. In her book, *Here's the Bright Side: Of Failure, Fear, Cancer, Divorce and Other Bum Raps,* she describes the positive things that have come from having cancer and other horrible or difficult problems.[2] Her book is filled with stories about people, including herself, who have benefited from—or even become happier after—a terrible experience. Her book is a retrospective look at the good that can come out of pain, disease, and other unfortunate events. We learn that we benefit even more if we couple a positive attitude with the knowledge that some good can come from even the worst experience. There is no guarantee that the road will be less rocky, but the gain for you and for others you touch can be that much better with a positive perspective.

By asking you to recall positive healthcare experiences, my intent is not to trivialize health problems or minimize problems that do exist in the healthcare system. Healthcare problems can be heart-wrenching, stressful, and painful. Norman Cousins was able to turn his own significant health problems around through his positive attitude. He said, "Laughter [a positive perspective] is a form of internal jogging. It moves your internal organs around. It enhances respiration. It is an igniter of great expectations."3 Many people have been jaded by the healthcare system. The negativity creates undue stress and may actually aggravate a chronic condition. Reflecting on pleasant prior healthcare experiences is an opportunity to recognize and celebrate the positive. This process helps lead you to be proactive, take control, and ask what you can do to improve your own healthcare experience.

Do It Now!

In the space below, describe three of your own happy times in healthcare, and why each was a positive experience for you.

My Three Positive Healthcare Memories

1. ____

____

____

____

2. ____

____

____

____

3. ____

____

____

____

VISION: WHAT IS MY VISION FOR MY HEALTHCARE AND HEALTH STATUS?

A personal vision is a picture of yourself in the future—of where you are going. It addresses all possible components about your future health status and your relationship with healthcare providers. Most people, even if only for preventive care, have some interactions with physicians and healthcare organizations. If you currently have a relationship with healthcare providers and the healthcare system, develop a vision that focuses on how you want to improve your current situation. If you do not currently have a relationship with healthcare providers and organizations, visualize what you would want your relationship to be like.

More empowered healthcare consumers make healthcare providers more accountable. This increased accountability results in a better healthcare system overall. Creating a health vision statement can help you be more prepared, more effective, more confident, and get the best results when you do interact with healthcare providers. The World Health Organization (WHO) defines health as " . . . a state of complete physical, mental, and social well-being, and the ability to lead a socially and economically productive life."[4] You may want to consider all of these components in your healthcare vision statement. You may also find it helpful to picture yourself and your lifestyle 10, 20, or 30 years from now.

My father-in-law, John Russo, is a good example of someone who uses a vision to help stay healthy. At 85 years old, he continues to have a disease-free, active lifestyle. His father died young of heart disease, his mother died of breast cancer, and his two brothers both died of kidney cancer. The only one left in his immediate family, he continues to defy the odds. One reason for his sustained wellness is likely his passion for baseball.

Recently, he, Emmalea, Joe, and I were watching one of my son John's baseball games at Limeport Stadium. It is a beautiful place that makes you feel like you are in a professional baseball stadium from the early 1900s. After we passed through the ticket gate, my father-in-law commented that he was charged the senior citizen's rate. He preferred to pay full freight and said to the ticket lady, "Inside this stadium, I am young. It's only out there that I am old." While my father-in-law has never actually told me this, I think he pictures himself sliding into home base and pitching batting practice to my son in another 10 or 15 years, when John has his own children. My father-in-law has pitched batting practice to my son John since my son could stand on his own. Whatever the weather or the season, my father-in-law would travel 40 minutes to our house every day for this exercise. I am sure that back then, almost 14 years ago, what my father-in-law saw in his mind was not a three-year-old, but a young teen slamming homeruns and fielding ground balls. And my father-in-law continually adjusts that vision to keep himself going.

Now, I cannot attest to the fact that my father-in-law has consciously created this vision, but we can all learn a real-life lesson from him. If he had created a health vision statement 10 years ago, I imagine it would have sounded something like this: "In 10 years, I will be able to run the bases as fast as I can today, and I will be able to pitch just as many balls to John as I can today." This vision, as simple as it is, implies a lot from a health perspective. It implies that he will be alive, well, and functioning at the same level of physical fitness or better. It also requires my father-in-law to be proactive about his nutrition, exercise, and maybe most important, his attitude (mental health).

Your health and healthcare are multi-faceted. They contain many different component parts, or categories. You may think in general or specific categories when creating your vision statement. Several of the *categories* you may want to include in your health vision statement are listed below (add to the list as you feel is necessary):

- Outcome
- Use of prescription drugs
- Diet and nutrition
- Physical fitness
- Healthcare provider relationships
- Knowledge of the system
- Health information or medical records
- Alternative care
- Healthcare settings

For example, the *categories* I included in my vision statement are:

- Physical fitness
- Diet and nutrition
- Preventive care
- Healthcare providers with whom I am collaborating
- Management of health information

After considering my categories, I crafted the following health vision statement:

I will be as physically, nutritionally, and emotionally fit as I am today, through my own actions and by enlisting a diverse team of healthcare professionals to track, measure, and share information on my health status.

The following vision statement is one that might be crafted by Jack LaLanne, 94, who still exercises daily. At age 70—using only his muscle power—he towed 70 boats loaded with 70 people in Long Beach Harbor, California for one-and-a-half miles, from the Queen's Way Bridge to the Queen Mary.[5]

By remaining physically fit and eating healthy, I will continue teaching as many people as possible to eat healthy, whole foods and to exercise daily to lead a healthier life.

Picture It!

A vision statement includes a picture in your mind of how you see yourself physically in the future. This visualization helps you achieve the vision statement that you have created. For example, the following is my own *picture of my future health*: (By the way, I currently have no grandchildren and neither of my kids is married.)

I am running through Central Park with my granddaughter, who is a member of her school's track team, and my grandson, who is a member of his school's baseball team.

Here is another example of a picture of future health from Lance Armstrong, as written in his book, *It's Not About the Bike: My Journey Back to Life. (*He had only one child when he wrote the book.)

To cross one last finish line as my wife and 10 children applaud.

Do It Now!

In the spaces provided below, list the topics you want to address in your vision statement. Then, draft your vision statement. As you do, cross off each of your categories to make sure all are included. Finally, write down the picture you see of yourself in the future.

Categories I Want to Include in My Vision Statement

1. ____

2. ____

3. ____

4. ____

5. ____

6. ____

My Health Vision Statement

____

____

My Picture of Future Health

____

____

____

Your vision statements may change over time just as values may change, so you will want to reassess your statement at least annually. Modify your statement to be consistent with any changes in your health, learning, or thinking.

WHAT IS MY HEALTH MISSION STATEMENT?

Vision is where you are going. *Mission* is how you will get there. Your mission statement weaves together your vision statement and your values. It specifically addresses how you will achieve your vision and become the person you see in your picture of future health. The mission statement is also the beginning of your daily plan.

As you begin to create your mission statement, have your vision statement with you. Refer to the contents of your vision statement to help you sketch out your mission statement. In many ways, creating your mission statement fills in the details of how you will achieve your vision. For example, here is my health mission statement:

I will be responsible and accountable for my own physical and emotional fitness and nutrition. I will exercise and meditate daily. I will continue to follow a raw vegetarian diet. I will secure relationships with my team of healthcare providers before I need them. I will keep abreast of new options in diet, preventive health, fitness, and healthcare in general by consulting with my team of healthcare providers and taking advantage of educational opportunities. I will access, read, and understand my health information. I will then coordinate and disseminate my health information in an electronic format to all individuals with a need to know.

I have used my vision statement, "I will be as physically, nutritionally, and emotionally fit as I am today through my own actions and by enlisting a diverse team of healthcare professionals to track, measure, and share information on my health status," as the basis for my mission statement. I have also incorporated my core values of collaboration, innovation, and growth. And I have included specific statements of actions I need to take, such as "continue to follow a raw vegetarian diet," "secure the best possible team of healthcare professionals before I need them," and "keep my health information in an electronic format."

Do It Now!

In the space below, write your health mission statement—a brief statement about how you will achieve your health vision.

My Health Mission Statement

____

____

____

Double-Check Your Mission Statement

Did you:

- ✓ Use your vision statement?
- ✓ Incorporate your values?
- ✓ Include specific actions?

Congratulations! You have created your health VVMS, a tremendous achievement. Pat yourself on the back, take a deep breath, and enjoy the moment. Now you can move on to creating your daily plan. You need to use the daily plan to turn your statements from words on paper and thoughts in your head to real accomplishments.

Where do you start? By using your VVMS as a guide, and then, to borrow a phrase from the motivational guru Tony Robbins, "chunk it out." In other words, break down your goals and plans into smaller pieces. This will help you prioritize your healthcare VVMS and give you a better chance of achieving your goals.

TOP PRIORITY FIRST

Identify what you will do beginning *today* to put your VVMS into action. Learn more about the healthcare system so you can be more confident? Understand diet and nutrition? Create a fitness plan? Start with your top priority. If it is learning more about the healthcare system or your health history, reading this book might be your first step toward achieving that part of your VVMS. If your first priority is fitness, what will you do to achieve that part of your VVMS?

For example, my top priority is meditation. I have often said I would do this activity, but have never practiced consistently. My commitment is to spend 10 minutes meditating daily.

DO IT NOW!

Write your top priority from all of the actions in your VVMS. Then, write what you will do, starting today, to put your VVMS into action.

My top priority is . . .

____

____

____

Today, I will . . .

____

____

____

Good job! By completing this exercise, you have really given some thought to your health VVMS. Pat yourself on the back, take a deep breath, and enjoy the moment. Next, you can move on to creating your daily plan. Figure 1.1 provides a sample plan to give you some ideas. Take a look at that and then create your own plan. (See figure 1.2.) You are on your way to achieving the healthcare and health status goals you have set for yourself!

Figure 1.1 Sample Daily Healthcare Plan

Vision Target	Daily	Weekly	Monthly	Yearly
Physical Fitness	Exercise for one hour daily.	Add variety at least once a week.	Do something physically challenging I have never done before.	Take an "exercise" vacation, such as cycling in Alaska.
Nutrition	Follow the principles of the raw vegetarian diet.	Try at least one new recipe.	Do a pure-juice fast for one day.	Attend an educational program on raw-food nutrition.
Health Information	Write in an online journal how I feel about my health today.	Look for trends in a health journal.	Update online health information (from healthcare professionals. lab tests, x-rays, etc.)	Review all health information to make sure my healthcare providers have the information they need.
Healthcare Professionals	Research which physicians and other healthcare professionals to create relationships with. Schedule appointments.	Discuss issues with team of healthcare providers as necessary.	Discuss issues with team of healthcare providers as necessary.	See primary care provider for annual checkup.
Preventive Care	Same as above.	Same as above.	Review preventive care plan, and schedule visits and tests as necessary.	Create a preventive care plan with primary care physician. Review my VVMS.

Do It Now!

To complete your daily healthcare plan, first fill in the *Vision Target* column. Refer back to your list of categories to include in your vision statement. These categories represent the specific areas important to your future vision of yourself. Next, write down what you can do every day, as well as every week, month, and year to achieve and maintain your vision.

Figure 1.2 My Daily Healthcare Plan

Vision Target	Daily	Weekly	Monthly	Yearly

REVISIT YOUR DAILY PLAN

Revisit your VVMS and your daily plan after you finish reading this book. You should be able to apply the information in the book to refine your VVMS. Before you read them, the pages in this book are just information. After you read them, they become knowledge, owned by you. Once you apply that knowledge, it becomes power for you to use as you see fit.

Creating a VVMS with or for Others

If you are a mentor, parent, friend, or child to someone who needs assistance creating a healthcare VVMS, be sure to use this book to help him or her do that. As we increase the number of successful healthcare visions, we increase the number of more knowledgeable, healthier people. *And that is a good thing.*

Key Highlights

To be a more confident, focused, and visionary healthcare consumer, create a statement of your own values, vision, and mission for your health and health status. Put your VVMS into practice in all of your personal health practices and your interactions with your healthcare providers. Then create a daily plan to ensure that your statements become reality. And remember to revisit and update your VVMS at least once a year.

Key Actions

- Create health values, vision, and mission statements (VVMS) to improve your healthcare and health status.
- Determine your three most important healthcare values.
- Visualize some "happy times in healthcare" and create a picture of yourself in the future to become a more positive and stronger healthcare consumer.
- Create an action plan to turn your VVMS into reality.
- Revise your VVMS regularly to help stay as healthy as possible.

Key Take-Away

Develop a clear understanding of where you want to go and how you will get there so you can move along a path that is satisfying and fulfilling for you.

Endnotes

---

[1] Armstrong, Lance. *It's Not About the Bike: My Journey Back to Life.* The Berkley Publishing Group, 2001.
[2] Rollin, Betty. *Here's the Bright Side: Of Failure, Fear, Cancer, Divorce and Other Bum Raps.* Random House, 2007.
[3] Cousins, Norman. *Anatomy of an Illness as Perceived by the Patient.* W.W. Norton & Company, 1979.
[4] Preamble to the Constitution of the World Health Organization as adopted by the International Health Conference, New York, 19 June–22 July 1946; signed on 22 July 1946 by the representatives of 61 States (Official Records of the World Health Organization, no. 2, p. 100) and entered into force on 7 April 1948. The definition has not been amended since 1948.
[5] From Jack LaLanne's Web site, *www.jacklalanne.com.*

CHAPTER

2

RECRUITING YOUR TOP TWO TEAM MEMBERS: PRIMARY CARE PHYSICIAN AND MEDICAL MENTOR

To succeed as a team is to hold all of the members accountable for their expertise. —Mitchell Caplan

Allison relies heavily on her primary care physician (PCP), Dr. Verma. Her relationship with him—as well as Dr. Verma's team approach to Allison's treatment—has been quite beneficial to her over the years. Allison has had her share of health struggles. She had been significantly overweight since the age of 14. Then, after getting married, she and her husband hoped for children, but Allison had problems conceiving. Because Allison trusted Dr. Verma, she and her husband decided to seek treatment from him for her infertility, instead of finding a specialist.

After many visits, strategies, and tests, Allison was diagnosed with polycystic ovarian syndrome (PCOS). In addition to numerous cysts on the ovaries—the definitive evidence of the condition—some of the other symptoms of PCOS are obesity, infertility, and abnormal menstrual cycles. The condition is treatable with medication, diet, and exercise, but it is not curable.

After the diagnosis, Dr. Verma had some ideas about treatment, but he recommended that Allison get a second opinion from an obstetrician/gynecologist (OB/GYN). He recommended a few good physicians to Allison and, once she made an appointment with one, Dr. Verma sent Allison's medical records to him. Allison was pleased with her visit to Dr. Hersh. He did not have an immediate solution for her, but he listened closely, provided some good information on PCOS, and ordered some additional tests. He told Allison he would work directly with Dr. Verma to design a treatment program for her in the next few days. Later that same day, Dr. Verma called her to see if she would be willing to meet with a nutritionist. She responded yes and made the appointment.

Allison dreaded the visit with the nutritionist because she knew that the entire discussion would be focused on her weight and eating habits, her two least favorite topics. To make matters even more difficult, the nutritionist was visibly pregnant. She introduced herself to Allison by her first name, Patty. Her pleasant demeanor and genuine caring attitude soon put Allison at ease. Their first trip was to the back corner of Patty's small office, where the scale was located. Allison stepped on the scale: 210. Next, her height: 5 feet, 4 inches. Next, Patty asked Allison a series of questions about her eating habits. Patty asked one very telling question about Allison's snacking: "After 5 in the evening, what would you estimate is the average amount of time between your snacks or between a snack and a meal?" Allison's response: "I don't really ever stop. The amount of food may vary, but really, I go from one thing to the next until bedtime." Using all of the information from their visit, Patty designed a nutritional program for Allison.

During Allison's next visit with Dr. Verma two days later, they discussed her treatment and reaffirmed her nutritional plan. Dr. Hersh prescribed medication to help regulate her menstrual cycles, and Dr. Verma monitored her every few weeks. Both doctors recommended a daily exercise plan. In six months, Allison lost almost 70 pounds and finally conceived her daughter, without taking fertility drugs. Allison and her husband could not have been happier. To this day, Allison credits the fact that her OB/GYN, PCP, and nutritionist worked together as a team to identify the problems and manage her treatment.

YOUR PRIMARY CARE PHYSICIAN AND YOUR MEDICAL MENTOR

Research shows that patients who, like Allison, have a good relationship with their doctors tend to be more satisfied with their care—and to have better results from their healthcare interactions. As you move forward to take control of your healthcare and achieve your VVMS, it is important to recruit the top two members of your team—your primary care physician (PCP) and your medical mentor. Both play a critical role in your healthcare plan.

While most people are familiar with the concept of a primary care physician, the medical mentor may be new, at least in title. Your PCP helps you maintain or improve your health and cares for your general medical needs. He will assist you in finding specialists if your condition warrants it. And he will generally coordinate all of the information and care among healthcare providers for you.

A medical mentor is usually a friend or relative. Your medical mentor helps you to, among other things, analyze treatment options, communicate fully with your healthcare providers, and organize treatment schedules. The choices you make and the partnerships you create can make a dramatic difference in your overall healthcare.

The book *Younger Next Year,* by Chris Crowley, a retired lawyer and patient in his 70s, and his PCP, Henry S. Lodge, tells an excellent story of a successful patient-physician partnership.[1] A very involved healthcare provider, Dr. Lodge helped Crowley to make significant lifestyle, diet, and other changes. Crowley is now leading a more active, healthy, and enjoyable life than he did when he was younger. And, because of their successes together, they decided to write a series of books to share their story with others. Most of us won't be so inspired by our relationships with our providers that we collaborate with them to write a book. However, we can read about relationships like the Crowley-Lodge association to learn what steps we should take to get the best possible healthcare.

Dr. Bernadine Healy, a physician and brain-cancer survivor, referred to *medical mentors* in one of her "On Health" columns in *U.S. News & World Report.*[2] An inspiration for many, she proposed the idea of securing a medical mentor as someone who provides a patient with personal support, advice, and guidance. Formerly director of the National Institutes of Health and president of the American Red Cross, she describes her own successful struggles as a patient in her book, *Living Time: Faith and Facts to Transform Your Cancer Journey.*[3] Some hospital programs have now established formal medical mentor programs. Many people have medical mentors, even though they may not use that specific term. From Dr. Healy's description and based on the many hospitals that have established formal medical mentor programs, the value and benefits are clear.

PCPs: FAMILY PRACTICE, INTERNAL MEDICINE AND OTHER PHYSICIANS

Today, more than ever, it is critical to rely on a PCP to coordinate healthcare options. Subspecialists are oriented toward research and care of patients who have highly specific problems. PCPs take a broader, more holistic perspective with patients, emphasizing both healthcare delivery and preventive medicine.[4] But when necessary, your primary care physician can and will guide you to a specialist.

Primary care medicine has its own subspecialties, so sometimes it is confusing to determine what type of doctor is best. (See figure 2.1.) Typically, PCPs are internal medicine physicians (internists) or family practice physicians. Both groups of physicians treat people of various ages, who have a wide range of conditions. Both groups also focus on preventive medical care. Five other types of physicians serve as primary care physicians. *Pediatrician*s treat children, generally from birth through 18 years of age. *Adolescent medicine physicians*, a newer specialty, care for teens and young adults. *Geriatric medicine physicians* treat older patients, generally 65 years and older, though some see patients in their 50s and early 60s.

Hospice and palliative care specialists provide primary care to patients who have life-limiting illnesses.

Obstetricians and *gynecologists* (OB/GYNs) may provide primary care for women, especially at certain points in their lives. Many doctors will not see or treat a pregnant woman without involving an OB/GYN. When I was pregnant, my dentist would not even see me for a toothache without my OB/GYN knowing about it. During menopause, and the time right before and after it, women may also feel more comfortable with an OB/GYN as their PCP.

There is no question that specialists outside of primary care medicine are important. But understanding their limitations and making sure the right ones are on your team of healthcare providers is critical. As Jim Collins says in his book, *Good to Great,* "You need to get the right people on your bus. And, once you have them on the bus, make sure they are in the right seats."[5] It is the same with your healthcare provider team. Moving forward without the guidance of a primary care physician is like embarking on a trip to a city a thousand miles away without a Global Positioning System (GPS), a map, or even a sense of direction.

New Types of PCPs: Hospitalists and Naturopathic Doctors

Hospitalists and naturopathic doctors are two newer types of primary care physicians. Let's take a closer look at who they are and what they do. *Hospitalists*, a term coined in 1996, are physicians who focus on general medical care for hospitalized patients. If your PCP admits you to a hospital that employs hospitalists, he may have the option (or in some cases be required) to have a hospitalist manage your care until discharge. Your PCP can still be available to you if you work with a hospitalist.

Academic medical centers have begun to develop hospitalist residency and fellowship programs, so the field is likely to grow. The Society of Hospital Medicine (SHM) describes some additional benefits of the hospitalist. The SHM Web site (*www.hospital medicine.org*) states that by focusing on the care of hospitalized patients, a hospitalist becomes experienced in the unique needs of a patient during a hospital stay. The SHM Web site identifies three main benefits of hospitalists' care for patients:[6]

- Since hospitalists practice only in the hospital, they are present whenever the patient or family member has a question regarding care. Patients no longer need to wait until their physician makes rounds to get answers.
- Hospitalists know how to expedite and improve care within the hospital. They are familiar with all of the key individuals in the hospital, including medical and surgery consultants, discharge planners, clergy, and others.
- Hospitalists can better facilitate connections with post-acute providers, such as home healthcare, skilled nursing care, specialized rehabilitation, and others.

Naturopathic doctors (NDs) are another new type of PCP. NDs can serve as PCPs in the 14 states that license them. A number of MDs in these 14 states employ NDs to integrate naturopathic medicine into their practice. This partnership offers patients more options. The 14 states that license NDs to practice medicine are: Alaska, Arizona, California, Connecticut, Hawaii, Idaho, Kansas, Maine, Montana, New Hampshire, Oregon, Utah, Vermont, and Washington.

The Association of Accredited Naturopathic Medical Colleges (AANMC) describes naturopathic medicine as "medicine that concentrates on whole-patient wellness. The medicine is tailored to the patient and emphasizes prevention and self-care." According to the AANMC Web site (*www.aanmc.org*) naturopathic medicine attempts to find the underlying cause of the patient's condition. NDs cooperate with all other branches of medical science, referring patients to other practitioners for diagnosis or treatment when appropriate.[7] (For more about the education, training, and philosophy of naturopathic doctors, see chapter 14.)

How a naturopathic approach made the difference. Tammy had danced since she could walk and all through college. When she had the opportunity to perform with a professional dance troupe in New York City evenings and weekends, she was thrilled. One night, after four years of flawless performances, Tammy suddenly forgot her steps in the dance routine. She had performed the same routine countless times before and suddenly, there in front of the audience and her troupe members, she stumbled through until the number was over. She was concerned, and thought the stress of working two jobs and not getting enough sleep had tripped her up.

A few days later at work while giving an important presentation, she could not remember what to say next. She became more concerned something was terribly wrong. She left the dance troupe because she was unable to finish most routines. Her primary care physician found nothing abnormal in her tests or physical exam and suggested she see additional specialists. When the specialists were also unable to identify a cause or treatment to resolve her continuing memory problem, she called her sister, Wendy, a naturopathic doctor on the West Coast.

Wendy immediately devised a strategy to identify the cause of her sister's symptoms. She ordered a series of blood tests, significantly more than, and different from, the previous traditional tests ordered. The new blood tests revealed that Tammy's mercury levels were extremely high, bordering on dangerous. Wendy asked Tammy questions about lifestyle and realized that Tammy's diet was the cause of the high mercury levels. Four months earlier, after reading about the benefits of salmon, Tammy began eating salmon every day. The farm-raised salmon Tammy had been eating had high levels of mercury. Once Tammy eliminated salmon from her diet, her memory problems disappeared. Tammy's recovery was a tremendous relief. She also realized the importance of taking a holistic approach to her health and to partnering with a clinical expert who could also be her medical mentor.

Figure 2.1 Types of Primary Care Physicians

FAMILY MEDICINE (MD or DO)

They treat	All general health issues, for all ages, and coordinate specialists' care. Focus is on prevention, diagnosis, and treatment.
Training	Three or four years of residency after medical school and board certification by the American Board of Family Medicine.
Common conditions treated	Asthma, allergies, childhood illnesses, diabetes, gastroenterology (GI) disorders, infections, and substance abuse.

INTERNAL MEDICINE (MD or DO)

They treat	Common and complex illnesses of adolescents, adults, and the elderly, and coordinate specialists' care. Focus is on diagnosis, treatment, and management of health problems.
Training	Three or four years of residency after medical school; board certification available by American Board of Internal Medicine, but not required.
Common conditions treated	Cancer; substance abuse; women's health; mental health; diabetes; heart disease; and common problems of the eyes, ears, skin, nervous system, and reproductive organs.

PEDIATRIC MEDICINE (MD or DO)

They treat	All general health issues of infants, children, and adolescents (newborn to 16–21 years old). Focus on prevention, diagnosis, and treatment.
Training	Three or four years of residency after medical school; 21 different certifications available through the American Board of Pediatrics, but not required.
Common conditions treated	Asthma, eating disorders, immunizations, tonsillitis, ear infections, pneumonia, and respiratory infections.

ADOLESCENT MEDICINE (MD or DO)

They treat	All general health issues of adolescents and young adults (ages 12–20), with a focus on developmental, sexual, behavioral, and medical concerns of this age group.
Training	Three or four years of residency after medical school, and two to three years of fellowship.
Common conditions treated	Eating disorders, including anorexia and bulimia; weight issues; sexually transmitted diseases; substance abuse; menstrual disorders; anxiety; and depression.

GERIATRIC MEDICINE (MD or DO)	
They treat	Problems and diseases of older adults; take a holistic approach to physical, psychological, and social factors; interact with other health professionals and organizations, such as home care agencies.
Training	Four years residency after medical school; one to three years of additional training; board certification available through the American Board of Internal Medicine and the American Board of Family Medicine, but not required.
Common conditions treated	Mood disorders, including depression; Alzheimer's disease; Parkinson's disease; arthritis; chronic heart and lung disease; osteoporosis; vision and hearing problems; and stroke.

HOSPICE AND PALLIATIVE MEDICINE (MD or DO)	
They treat	Serious, complex illnesses; focus on alleviating pain, managing symptoms, and improving quality of life.
Training	Four years of residency after medical school; one to two years of additional training; board certification available, but not required to practice.
Common conditions treated	Amyotrophic lateral sclerosis (ALS), multiple sclerosis (MS), end-stage renal disease, AIDS, and cancer.

OBSTETRICS/GYNECOLOGY (MD or DO)	
They treat	All general health issues of women, with a focus on preventive care, pregnancy care, and disorders of the reproductive system.
Training	Four years of residency after medical school; three years for subspecialties; board certification available through the American Board of Obstetrics and Gynecology, but not required.
Common conditions treated	Pregnancy, infertility, endometriosis, uterine fibroids, breast disorders, and sexually transmitted diseases, cancer of the female reproductive system.

HOSPITALISTS (MD or DO)	
They treat	Medical conditions of hospital patients; take over for patients' regular primary care physicians; coordinate specialists' care.
Training	Four years of residency after medical school; physicians may obtain a certification depending on their residency training, through the American Board of Internal Medicine or the American Board of Family Medicine, but not required; no hospitalist certification is available.
Common conditions treated	Pneumonia; stroke; heart failure; chest pain; diabetes; and problems of the esophagus, stomach, and other digestive organs.

NATUROPATHIC DOCTORS (ND)

They treat	Medical and minor surgical problems, with a focus on taking a natural approach to identify the cause of symptoms and avoid invasive treatment.
Training	Four years of medical school at a naturopathic medical college, clinic training, and state licensure (Currently only 14 states license NDs.)
Common conditions treated	Fatigue, menstruation and hormone issues, allergies, depression, insomnia, thyroid problems, weight and appetite issues, cholesterol issues, headaches and migraines, and fibromyalgia.

How to Find a PCP

Many methods and resources are available to find a primary care practitioner. Referrals are important, but it is helpful to first identify criteria to select your physician. The following is a good strategy:

1. Identify what is important to you in a PCP. (Review your VVMS created in chapter 1.)
2. Identify which physicians accept your insurance.
3. Create a list of credible resources to identify possible physicians.
4. Create a "short list" of physicians that may include your top three to five choices.
5. Create a list of questions to ask the physician or office staff.
6. Call the physicians' offices and narrow your list based on responses.
7. If possible, visit the doctor's office for an inspection.
8. Choose a doctor and schedule a wellness visit to establish yourself as a new patient.

Your choice of resources to help you find a PCP depends on what works best for you. The Internet resources in figure 2.2 are all referenced by more than one source, usually a health insurance company and a U.S. health agency. Other resources include local magazines, hospitals, and, of course, friends and family members you trust. You may want to use two or three different sources to verify that the physicians on your list are rated highly by multiple sources.

Figure 2.2 Sources to Help Find a PCP

Internet-based rating services	• American Board of Medical Specialties (*www.abms.org*) • HealthGrades (*www.healthgrades.com*) • Administrators in Medicine's DocFinder (National Organization for State Medical and Osteopathic Boards) (*www.docboard.org/docfinder.html*)
Local magazines and organizations	• Your preferred hospital • City or regional magazine's list of top doctors • Local or state medical society • Your health plan
Associations and agencies	• American Academy of Family Practitioners (*www.aafp.org*) • American College of Physicians-Internal Medicine (*www.acponline.org)* • American Medical Association "physician select" (*www.ama-assn.org/aps/amahg.htm*) • National Institutes of Health (*www.nccam.nih.gov*) • The Association of Accredited Naturopathic Medical Colleges (*www.aanmc.org*)
Personal referrals	• Physicians you know • Friends, relatives, business associates

Questions to Ask Your Potential PCP

First, go back to your VVMS and review your top three values. Reviewing your values helps ensure that your healthcare decisions align with your values. When values and decisions align, you are more likely to make better decisions, such as choosing a primary care physician who is right for you. Next, you want to ask several questions of potential PCPs to help you find the one that most closely aligns with your values. (See the following list of questions and items to check.)

- ✓ Do you accept my insurance?
- ✓ What is the size of your practice? (How many other physicians do you practice with?)

- ✓ What are your office hours? Any hours on evenings or weekends?
- ✓ Are you affiliated with an academic medical center?
- ✓ Which hospitals do you have admission privileges to?
- ✓ How long have you been in practice?
- ✓ How many patients do you currently manage?
- ✓ How much time do you spend with patients on their first visit? Follow up visits?
- ✓ Do you use any CAM or holistic approaches?
- ✓ How do you feel about patients seeking second opinions?
- ✓ What is your network of specialists like? How many do you work with regularly?
- ✓ Do you give advice via the phone or e-mail for common medical problems?

Additional Items to Check

- ✓ Is the lobby clean?
- ✓ Is the lobby welcoming?
- ✓ Is the physician's staff friendly?
- ✓ Is the physician's staff helpful?
- ✓ How long, on average, do patients need to wait to be seen?
- ✓ Is there any written material (brochures, newsletters) available for patients in the lobby?
- ✓ Are there any educational programs (videos) playing in the lobby?

A strategy for finding the right PCP. At the age of 70, Ed decided he needed a new primary care physician. He was in good health and had never been hospitalized for a serious or acute illness. He had worked his way up from a salesman at IBM in the 1960s to owner of his own software consulting firm 20 years later. He had worked his way through many complex organizations and was always able to achieve his goals. Still working in the information technology industry, but now with a firm in Princeton, New Jersey, things were not to be any different. Ed had always been the kind of guy to make sure he got the best possible value for every dollar he spent, and he was not about to let a change in his healthcare insurance coverage get the best of him.

He picked his healthcare providers the same way he did business. Create a plan with a goal, conduct the necessary research, have some personal interaction, take a test drive, and then, make the final decision. First, his criteria: an MD, not too young, and male. Second, to avoid out-of-pocket expenses, he compared the list of participating physicians from his health plan with information he was able to find about physicians in his area. Third, he conducted some additional research, checking out doctors on the Internet and calling doctors' offices. He rated the telephone interactions he had with each office assistant. Physicians whose office assistants were friendly, polite, and willing to answer his questions stayed on the list.

Fourth, he visited the offices. From his many years in business, he had found that the lobby or reception area is where you get your first impression. If it does not evoke the feeling that you are looking for, then look in another place. Ed's preferences: immaculately clean, neat, a comfortable waiting area, not a lot of people sitting there for a long time. How do you know if they have been sitting for a long time? You ask them. Fifth, he asked to speak with the physician for a few minutes, either in person or on the phone, to interview him. Ed wanted to know how thorough the physician is, what his philosophy on drug prescriptions is, how much time he typically spends with patients, and whether he is a nice guy. After all these steps, Ed made his final decision.

About a week after he began his search, Ed had his first visit with his new physician, Dr. Campbell. He felt best about the amount of time the doctor spent with him and that the doctor really listened to him. And Ed very much appreciated getting several brochures on different health issues, even though he does not have any health issues to be concerned about. He and his wife Helen take 20-mile bike rides a few times a week, eat well, and keep each other mentally stimulated. So, it wasn't Dr. Campbell's treatment style that made a difference to Ed. He was in good health. What he needed, and got, from Dr.

Campbell was a healthcare partner who now has his health information (yes, he took it with him), readily available should the need arise.

Defining the Role of Your PCP

To the primary care physician, the patient is as important as the disease. In his book *Doctoring: The Nature of Primary Care Medicine,* Eric J. Cassell, MD, discusses how patients' knowledge and power influence primary care medicine. He points specifically to the use of phrases like "patient-centered medicine," "patient as partner," and "patient as director of care."[8]

Every healthcare consumer could do well to heed Dr. Cassell's description. To get your best primary care, you must take a proactive role. You can start by defining the role you would like your primary care practitioner to take in your life and healthcare management. Some functions may include:

- Devising a plan to maintain wellness
- Being the first contact for health issues
- Managing multiple medications
- Recommending and referring specialists
- Coordinating care
- Informing specialists about test results to avoid duplicating tests
- Providing diet and nutrition guidance
- Providing guidance for physical fitness planning
- Offering strategies to reduce stress

Ronald L. Hoffman, MD, also notes the importance of patient responsibility. In his book *How to Talk with Your Doctor*, he urges you to assume ultimate responsibility for managing your condition and working with your doctors to set goals and expectations.[9] You can begin by determining exactly the areas where you would like your PCP to provide you direction, guidance, and care.

One way to take this list of care areas to the next level is to create your "Primary Care Project Plan." Project management is an important part of all of our lives at some point. If you were planning an important event such as a wedding, you might consider hiring entire teams of people, led by a wedding planner, to ensure the best outcome. As part of the planning process both you and the wedding planner would begin with a documented plan of what needs to be accomplished and how much it will cost. Then you would check off the items as they were completed. There would be responsibilities on both sides. The same is true for someone building a house or an addition to an existing house. In this example, as the owner, you would likely need the expertise of architects, builders, and designers to achieve your goal.

What is more important than your health? Have you ever co-designed a project plan for your health with your primary care physician? Perhaps it's time to start to at least consider the concept. Figure 2.3 is a simple project plan form. You can modify it to meet your needs. You may even want to create a document together with your PCP, based on documents she uses in her current records. The plan keeps you both accountable. At every visit, you should receive an updated copy of your Primary Care Project Plan.

Figure 2.3 Sample: Primary Care Project Plan

Patient:__________________________ **Physician:** _________________

Date:__________

Plan period:______________________ **to** ________________________

The following topics are to be addressed as part of the primary healthcare for ________________provided by_____________________. This health plan is not a contract for services. The patient and physician will discuss this plan during each visit and update it as necessary. In the spaces provided under each year, the physician can document the date that he discusses a specific topic with the patient. The patient can then initial the area. This document is to supplement the patient's medical record, not replace it.

Topics to review	Frequency	2008	2009	2010	2011
Preventive maintenance: • Blood tests • Chest x-ray	Every 2 years				
Preventive maintenance: • Mammogram • Colonoscopy	Annually				
• History and physical	Annually				
• Medication management	Every 2 months				
• Referrals to specialists	When necessary				
• Health information management	Copies to patient after every visit				
• Diet and nutrition planning	Every quarter				
• Physical fitness discussion and planning	Every quarter				
• Stress reduction	Every quarter and as needed				
Comments					

What if we planned for our healthcare like Joe planned for his pond? My husband Joe dreamed of having a pond all his life. He wanted a pond that contained the entire food chain of the fish family, from minnows to bass. When we bought a house on five acres, Joe decided it was time to make his dream come true. He bought libraries of books about fish and fresh-water ponds. He taught himself details about fish and plant co-habitation and became an expert in pond life. Then he hired a designer to create a blueprint for the pond. He priced it out and searched for the right excavators, designers, and fish experts.

Then, about three years later, when we were able to afford it, Joe put his plan into action. As the final truck from the fish hatchery gently dumped the last load of minnows, we all cheered. The pond was complete. Joe's ongoing care and maintenance ensured we all could continue to enjoy the pond. We generally do not plan for healthcare the way Joe planned for his pond, but what if we did? Perhaps healthcare systems and processes would be a familiar part of everyday life, rather than something unfamiliar that we only confront when we are sick.

MEDICAL MENTORS

I interviewed many patients while I was writing this book. Most of them spoke about one person in particular who helped them through their illness. This person was not the spouse or domestic partner (who usually focused on providing emotional support), although this individual was often a family member. This person helped the patient with decision making, research, physician discussions, analysis of medical bills, and other challenges the patient was not able to address alone. This person was the patient's medical mentor.

The *Oxford English Dictionary* defines *mentor* as "an experienced and trusted advisor." The "trusted advisor" part of this definition is probably most important. Whether a mentor is a healthcare professional may be irrelevant. In the interviews I conducted, sometimes the mentors were healthcare professionals who were able to use their healthcare knowledge to simplify information from the healthcare provider. In most cases, though, the mentors were not healthcare professionals. Many of the mentors had experiences similar to the patient's. Some had a knack for analyzing information and communicating with doctors. You may feel at a disadvantage when communicating with your doctors. Sickness may create an even greater imbalance in the physician-patient relationship. Having a medical mentor to lend support and guidance can be life saving.

When Do You Need a Medical Mentor?

You will probably need a medical mentor if you are newly diagnosed with a condition or are managing a chronic illness. The role of a medical mentor can vary based upon the seriousness or acuteness of a condition. Whatever their illness, the patients I interviewed did not discuss the role of medical mentor with a particular person prior to becoming ill. Most people do not. This is partly because people do not tend to think about getting sick when they are healthy, and partly because the concept of a medical mentor is relatively new. In each case, the medical mentor "stepped up to the plate" when needed. It was almost an automatic response for the mentor.

You may want to have a discussion with someone about being your medical mentor in the event you need one. At a minimum, it is a good idea to think about whom you would want to lean on as your "experienced and trusted health advisor." If you decide to have a conversation with your potential medical mentor, or if you are currently in need of a medical mentor, you can use the information below to help you select someone and to guide your discussion.

Who is a Good Medical Mentor?

Every medical mentor I interviewed shared the following characteristics: (1) cared deeply for the patient and had a close relationship, (2) had the ability to influence the patient, (3) had good research and note-taking skills, (4) had good communication skills, and (5) was not intimidated by the medical profession or doctors.

Two interactions are important to consider when selecting your medical mentor. The first is the person's interaction with you. The second is how he or she is likely to interact with your physician and other healthcare providers. Of course, your medical mentor must also be willing to take on the responsibility of guiding and advising you. Dr. Bernadine Healy describes her ideal medical mentor as someone who is informed and experienced, trustworthy, a good listener and empathetic.[10] Ultimately, it is important that you and your medical mentor agree to move forward together because it is the right thing for you both.

You may want to serve as a medical mentor yourself. It is a rewarding experience to be able to help someone through the complexities and emotions of managing an illness. Taking on the role of medical mentor for someone else can enable you to have a greater appreciation for the responsibilities should you or one of your family members need a medical mentor.

In addition to providing personal medical mentors, some hospitals also have medical mentor programs specifically for cancer patients or organ-transplant patients. Many hospitals have found that training former patients to be medical mentors provides emotional support for the current patients, as well as more efficient and improved outcomes. Vanderbilt-Ingram Cancer Center in Nashville has developed a Clinical Trials Mentoring program.[11] This program trains cancer survivors who have participated in clinical trials to discuss the basics of clinical trials and their own experiences with patients considering a trial. Another medical mentor program, which the Consumer Health Information Corporation (CHIC) designed, trains mentors for transplant patients.[12] Participating medical centers choose former transplant patients to participate in the 12-part training program.

Cyclist Lance Armstrong has described the role his mother played in coordinating his healthcare and providing him with constant support and advice.[13] Although he does not actually call her his "medical mentor" in his book, it appears that she did indeed play this role. Among other things, she organized and carried his medical records from physician to physician. She designed schedules for visitors so he would not get too fatigued during treatment. She visited every physician and hospital with him when he was seeking second and third opinions.

In analyzing your criteria for a medical mentor, go back again to your VVMS. As with all your healthcare decisions, aligning your decision making with your values will more likely result in the best possible healthcare for you. Use the space below to list what qualities your medical mentor needs to have and individuals you would consider as your medical mentor.

What Qualities Am I Looking For in a Medical Mentor?

____

____

____

Who Might be a Good Medical Mentor for Me?

____

____

____

____

A Natural Medical Mentor Match. MaryAnn is one of six children. Everyone in the family turns to her when they need a medical mentor. Nobody actually calls her a medical mentor, but she fits the role. MaryAnn herself has had some challenging health issues that she managed to work through. Smart, confident, articulate, and particularly adept at negotiating contracts, her qualities come in handy when she needs to review a family member's medical records, do some research, and discuss concerns with physicians.

It was no surprise, then, that when her sister Vera was diagnosed with breast cancer, MaryAnn was right beside her, yellow pad in hand, doctor visit after doctor visit. As I talked to Vera about her experience with cancer, MaryAnn's name was mentioned in almost every sentence. MaryAnn helped Vera research physicians and hospitals. She helped her make the decision about where to get treatment. She sat next to Vera at every doctor appointment. Before the appointments, they discussed questions to ask and what they wanted to achieve.

During doctor visits, MaryAnn asked many of the questions. In fact, she took notes so intensely that one of Vera's physicians asked her to stop. It made her nervous, the physician explained. At the end of the visit, MaryAnn summarized all of the information and made her notes part of Vera's permanent personal medical record.

The role MaryAnn took on during Vera's cancer diagnosis and treatment was different from that of anyone else in the family. She was Vera's medical mentor. Vera knew she would be likely to manage the ordeal more effectively and have a better outcome with MaryAnn acting as her medical mentor throughout the process. And, MaryAnn stepped up to the role of medical mentor without thinking twice.

Key Highlights

Your primary care physician (PCP) is the healthcare practitioner who coordinates your care and takes a holistic approach with a focus on prevention. Many options are available to explore and determine what type of PCP works best for you. Use resources on the Internet and in your local area, including friends and family, to find the best doctor for you. Your medical mentor is someone who helps you with decision making, research, physician discussions, analysis of medical bills, and other challenges you may not be able to address alone when facing a health crisis.

Key Actions

- Revisit your VVMS to determine what is important to you in a PCP.
- Conduct adequate research to find the right PCP for you. Use available Internet resources. Call or visit the office and ask questions.
- Play an active role in your relationship with your PCP and define the role you want your PCP to take in your life and healthcare.
- Work with your PCP to create a primary care health plan.
- Select a medical mentor.
- Consider being a medical mentor yourself.

Key Take-Away

You and the top two members of your healthcare team, your primary care physician and your medical mentor, will determine the effectiveness of your healthcare.

Endnotes

[1] Crowley, Chris and Lodge, Henry. *Younger Next Year*. Workman Publishing, 2006.
[2] Healy, Bernadine, MD. "Find a Mentor: Not just a companion, but a trusted medical guide," *U.S. News & World Report,* health.usnews.com, posted October 31, 2004.
[3] Healy, Bernadine, MD. *Living Time: Faith and Facts to Transform Your Cancer Journey*. Bantam, 2007.
[4] Myerburg, Robert J., MD. "Departments of Medical Specialties: A Solution for the Divergent Missions of Internal Medicine?" *The New England Journal of Medicine* 330 (1994): 1453-56.
[5] Collins, Jim. *Good to Great: Why Some Companies Make the Leap . . . and Others Don't*. HarperCollins, 2001.
[6] Society of Hospital Medicine, *www.hospitalmedicine.org*
[7] Association of Accredited Naturopathic Medical colleges, *www.aanmc.org*
[8] Cassell, Eric J., MD. *Doctoring: The Nature of Primary Care Medicine*. Oxford University Press, 2002.
[9] Hoffman, Ronald L., MD. *How to Talk with Your Doctor*. Basic Health Publications Inc., 2006.
[10] Healy, Bernadine, MD. "Find a Mentor: Not just a companion, but a trusted medical guide," *U.S. News & World Report,* health.usnews.com, posted October 31, 2004.
[11] Vanderbilt-Ingram Cancer Center, *www.vicc.org*.

---

[12] Consumer Health Information Corporation, *www.consumer-health.com.*
[13] Armstrong, *It's Not About the Bike: My Journey Back to Life.* The Berkley Publishing Group, 2001.

CHAPTER

3

Paying for Healthcare: When You are Insured—and When You Are Not

Decide what you want. Decide what you are willing to exchange for it. Establish your priorities and go to work. — H.L. Hunt

Clyde and JoDee were in their early 60s. They had been married for 40 years and both were in relatively good health. Shortly after her 62nd birthday, JoDee had chest pains that became so intense Clyde took her to the emergency room of their local hospital. After hours of testing, poking, and prodding, the ER doctors recommended she see a cardiologist. A few days later at the cardiologist's office, she had an electrocardiogram (EKG) and stress test. Both were abnormal. The doctor sent her back to the hospital for a cardiac catheterization, which revealed a 93 percent blockage of one of her coronary arteries. The doctor immediately performed an angioplasty, inserting a stent to open the artery. After some unexpected complications and a return trip to the ER, Clyde and JoDee were relieved her problem was resolved successfully.

Then the bills started coming in. Lots of them. Bills came from radiologists, emergency room physicians, pathologists, and the cardiologist. The biggest one came from the hospital. As Clyde looked over the bills, he was shocked to find the insurance company had denied many charges. Determined to discover the root of the problem, he scrutinized all the bills. The first bill denied was for the radiologists in the ER. As it turned out, the ER was in the health plan's network, but the radiologists were not in the plan. "They said it was our responsibility to request a radiologist in our network. That's the last thing on your mind in a situation like this," Clyde said. "But the radiology group was nice when I called them. They waived all the fees." That saved Clyde and JoDee $222. Pleased with his results, Clyde's persistence strengthened.

The next denied bill came from the ER physicians, an independent group the hospital contracted with. All of the hospital's contracted employees were supposed to be covered by the plan's network. However, after much investigation and several conversations, Clyde discovered a technical, but complex conflict that prevented payment for the bill. It seemed inevitable to him that he would have to pay the very high bill out of his own pocket. Despite this, Clyde refused to give up. After several additional calls, letters, and e-mail messages, Clyde managed to get the insurance company to pay $797 of the bill. Reluctantly, the ER group waived the additional $220 of patient charges.

Next, Clyde scrutinized the small pathology bill and the enormous cardiology bill. He had a few questions about those, which the healthcare providers answered to his satisfaction. As a result, he agreed to pay the patient portion of these bills, since the charges met his health plan's standard practices. Clyde then tackled the hospital bill. Many pages long, it detailed every piece of equipment, every nurse's visit, and all medication the healthcare team gave to JoDee during her overnight stay and ER visits. The total bill was $62,549. Under their plan, JoDee and Clyde were responsible for $6,913 of the bill. "I went to the business office [of the hospital] and asked for help understanding the bill," Clyde said. But no one was able to provide Clyde with any helpful assistance.

The hospital was part of a large, for-profit, national chain. Clyde called the national headquarters and received help immediately. The professional he spoke to offered him a 25 percent discount if he paid the bill in cash. Clyde was satisfied and sent in the payment for

$4,913 immediately—saving $2,030. Overall, Clyde was able to avoid paying $3,500 to the providers. Paying for healthcare can present genuine financial hardship, even when you have health insurance. Clyde and JoDee's story teaches us the lesson that questioning everything and being as thorough as possible in your investigation—especially when you're hit with thousands of dollars worth of bills—can lighten your financial burden.

DO YOU HAVE PRIVATE OR PUBLIC INSURANCE?

If you are part of the 85 percent of the U.S. population with health insurance, you have either public (government-sponsored) insurance or private insurance. The criteria for public insurance is age, in the case of Medicare and economic status in the case of Medicaid. Medicare primarily covers individuals 65 years and older. Medicaid covers individuals who are at or below state-determined maximum income levels. Both the federal and state governments fund Medicaid, but each state administers it. Since 1997, Medicaid also covers children through the State Children's Health Insurance Plan (SCHIP). The third type of government-sponsored health insurance is for federal or state government employees. Health insurance coverage for federal employees is different from Medicare or Medicaid. It is similar to private insurance but with more choices for employees.

If you have private health insurance, you have most likely received it through your employer's benefits package or you've purchased it yourself. If you are covered by an insurance plan through your employer, you may or may not have a choice in insurance companies. Smaller firms tend to have one healthcare plan, while larger firms may have several. In some larger private firms, the firm and its employees are self-insured. This means the firm acts as its own insurance company. These companies take a risk by assuming that the cost of care will be less than the health insurance premiums they charge employees.

Individual health insurance programs generally are available to anyone who wishes to purchase the plan, such as self-employed individuals, early retirees, students, and people whose employers do not offer health benefits. Individual policies are usually much more expensive than group policies. However, if you are strategic, there are a number of ways to save money. Some organizations, such as unions, professional associations, chambers of commerce, or other social or civic groups offer health plans for members. For example, if you join the Greater Lehigh Valley Chamber of Commerce, you can participate in one of four health plans for about the same rate you would pay if you were an employee of a larger firm.

Most insured Americans have private, employer-sponsored insurance (almost 60 percent), although this percentage has decreased slightly each year since 2001. Meanwhile, the percentage of people insured under the Medicaid/SCHIP programs has increased slightly each year since 2001. (See figure 3.1.)

Figure 3.1 How Americans are Insured[1]

Year	Employer-sponsored	Individual purchase	Military healthcare	Medicare	Medicaid/SCHIP
2005	59.5%	9.1%	3.8%	13.7%	13.0%
2004	59.8%	9.3%	3.7%	13.6%	13.0%
2003	60.4%	9.2%	3.5%	13.7%	12.4%
2002	61.3%	9.3%	3.5%	13.4%	11.0%
2001	62.6%	9.2%	3.4%	13.5%	11.2%

A Web-based Tool to Help You Purchase Insurance

MostChoice is a Web-based insurance broker (*www.mostchoice.com*) that will provide you with several health insurance quotes. For example, when I inquired about insurance quotes, the site asked me to provide basic demographic information about my family and me. It also asked if anyone in the family had any of the following conditions: diabetes, asthma, epilepsy, depression requiring medication, heart condition or stroke, lupus, cancer, HIV/AIDS, or sexually transmitted diseases (STDs). As an exploratory exercise, I first answered the site's health questions as if no family members had any of the conditions listed. Then I checked to see how the prices changed with "yes" responses to one or more of the health conditions. The quotes, in most cases, almost doubled. Be aware that the quotes are estimates only, and insurers require verification of your health status, which may affect your final cost.

For a family of three, MostChoice listed 76 plans through six insurance companies. These plan types include managed care plans, such as health maintenance organization (HMOs), preferred provider organizations (PPOs), and point-of-service (POS) plans, as well as indemnity (or fee-for-service) plans. (I explain more about these plan types a little later in this chapter.) The fees ranged from $273 to $1,095 per month. (See figure 3.2.) Just like with car insurance, the rates vary depending upon deductible and co-insurance amounts. The higher the deductible amount and co-insurance (a greater economic burden on the insured), the lower monthly rate you pay.

Figure 3.2 Sample: MostChoice Search and Results 2007[2]

Search Category	Result
Numbers of plan choices	76
Health insurance plan providers	Assurance, U.S. Healthcare, Aetna, Health America, Celtic, Significa
Types of plans	HMO, PPO, Network
Monthly fee range	$273 to $1,095
Deductible range	$0 to $10,000 (variances driven by plan type, with some HMOs at $0 deductibles)
Co-insurance/patient co-pay	0% to 50%
Office visit (amount insured pays)	$0 to $35

Please note that I am not endorsing any of these health plans. The real power of this type of Web site service is the amount of information that is immediately available to you. MostChoice also provides consumer feedback to help you choose a plan. MostChoice has its own internal rating system created by more than one million consumers who have obtained insurance on the site. Nearly every plan is rated extensively, based upon customer service, doctor selection, and benefit coverage.

Plan Types: How do They Differ?

Today, most Americans who have health insurance are enrolled in some kind of managed care plan, an organized way of both providing services and paying for them.[3] Different types of managed care plans work differently and include preferred provider organizations (PPOs), health maintenance organizations (HMOs), and point-of-service (POS) plans. The other type of health insurance plan, rarely available today, is known as "indemnity" health insurance, also called "fee-for-service." Different types of managed care plans vary in the following three key areas:

1. **Your choice of providers.** Many health plans have a network of "participating providers." As a member of a health plan, you will receive the best coverage when you use participating providers. However, if you choose a doctor who is outside of that network, you will probably have to pay a larger portion of or even the entire bill. Generally, HMOs have the greatest limitations on choices. PPOs and POS plans also limit your choices, but not as much as an HMO.
2. **Your out-of-pocket costs.** Generally, your costs will be lower with a plan that offers you fewer choices in healthcare providers. For example, with an HMO, you may have very few doctors to choose from, but you may not have to pay anything when you see the doctor. PPOs and POS plans usually require you to pay a co-pay of 5 dollars to 20 dollars per visit.

3. **Your financial paperwork (or how your bills are paid).** Less choice means less paperwork. PPOs and POS plans require minimal paperwork if you receive your care from in-network providers. If you use an out-of-network provider, you are likely to be deluged with paperwork to get your bills paid. An HMO will send you little to no paperwork.

Three types of managed care plans

The three types of managed care plans are HMOs, PPOs and POS plans. Let's take a closer look at each one.

Preferred Provider Organization (PPO)

A PPO has arrangements with doctors, hospitals, and other healthcare providers, who agree to accept lower fees from the insurer for their services. As a plan member, your costs are lower if you choose providers within the PPO's network. If you go to a doctor within the PPO network, you will pay a copayment (a set amount for certain services—say $10 for a doctor's office visit or $5 for a prescription). Co-insurance, the amount the insurance company pays, will be based on lower charges. Out-of-network providers' fees will be higher than those of in-network providers. Therefore, if you go outside the network, you have to meet the deductible and also pay additional fees because the co-insurance the plan pays will not cover as much of the provider's charges.

Health Maintenance Organization (HMO)

HMOs are the oldest form of managed care plan. They offer members a range of health benefits, including preventive care, for a set monthly fee. There are many kinds of HMOs. If doctors are employees of the health plan, and you visit them at central medical offices or clinics, it is called a "staff model HMO" or a "group model HMO." Other HMOs contract with physician groups or individual doctors who have private offices. These are called "individual practice associations" (IPAs). HMOs will give you a list of doctors from which to choose a primary care doctor who coordinates your care. Generally you must contact your primary care doctor for a referral to a specialist. Some HMOs require a copayment, usually ranging from $5 to $25 for various services; other HMOs have no out-of-pocket costs.

Point-of-Service (POS) Plan

POS plans provide more flexibility in choosing healthcare providers than HMOs, but not as much flexibility as PPOs. The primary care doctors in a POS plan usually make referrals to other providers in the plan. As a member, you also can refer yourself outside the plan and get some coverage. If your doctor makes a referral out of the network, the plan pays all or most of the bill. If you refer yourself to a provider outside the network, you will usually have to pay a higher percentage of the bill than if you saw a participating provider.

Your Choices in Public Health Insurance: Medicare and Medicaid

The choices available in public insurance are limited and vary based upon state and section of the country. In many areas, if you are covered under Medicare you now can choose between managed care and indemnity plans. You can also switch your plan for any reason. Because the policies may change frequently, it is best to contact your local Social Security office or the state office on aging. In some states, Medicaid recipients are required to join managed care plans. Insurance plans and state regulations differ, so check with your state Medicaid office to learn more. (For more details about Medicare and Medicaid guidelines, see chapter 7.)

Your Choices in Private Health Insurance

In choosing a health plan, you first have to decide what is most important to you. Factors to consider include services, choice, location, and costs. All plans have tradeoffs. Here is another place where you can apply your VVMS. You may want to ask yourself the following questions in deciding what plan is best for you and your family.

Services

- How comprehensive do you want coverage of healthcare services to be?
- What services are limited or not covered?
- Is there a good match between what the plan provides and what you think you will need? For example, if you have a chronic disease, is there a special program for that illness?
- Will the plan provide the medication and equipment you need?
- Does the plan pay for preventive care?
- If alternative or holistic treatment options are important to you, does your plan cover them?

Location

- How close to your home do you need your providers to be?
- Are you willing to drive long distances to see your provider of choice?
- Do you need your provider to be near public transportation?

Choice

- How do you feel about limits on your choice of doctors or hospitals?
- What doctors, hospitals, and other medical providers are part of the plan?
- Are there enough of the kinds of doctors you want to see?
- If you want to see a specialist, do you need a referral from your PCP?
- Does the plan require prior approval before going into the hospital or getting specialty care?

Costs

- How much are you willing to spend on premiums and other healthcare costs?
- How do you feel about paying up front for healthcare services?
- Are you willing to pay more to see the provider of your choice?

- Are you willing to give up some freedom of choice to save money?

No health insurance plan will cover every expense. To get a true idea of what your costs will be under each plan, look at how much you will pay for your premium and other costs. If you have a health issue that involves a hospital stay or surgery, your health insurance may cover a high percentage of the bill, but your out-of-pocket costs could still run into thousands of dollars. Keep this in mind when choosing your plan.

Is One Insurer Enough?

Physician fees, prescriptions, and other non-covered costs can be significant if you have a catastrophic illness. Depending on your situation, you may want to purchase a secondary health insurance policy. Commercial insurance companies offer secondary insurance for anyone with a specific type of disease or healthcare need. For example, Aon (*www.aon.com*) offers secondary insurance for several conditions including cancer, heart attack, stroke, and heart surgery. Secondary health insurance is available for children with special needs through Medicaid. These insurance plans cover services that are not covered or only partially covered by the primary insurer, such as special therapies, medical equipment, supplies, devices, and transportation. You should consider secondary insurance if your out-of-pocket costs are too high (measured against the additional premium payment), or if you have a significant acute or chronic condition.

Secondary insurance policies are usually purchased by Medicare patients who are not HMO members. These patients purchase something called a *Medigap* insurance plan that covers costs they would otherwise need to pay out-of-pocket. In general, to purchase a Medigap plan, you must have Medicare Part A and Part B. Many private insurance companies offer Medigap plans, all of which must be standardized and follow strict federal and state laws designed to protect you. Medicare offers an informational booklet through its

Web site (*www.medicare.gov*) to help you choose the best Medigap plan for you.[4]

MAKING SURE YOUR HEALTH PLAN PAYS

Once you've chosen your plan, you still have more work to do. Health plans are complicated and you have to keep track of your health plan's payments. The insurance company sometimes stands between you and your doctor. Occasionally, the insurer refuses to approve a test or treatment. Other times, you may receive treatment, but the insurance company later denies payment because you did not follow one or more of its rules.

There are at least three areas where things could go wrong with your healthcare insurance process: (1) between you and the insurance company, such as if you select an out-of-network provider, perhaps from an outdated list, (2) between you and the provider, such as when you give the provider incorrect insurance information during registration, and (3) between the provider and insurance company, such as when the provider submits a bill with missing information. If you had a direct relationship with the provider, there would be only one place for these types of things to possibly go wrong—between you and the healthcare provider. Unfortunately, it's not that simple. However, there are many basic steps you can take on your own—most won't take much time—to prevent problems.

You and Your Health Plan: Three Strategies You Can Take

Good communication is key to maximizing your health plan's benefits. Here are three strategies to consider:

1. **Make sure you understand your health plan's rules.** If you have single coverage, take responsibility for being familiar with as many plan details as you can. If you have family coverage, be sure one family member is the health plan expert. Your medical mentor may also be able to help. Today, most plans have significant resources to explain plan operation and coverage, available

through both printed materials and the Internet. Also, many practitioners are familiar with the health plans they accept. Sometimes they can offer tips about navigating the system. If your insurance is through your employer, your human resources administrator should be able to explain your plan or, if not, to direct you to other resources. Calling your insurance company representative can also help clarify specific coverage benefits. Whatever resources you use, the more informed you are, the more likely you will be able to maximize your benefits.

2. **When you receive a request from your health plan, respond to it.** Health plans make requests because they lack some information about you. Often this information is necessary to pay a claim. Unanswered requests do not just fade away. They can result in denied payments or delays that end up costing you money. Sometimes, they can even delay your treatment.
3. **Develop a relationship, if possible, with a plan representative.** Telephone contact is usually available with most plans. If you can develop a relationship with one particular person, it may be easier in the future to resolve any issues. If that doesn't work, then be sure to get any correspondence with the health plan in writing. Before you call, gather important information, such as your insurance card, policy booklet, or recent bill. When you receive answers to your questions over the phone, ask the individual to e-mail you the response. Also ask for his full name, title, and direct phone number. Document your conversation in writing. Include the individual's name, number, and date of the call, in case disagreements arise later.

You and Your Healthcare Provider: Three Strategies You Can Take

The minute you walk in your provider's door, you begin giving information that eventually ends up on the bill to your insurance company. You have no control over some information, such as the list of services provided and payment codes submitted. However, you can control other pieces of information. Use these three strategies:

1. **Provide complete and detailed information during registration.** Your input is the primary, and usually the only, source of information at registration. Therefore, it's important that it is detailed, accurate, and complete.
2. **Provide valid, current insurance information.** When something changes in your insurance plan, let your healthcare provider know immediately. If you don't, your doctor or hospital will continue to use your old information. This will result in initial denials and hassles as your provider resubmits requests for payments.
3. **Make sure your physician is a participating provider.** If you have a new physician, check the plan directory and call the physician to confirm her participation in your plan. If you have not been to your doctor for some time, reconfirm her plan participation before you make your next appointment.

Your Providers and Your Health Plan: Three Strategies You Can Take

When it comes time for your insurer to pay the bill that your doctor or hospital submitted, completeness of information is key. The steps that you take in providing your doctor or hospital with complete and accurate information can help make the process run smoother. At this point, you should do three things:

1. **Examine the explanation of benefits (EOB) statement your insurer sends to you.** Every health insurer is required to send you an Explanation of Benefits (EOB) when your healthcare provider has submitted a bill to them for services. The EOB must include at least the following: name of the healthcare provider; date of the service; what service was provided; the provider's charge for the service; the amount payable after deductibles; co-payment and any other reduction of the billed amount; an explanation of any denial, reduction, or any other reason for not providing full reimbursement for the amount claimed; telephone number or address where an

insured may obtain clarification; and information on how to file an appeal of a denial of benefits including the applicable time-frames to file. Make sure to review your EOBs for accuracy.

2. **If you think the EOB is not accurate, notify your provider.** Because of the coding systems used, sometimes the information on the bill may appear inaccurate but is not. The codes used represent the best description of your treatment. However, in some cases, a short discussion with your healthcare provider's office staff can reveal a mistake. The staff can then correct it and resubmit the bill.
3. **If, after you speak with your provider, you still determine that the bill is inaccurate, notify your insurer of your concern.** E-mailing and copying the appropriate individuals at your doctor's office and your health plan is the best way to cover all bases. It's also a good idea to follow up with a phone call to make sure the intended recipients received the e-mail.

The power of having a health advocate to get your bills paid. When Natasha found out she was expecting her second child, she was ecstatic but calm. Her first pregnancy had been smooth sailing and Ewan a beautiful, healthy baby boy was born. Confident that they were prepared for any and all emergencies, Natasha and her husband Dave believed the second time would be no different. However, during her fourth month of pregnancy, the obstetrician saw an irregularity on Natasha's ultrasound and referred them to the perinatal center. Concerned, but optimistic, they booked the appointment immediately. Once there, the neonatologist diagnosed a heart murmur and referred them again, this time to the experts at Children's Hospital of Philadelphia (CHOP). Panic began to set in as they sat through another battery of tests and examinations. Finally, the pediatric cardiologist at CHOP told Natasha and Dave the news they had been dreading: their soon-to-be-born daughter, Ainsley, had a rare congenital heart defect called transposition of the great arteries (TGA). The young parents were devastated. Numb, they listened while the specialist explained more about TGA. "With TGA," he said, "the aorta and pulmonary artery are connected to the wrong ventricles on the heart. As a result, blood from the body never reaches the lungs and the body is starved of oxygen."

Just as Natasha and Dave were beginning to catch their breath, the doctor then informed them that immediately after birth, Ainsley would require open heart surgery. The doctor and a nurse talked them through the procedure, how it would work, how the delivery would be handled, and a host of other details. The nurse also informed them that the physician group was not a participating provider in Dave's health insurance plan. This seemed like an insignificant detail to Dave and Natasha, since all they could think about was making sure their baby would survive and thrive. Thankfully, Ainsley did just that. Natasha and Dave's daughter came through surgery successfully and had no serious consequences. Today, she is a happy, healthy toddler and has a baby sister, Chloe.

The day after that first visit to CHOP, Dave started going through the details of his insurance plan. Since the doctors were not participating providers in his Horizon Blue Cross and Blue Shield PPO plan, he would have a $5,000 deductible to pay out of his own pocket. After that, the policy said the insurance company would cover 80 percent of the *cost*. This seemed inconsequential to Dave—managing the economics of the process dwarfed in comparison to his concerns about his daughter's life and health. As Dave continued to study the health plan, he realized the deductible was per person. This meant his initial up-front cost would actually be $10,000. Dave was flabbergasted by the amount—it was much, much more than he expected. However, the worst was yet to come. The 80 percent payment, it turned out, was applied to the plan's approved *reasonable cost* and not the *actual billed amount* from the provider. This meant that his insurance plan would only cover about 15 percent of the actual bills. That difference would be Dave and Natasha's responsibility.

On a suggestion from the doctor at CHOP, Natasha immediately called Horizon to request a caseworker. Once Natasha explained the seriousness of the situation, Horizon immediately assigned Danielle, one of their health advocates, to coordinate all of the care and provide a single point of communication for them. The first issue at hand was the 10,000 dollar deductible. When Natasha explained that there was no alternative care for Ainsley within the plan's coverage, Horizon waived the entire deductible.

Next came the doctor bills, which were sent directly to Dave. For months after Ainsley's birth, usually three or four bills arrived daily, some of them hundreds of pages long. Dave and Danielle worked out a complex, but necessary, process. Dave sent every doctor bill he received to Horizon. The company would then send either a check for the reduced amount or a denial of payment and the explanation of benefits (EOB). Then, Dave would send all of the denials and EOBs to Danielle. She was *usually* able to get the remainder of the bill approved, and the insurance company would then send Dave a check. After depositing the checks, Dave would pay the doctors' bills.

In the end, the insurance company paid almost all of the bills, even though the costs were far above and beyond what the plan covered. The final bill for all of Ainsley's and Natasha's care was about $600,000. According to the plan's policy, Dave and Natasha would have been responsible for paying about $511,000 of the bill. Instead, they paid $9,000 from their own pockets. Dave and Natasha took an active role in the payment processes and procedures. Danielle, Horizon's health advocate, made the road less rocky for them. They would not have been able to figure out all of the financial details without her guidance and for that, as well as for their daughter's continuing good health, they are eternally grateful.

What Happens If I Have a Pre-Existing Condition?

A pre-existing condition is any medical condition diagnosed or treated before you join a new health plan. The Health Insurance Portability and Accountability Act (HIPAA) limits health plans from denying payment for care for a pre-existing condition. In the past, health plans required a waiting period before paying for pre-existing conditions for new members. These waiting periods were costly and detrimental to the member's health. Under HIPAA, when you join a new group plan, any pre-existing condition is covered without a waiting period, *as long as* you have been insured without interruption during the previous 12 months. This means that if you remain insured for 12 months or more, you will be able to go from one job to another, and your pre-existing condition will be covered. In the event that your coverage lapsed and you have a pre-existing condition, the longest you have to wait before you are covered for that condition is 12 months.[5]

What about Coverage for Mental Health Conditions?

Some health plans treat individuals who have mental health disorders differently. Coverage for mental health conditions in the U.S. has traditionally not been on par with coverage for medical or surgical conditions. For this reason, the Mental Health Parity law was passed in 1996. This law provided parity, but only for annual and lifetime limits between mental health coverage and medical surgical coverage. The current version of this law is looking to expand parity by including deductibles, co-payments, out-of-pocket expenses, coinsurance, covered hospital days, and covered out-patient visits. While this law, when it is passed, is likely to increase mental health coverage even more, legislatures will probably need to continue working to amend and clarify provisions of the act for years to come. The joint committee of the Senate and House of Representatives continues to work to eliminate this bias. Former First Lady Rosalynn Carter is a proponent of this legislation and works tirelessly with the committee to promote it. You should check your plan's policy to determine whether you have any limitations on coverage for mental health conditions.

What Does the Healthcare Provider Charge for Services?

When you purchase something, one of the first questions you ask is, "What will this cost?" However, if you're like most people, you probably don't ask that question of your healthcare providers. You may not be inclined to ask if you are insured, since you are not primarily responsible for the payment. However, because you may have to pay a percentage of the charge, it is important to question the cost for each procedure.

Despite the importance of knowing costs ahead of time, getting an answer is not so easy. Hospitals, doctors, and other healthcare providers use a specific strategy for pricing their services. First, they determine charges for every service they provide using a strategy that includes all of their direct and indirect costs to provide the service. For a hospital, this includes items such as running the building and staffing, just like any business. Charges vary based upon the location of the hospital and the types of services they provide. For example, it will cost more to run a 1,000-bed teaching hospital in the Northeast than to run a 200-bed community hospital in the rural Midwest.

Every hospital has an official *charge master* document that lists every service and procedure and the charge for them. The hospital uses this document to negotiate payments with private health insurers for various services. Medicare and Medicaid, on the other hand, publish their own reimbursement rates. These government insurers tell the healthcare providers how much they will pay for each service. Hospitals have no bargaining power here. They must accept the Medicare and Medicaid rates.

With private insurance companies, hospitals generally negotiate contracts every few years. Certain key factors play an important role in how the negotiations turn out. Generally, larger hospitals with a bigger patient population are in a better position to negotiate for higher fees than smaller hospitals. Larger insurers are in a better position to negotiate lower rates. Because contracts differ with each individual health plan, hospitals may receive different payments for the same services, depending on the insurer. In fact, one New York City hospital had 55 different rates for each procedure because its patients used 55 different health plans. That number could change during any given month, year, or even day. Negotiated rates with private insurers are proprietary information and held close to the vest in every hospital.

In one of my Internet-based surveys of healthcare consumers, I asked what their top three questions were about healthcare. Of the

2,000 responses, one of the most common questions was, "Why do hospitals charge much more for patients who don't have insurance to get hospital care than for patients who do have insurance?" Many respondents added that it wasn't fair that they were charged more for the same services just because they were not insured. I agree. It isn't fair. However, as long as hospitals continue to negotiate different payments with every health plan inconsistent billing will likely continue.

Figure 3.4 highlights the difference between the rates that a hospital charges, what its direct cost for the service is, and what it is paid. The data is for a 500-bed teaching hospital in a suburban area.[6] It shows that of the top 14 services provided to patients in the outpatient setting, the hospital makes money on nine of them (in the gray boxes in the far right column) and loses money on five of them. And, in some cases, like medication injections of the drug Epoetin, the most common service, the hospital loses about $350,000 per year. If any other business were not making money for a service, it would discontinue the service. This, of course, is not a possibility in healthcare.

Figure 3.4 Services, Charges, Costs, and Payments for a Suburban Pennsylvania Teaching Hospital with 500 Beds

Outpatient Service, Procedure, or Drug Administration	Units of Service	Average Direct Charge	Average Cost	Average Payment
Injection of Epoetin (drug for anemia, for patients on dialysis)	171,222	$68	$13	$11
X-ray, level 2	11,137	$753	$150	$118
Cardiac catheterization	558	$4,134	$731	$1,977
Colonoscopy	1,806	$1,698	$367	$444
Injection of Rituximab (drug for rheumatoid arthritis & lymphoma)	1,587	$1,898	$377	$436
Radiation therapy	7,566	$404	$80	$90
Injection of Pegfilgrastim (drug used for cancer chemotherapy patients with low white blood cell counts)	260	$7,881	$1,566	$2,401
Injections into the nerves (for pain relief)	1,600	$866	$242	$317
Injection of Zoledronic Acid (drug for cancer patients with high levels of calcium in their blood)	2,547	$906	$180	$196
Infusion, IVIG non-lyophil (cancer chemotherapy drug)	5,759	$244	$48	$80
X-ray, level 1	10,456	$278	$36	$42
Radiation therapy (IMRT type)	1,480	$3,993	$798	$292
Emergency visits, complex	1,816	$826	$226	$223
Computerized axial tomography (CT Scan)	1,885	$1,447	$176	$161

Are Hospital Fees Negotiable?

Hospitals negotiate fees with health plans continuously. A similar strategy may work for you, especially if you are uninsured. If you have no insurance coverage or need to pay some hospital fees, it will be helpful to speak with the hospital business office or finance department. Either you or your medical mentor can have the discussion. First, let the hospital know you are aware that their published charges are not the same as the rates the insurance companies pay them. And, as a customer, you expect at the very least, to be charged no more than the average rate a health insurer would reimburse the hospital for the service. Before the discussion, look up the average cost on the American Hospital Directory Web site (*www.ahd.com)*, which provides hospital information through free and subscription-based services.

The fact that hospitals charge uninsured patients the rate on their *charge master* is not malicious. Federal law actually requires the hospital to charge you its published fee—unless you, the patient, initiate negotiations to reduce the fee. You can and should use this information to negotiate the price for your healthcare services.

WHAT IF I CAN'T GET INSURANCE? TEN RESOURCES TO TAP

For the 15 percent of Americans (almost 47 million people) who are not currently insured, there are many resources to tap. These resources may also be available if you have insurance, but you likely will have certain limits or exclusions. Some of these resources, like participating in clinical trials, are available to anyone who meets the clinical criteria, regardless of ability to pay.

1. Your State Medical Assistance Program

Most state medical assistance programs provide some level of healthcare funding assistance even if you do not qualify for Medicaid under the economic criteria. For a list of all state medical assistance Web sites, see the National Association of Health Underwriters (NAHU) Web site at *www.nahu.org.*

Medicaid also has a little-known program, the Health Insurance Premium Payment (HIPP). This program serves patients who have chronic and severe illnesses, such as heart problems, congenital birth defects, cancer, and AIDS.[7] These patients are, or were, covered through their employers, but are at risk of losing their coverage due to inability to pay their premiums. Medicaid considers paying the premiums when the cost of the premium, deductible, and co-insurance are less than the cost of providing Medicaid coverage.

2. Federal Free Clinics

The Health Resources and Services Administration (HRSA), a division of the federal government's Department of Health and Human Services, runs free clinics nationwide.[8] Their Web site provides addresses and contact information for clinics that offer primary medical, obstetrical, gynecological, mental health, substance abuse and dental care and support services. To learn more, visit *www.ask.hrsa.gov/pc.*

3. Free Clinic Foundation of America

The Free Clinic Foundation of America is a network of independent free clinics located throughout the country.[9] These free clinics are different from the federal free clinics mentioned above. To find a free clinic in your state visit *www.freeclinicfoundation.com.*

4. Hill-Burton Act Patient Benefits

In 1946, the U.S. Congress passed a law giving hospitals and other health facilities grants for construction. In return, the facilities agreed to provide a reasonable volume of services to individuals residing in the area and unable to pay for healthcare. About 250 healthcare facilities nationwide are still obligated to provide free or reduced-cost care. The steps to apply for Hill-Burton free or reduced cost healthcare are the following:[10]

1. Find a Hill-Burton facility from the list at www.hrsa.gov/hillburton/hillburtonfacilities.htm.
2. Obtain a copy of the *Hill-Burton Individual Notice* from the facility's admissions department. The *Individual Notice* will tell

you what income level makes you eligible for free or reduced-cost care and what services might be covered.

3. Go to the office listed in the *Individual Notice* and say you want to apply for Hill-Burton free or reduced-cost care. You may need to fill out a form.
4. Provide the facility with any other required documents to prove income eligibility.
5. If the facility asks you to apply for Medicaid, Medicare, or some other financial assistance, you must do so.
6. When you return the completed application, ask for a *Determination of Eligibility*. Check the *Individual Notice* to see how much time the facility has before it must tell you whether you will receive free or reduced-cost care.

The Hill-Burton law only covers facility costs, not private doctors' bills. Hill-Burton facilities must provide a specific amount of free or reduced-cost care annually, but can stop once they have given that amount. Obligated facilities publish an *Allocation Plan* in the local newspaper each year. The *Allocation Plan* includes the income criteria, types of services covered, and amount of free or reduced-cost services the facility will provide for the year.

5. Clinical Trials

If you need treatment, you may be able to take part in a research study called a *clinical trial*. Clinical trials are used to find out whether new drugs or treatments are safe and effective. The Web site for the National Institutes of Health (NIH) lists many clinical trials that are in progress. Visit the site (*www.clinicaltrials.gov*) to learn if a clinical trial is underway for your condition and whether you might be able to take part in it.[11] Additional clinical trials are listed at the CenterWatch Web site (*www.centerwatch.com*). This site lists more than 41,000 clinical trials.[12]

The entity conducting the study covers the cost for care provided under a clinical trial. If you are interested in participating in a clinical trial, you will be provided with a significant amount of information. This will help you understand everything that is involved, including the risks or possible side-effects, before you consent to participate. You will also have opportunities to ask questions and can remove yourself from the study at any point in time. (For more details on participating in medical research, also known as clinical trials, see chapter 11.)

6. The Free Medicine Program

The Free Medicine Program helps patients obtain prescription medications absolutely free of charge.[13] The program was established by volunteers and has helped countless families across the nation substantially reduce or completely eliminate their prescription drug bills. The majority of applicants have too much income to qualify for government prescription-assistance programs, but not enough to purchase private prescription drug insurance coverage. For more information, visit *www.freemedicineprogram.org.*

7. Pharmaceutical-Sponsored Medication Programs

Pharmaceutical companies also run programs to provide free medications to people who cannot afford to buy their medicine. For information about how to apply for assistance with prescription costs, visit *www.rxassist.org*[14] and *www.cancersupportivecare.com/.*[15]

8. Federal Healthcare Tax Credit Program

The Federal Healthcare Tax Credit Program (HCTC) provides a refundable tax credit to help eligible individuals purchase health insurance from a number of different sources.[16] Those who have suffered a job loss due to a trade-related event, or receive pension benefits from the federal Pension Benefit Guarantee Corporation are eligible. HCTC recipients must use their tax credit monies to purchase specified types of health insurance policies. For more information, visit *www.nahu.org/consumer/healthcare/topic.cfm?catID=95.*

9. Academic Medical Center (AMC) Clinics and Free Care

U.S. medical schools and teaching hospitals provide free or low-cost community-based programs, such as wellness programs, preventive and primary care medicine, health education initiatives, and emergency care.[17] These services are designed to help the uninsured and underinsured. For a listing by region of AMC services, visit *www.aamc.org/uninsured/start.htm.*

10. Local Hospitals

All hospitals have some level of obligation to provide services and charitable care to their community. Hospitals that have a nonprofit status are under a greater obligation than for-profit hospitals. You can determine your local hospital's profit or nonprofit status by looking it up on the American Hospital Directory Web site at *www.ahd.com.* Contact the hospital's public relations or financial departments to inquire about special programs for patients with economic needs. Most hospitals identify uninsured patients, determine whether they qualify for Medicaid coverage, and assist them in completing the application.

The American Hospital Association (AHA) provides a brochure, *Patient Care Partnership,* to member hospitals. This brochure explains how hospitals will help uninsured patients. The following is an excerpt from the AHA brochure:[18]

Our staff will file claims for you with healthcare insurers or other programs, such as Medicare and Medicaid. They also will help your doctor with needed documentation. Hospital bills and insurance coverage are often confusing. If you have questions about your bill, contact our business office...If you do not have health coverage, we will try to help you and your family find financial help or make other arrangements. We need your help with collecting needed information and other requirements to obtain coverage or assistance.

Being a nonprofit organization means, among other things, that the organization does not have to pay taxes on any profits it makes. The government expects, however, that the organization will give some portion of profits back to the community or use the monies for charitable care. The more money a nonprofit makes, the more the federal government watches for potential slip-ups. A few hospitals have lost their nonprofit status for failing to fulfill their charitable and community obligations. As a result, every nonprofit hospital has a significant incentive to serve its community.

Figure 3.5 Free and Reduced-Cost Healthcare Resources

Free and Reduced-Cost Healthcare Resources	Only Available to the Economically Needy?
1. State medical assistance	1. Yes
2. Federal free clinics	2. Yes
3. Free Clinic Foundation of America	3. No (sliding-scale payments)
4. Hill-Burton Act hospitals and healthcare organizations	4. Yes
5. Clinical trials	5. No
6. Free Medicine Program	6. Yes
7. Pharmaceutical-sponsored medication programs	7. Yes
8. Federal Healthcare Tax Credit Program	8. Yes
9. Academic medical center free clinics and other free care	9. Yes
10. Local hospital assistance	10. Yes

OTHER ASSISTANCE INFORMATION

The following patient advocacy organizations also provide financial aid for medical care: Families USA (www.familiesusa.org),[19] National Patient Advocate Foundation (npaf.org),[20] Association of Maternal and Child Health Programs (www.amchp.org),[21] and Patient Advocate Foundation (www.patientadvocate.org).[22]

Key Highlights

Paying for healthcare can be complicated, especially if you have no insurance. If you do have health insurance, you have either private insurance or public (government-sponsored) insurance. If you are self-employed or your employer does not offer health benefits, resources are available to help you find affordable health insurance. Organizations, such as unions, professional associations, or chambers of commerce, may be able to help. If you are uninsured, resources are available to help you access healthcare. These include state medical assistance, federal free clinics, and the Free Clinic Foundation of America. In addition, you can find financial aid information for medical care from several patient advocacy organizations, including Families USA and National Patient Advocate Foundation.

Key Actions

- Understand how your insurance plan works and be as proactive as possible to maximize your benefits.
- Research all options, including professional or civic organizations, if you need to purchase your own health insurance.
- Identify what is important to you when determining what type of insurance to purchase.

Key Take-Away

Whether you are insured or uninsured, healthcare resources are available for you to use.

Endnotes

[1] From the U.S. Agency for Healthcare Research and Quality, *www.ahrq.gov.*
[2] From MostChoice, *www.mostchoice.com.*
[3] The U.S. Agency for Healthcare Research and Quality, *www.ahrq.gov*, is the source for the information on and definitions of health plans.
[4] Centers for Medicare and Medicaid Services, *2007 Choosing A Medigap Policy: A Guide to Health Insurance for People with Medicare.*
[5] HIPAA is Public Law 104-191, passed by the 104th Congress. The rules regarding pre-existing conditions are under Title I of HIPAA.
[6] Taken from publicly available records hospitals must file annually through the *Medicare Cost Report* (*www.ahd.com*).

---

[7] The Health Insurance Premium Payment program was enacted as part of the Omnibus Budget Reconciliation Act of 1990, Public Law 101-508.
[8] Health Resources and Services Administration, *www.hrsa.gov.*
[9] Free Clinic Foundation of America, *www.freeclinicfoundation.com.*
[10] Health Resources and Services Administration, *www.hrsa.gov/hillburton.*
[11] National Institutes of Health list of clinical trials, *www.clinicaltrials.gov.*
[12] Center Watch list of clinical trials, *www.centerwatch.com.*
[13] The Free Medicine Program, *www.freemedicineprogram.org.*
[14] RxAssist, *www.rxassist.org.*
[15] Cancer Supportive Care, *www.cancersupportivecare.com.*
[16] National Association of Health Underwriters, *www.nahu.org.*
[17] Association of American Medical Colleges, *www.aamc.org.*
[18] American Hospital Association. *The Patient Care Partnership: Understanding Expectations, Rights, and Responsibilities.* AHA, 2003. To download a copy of this brochure, go to *www.aha.org/aha/issues/Communicating-With-Patients/pt-care-partnership.html.*
[19] Families USA, *www.familiesusa.org.*
[20] National Patient Advocate Foundation, *www.npaf.org.*
[21] Association of Maternal and Child Health Programs, *www.amchp.org.*
[22] Patient Advocate Foundation, *www.patientadvocate.org.*

STEP

2

OWN YOUR STORY

CHAPTER

4

Playing an Active Role in Creating Your Healthcare Story

Heirlooms we don't have in our family. But stories we've got.
—Rose Cherin

My maternal grandfather, a legend in our family, died when I was less than a year old. We heard many stories about his athletic feats as a Villanova University football star and his days as a beloved, small-town football coach. As a husband and father of four, he was an enthusiastic entrepreneur of the 1940s. In all the pictures I have ever seen of him, he looks dashing: full head of white hair, flawless profile, sharp eyes, and always the perfect smile. As I was growing up, looking through my parents' wedding album for a peek at my grandfather, I never imagined my most intimate encounter with him would be through his medical record.

On my first day of work in a local hospital medical record department, I was charged with finding records for a study of patients treated within the past 25 years. Once I located all current patients' records, I headed to the sub-basement of the hospital, commonly referred to as *the dungeon,* to review archived paper records. When I finished with the archived records, I looked at the oldest, microfilmed records. As I turned the knob on the side of the microfilm machine, there it was—my grandfather's name. His entire medical record—all 54 pages of it—was right in front of me. One by one, I printed off each page for the study. As I waited, I read the contents. I can still remember certain phrases like, "pleasant 47-year-old man," "worked around the production of rubber," "known the family for the past 20 years." I devoured every piece of information. It was a wonderful opportunity to get to know the grandfather I had never really met. Reading his medical record did a few things for me. First, it made me feel like I knew him, or at least was able to share in some small piece of his past, more so than the typical family album. Second, it filled in some gaps about what diseases were or were not a part of my own heredity.

More than 20 years later when the doctors were diagnosing my daughter Emmalea's juvenile myoclonic epilepsy, one of the first questions they asked was whether epilepsy ran in the family. Both my husband and I responded no. As it turned out, Emmalea's symptoms and test results were strong enough to support the diagnosis of JME, a hereditary condition. My mother investigated and was surprised to find that her aunt, uncle, and grandmother all had epilepsy. Two years later, also to our surprise, we found out that one of my father's uncles had epilepsy.

We could not possibly have expected these ancestors to pass along the information about their conditions, which may have impacted a third generation. What we can hope for today, with all of the technology and resources that are available to us, is a way to share health information that will be helpful to future generations. Understanding the information that is collected and documented on each of us by physicians and other healthcare providers, and obtaining access to our information and that of our loved ones, are steps in the right direction.

YOU HAVE A STORY, TOO

Everyone has a story. In addition to our life story, we each have a healthcare story, a story healthcare providers preserve and document. While this story may not be the one you love to tell, it is important to know it and share it—not only for your own well-being, but for that of your descendents. In technical terms, this story is your *medical record* or *health information.* You are the owner of your health information—your healthcare story. Would you like to know where it is, what it says, what it means? Would you like to have a copy of it? Would you like to know what health information you are leaving behind for the benefit of future family members? You may not plan to share your medical records like the family photo album, but with the increasing use of computerized information and growing interest in genetic predisposition to disease, examining our ancestors' medical records could become commonplace someday. If you have access to this kind of information, you can create a family health history on the U.S. Surgeon General's Web site, My Family Health Portrait (*www.familyhistory.hhs.gov*).

This chapter explores how and why your healthcare story is created. The focus here is specifically on the part of your medical record called the *history and physical,* since it is the first clinical document created in your record. It is one of the most important documents in your medical record. (For more details about how to read your medical record, please see Appendix 1.)

You may have never reviewed your medical record, yet you can get a copy any time, for any reason. You will learn how to be proactive in the creation of your healthcare story. Each of our conscious contributions to the content of our healthcare story will make a difference to the quality and reliability of information for our future generations, others and us.

How Your Healthcare Story Is Created

Before your doctor becomes acquainted with you, he becomes acquainted with your medical record. Your story starts the minute you encounter the healthcare provider setting, even before you see the doctor, usually at the time you register, sign in, or show up for an appointment. Some information you may provide by completing forms. Then, your physicians, nurse, and other clinicians add information in your record based on conversations with you about your health status. Finally, information comes from various procedures and diagnostic tests such as x-rays, MRIs, and blood analysis.

Chances are you will repeat a lot of historical information every time you visit a healthcare provider for the first time, lending to slight, but sometimes significant, differences in your record. Each doctor and hospital you've visited over the years has created a separate medical record for you. Even if you give permission to transfer your information from one place to the next, each healthcare provider creates his or her own version of your medical record.

This scattering of information creates numerous healthcare disadvantages, yet it is quite common. However, if you, the owner of your healthcare story, obtain and keep copies of your own medical records from your healthcare providers, you can diminish these disadvantages and be a stronger partner with your healthcare team. You'll be in a better position to check the accuracy of information, ask questions regarding that information, and share your information, when appropriate, with your team members or relatives.

The federal government is developing an alternative to the fragmentation of healthcare information—a universal health record number for every American. This would be one number, similar to a social security number, assigned to each of us for healthcare information. Your healthcare providers would use the number to access old records and document new information. Ideally, all of your health information would be stored in one, electronic location. It may take decades for the government to put this concept into practice. In the meantime, you have the power to obtain and maintain all of your medical records yourself.

MEDICAL RECORD: THE RECORD *YOUR HEALTHCARE PROVIDERS* MAKE WITH YOUR FEEDBACK

To some degree, you control the quality of care you receive by providing detailed, accurate, honest, and complete information about your condition. Your description of your problem, in part, guides your physician's initial decisions. Without it, your physician may have difficulty diagnosing any problem. A skillful physician asks clarifying questions, but the more accurately you describe your symptoms, the more accurate your diagnosis is likely to be.

Figure 4.1 Example: Information to Tell Your Healthcare Provider about Chest Pain

Quality	Description
Detail	Specific to the pain, tell the length of time, severity, and quality (sharp, dull).
Accuracy	Be as factual as possible. Ask yourself: "Are my emotions making my description inaccurate?"
Honesty	Do not omit any details, even if you feel embarrassed or did something your physician warned you not to do. Specify what you ate, drank, and did before the pain began (e.g., running vigorously, fighting, or some other stressful activity).
Completeness	Bring in all facts that could possibly help the physician better diagnose and treat you, including a list of current medications and dosages, prescription and over-the-counter. Describe habits, general diet, exercise (or lack thereof), relationship issues, and other symptoms or conditions you have.

Do It Now!

Think about the last time you had a doctor's appointment. What did you have to describe to her? Ringing in your ears? Numbness in your foot? Stomach pain? Whatever it was, how did you describe it and how might you have described it better? Also, if you are experiencing non-emergency symptoms over a period of time, write them down, providing as much detail as you can.

My Description of Symptoms

____

____

____

____

____

____

What Else Comes from You: Your Medical History

The history and physical section is one of the most important parts of your health record. You are the sole supplier of information in your medical history. Your medical history is documented by the physician, but in the words that you use. The physician, with your input, documents your physical exam in his words. In the physician's office, the history and physical section is the main part of your medical record. In the hospital, this section is just one of many different forms and pieces of information in your record. Even then, your history and physical is a primary document every clinician you see refers to and relies upon for accurate and safe coordination of your care.

Just as you rely upon the expertise of the healthcare practitioner to ask the right questions and make the best decisions, she relies on you to provide accurate, honest, and complete information. In addition to your medical history, you provide information for your medical record when you answer your doctor's questions during a physical exam. Often patients give only "yes" or "no" answers. Instead, try to give more detailed descriptions to help your doctor make a concise diagnosis. For example, when describing pain, you may want to specify its intensity on a scale from 1 to 10, if that is helpful to your doctor. If you are not sure how to respond to a question, ask for clarification. Some details may seem unimportant to you, but could potentially lead to a more accurate diagnosis and better treatment.

Tests: Gathering Evidence for a Diagnosis

The physician's process to correctly diagnose your condition is something like that of an investigator searching for clues to solve a crime—evidence is key. The physician gathers evidence when you are relating the history of your problem and when he performs his physical exam. He makes a list of possible diagnoses (also known as differential diagnoses) and orders tests to either confirm or rule out the diagnoses.

For example, a patient arrives at the emergency room, complaining of chest and upper abdominal pain. The doctor orders an EKG to rule out a heart attack or myocardial infarction. If the doctor is able to exclude a heart attack, he may then ask additional questions and request several lab tests as well as x-rays, an MRI, and/or CT scan of the patient's abdomen and chest. Figure 4.2 provides an example of a radiologist's interpretation of a chest x-ray. The emergency room doctor analyzes the results of the chest x-ray, as well as other tests, to arrive at the diagnosis or cause of the patient's pains.

Figure 4.2 Sample Chest X-Ray Medical Record

Patient name: _______________ **Medical Record #** ________________

Date: ________________

Exam: Portable chest x-ray

Ordering physician: Dr. Smith
Reason for exam: chest pain, shortness of breath, and fever
FINAL REPORT

Interpreted by: Dr. Jones

An upright view of the chest was obtained. There is opacity at the right lung base and pneumonia cannot be excluded. There is prominence of the pulmonary vessels, consistent with pulmonary edema. Midline sternotomy wires are seen in the stable position.

Impression: pneumonia, congestive heart failure, status post-coronary bypass surgery
Dr. Jones
(electronic signature)

Your Diagnosis

Determining and documenting your definitive diagnosis is a key part of your visit to your physician. Based on the patient's symptoms (fever) and x-ray results (pneumonia) in figure 4.2, it is likely that he has pneumonia. However, it appears that he may also have some cardiac problems, including heart failure. This may be a case where the emergency room physician cannot determine the patient's diagnosis based solely upon preliminary test results. This patient may need additional testing or a consultation with a cardiologist to determine his definitive diagnosis.

Your physician considers your responses to her questions, your test results, and your health history to determine your diagnosis. The diagnostic process can be straightforward or complex. When a physician sees a patient who has a sore throat and tests positive for strep, the diagnosis is straightforward. However, a patient who has a positive strep culture and a recent history of breast cancer and chemotherapy requires a more complex decision-making process. Chemotherapy may have compromised the patient's immune system, so the physician must consider issues besides the immediate complaint of sore throat. Whether your case is simple or complex, it is important for you to be as accurate, detailed, and complete as possible in your communications with your physician.

Your Treatment

When your physician recommends a treatment or action plan, it is important for you or your designated medical mentor if you are too ill, to be as proactive as possible. Ask questions and clarify information. Treatment may include medication or one or more procedures. An action plan may include follow-up tests, appointments, or therapy. The physician will document your treatment and action plan in your health information.

Many physicians provide a written statement of the treatment plan and follow-up activities they discussed with you. However, if your physician or healthcare provider does not do this, don't assume you will remember everything. If you misinterpret your treatment plan, you may harm yourself. If you are given prescriptions, for example, ask the doctor to write down the instructions and possible side effects. It is your doctor's responsibility to provide you with the best treatment and care, but it is *your* responsibility to obtain, apply, and maintain this information.

The Difference between Physician Office Records and Hospital Records

The physician office record is quite different from a hospital record. Part of the reason for this difference is that the record for one hospitalization can include as many as 10 or more days' worth of documentation, testing, and diagnosing by many different physicians and clinicians. Each visit to the hospital marks the beginning of a new medical record. In the physician office, your physician documents a short, dated entry (also known as a progress note) for each visit. He is usually the only clinician documenting in your office record.

With your input, your physician initially documents and then updates your history and physical every 30 days, or whenever your next visit or phone call occurs. He will generally provide you with a discharge slip that contains your diagnosis, length of visit, and amount of the bill (since this form often serves as the copy of the bill for you). Other documents your physician may keep in your clinic or office medical record include reports from consultants who have seen you, test results, applicable surgical reports, and second opinions.

PERSONAL MEDICAL RECORD: THE RECORD *YOU* MAKE

A personal medical record is a collection of information relevant to your health that you keep. It is separate from, and in addition to, the records your physicians create for you. Creating your personal medical record does not have to be an overwhelming process. You can start out brief and focused, and add detail as you go.

Benefits of the Personal Medical Record

Creating and maintaining a personal medical record requires time and diligence, but it is worth the effort, as it serves many purposes, including to:

- Serve as a reference to remember vital health details, such as the last time you got a tetanus shot.
- Provide documentation to your doctor to avoid unnecessary paperwork.
- Aid your physician in providing better care because he has the information he needs at hand, and can be more informed, focused, and complete in treating you.

- Reduce unnecessary testing because you will have a record of previous test results. This benefits you, your physician, and the healthcare system, since fewer unnecessary tests reduces the cost of healthcare.

Start Small

Two nonprofit healthcare associations, the American Health Information Management Association (AHIMA)[1] and the American Medical Informatics Association (AMIA),[2] address the essentials of what to include in your personal medical record. They recommend the following contents:

- ✓ Personal identification, including name and birth date
- ✓ People to contact in case of an emergency
- ✓ Names, addresses, and phone numbers of your physicians, pharmacist, dentist, and specialists
- ✓ Health insurance information and phone numbers
- ✓ Living wills, advance directives, or medical power of attorney
- ✓ Organ-donor authorization
- ✓ Significant illnesses and surgical procedures, and the dates they occurred
- ✓ Current medications and dosages, both prescription and over-the-counter
- ✓ Immunizations and dates received
- ✓ Allergies or sensitivities to drugs, food, or materials, such as latex
- ✓ Important events, dates, and hereditary conditions in your immediate family history
- ✓ Results from a recent physical examination
- ✓ Opinions of specialists
- ✓ Test results
- ✓ Eye and dental records
- ✓ Correspondence between you and your practitioner

You can learn more about developing your own record at this AHIMA-sponsored Web site: *www.myphr.org.*

Grow Your Record

Ideally, your personal medical record should consist of your basic health information and a copy of every medical record created by every healthcare provider who has ever cared for you. Because collecting all of these pieces to your medical record can be a daunting task, you may want to prioritize your requests for your health information based on importance and your most recent visits.

How we addressed the personal medical record need. Within three months of Emmalea's diagnosis of epilepsy, she had been to see three different physicians and had been in three different hospitals. Another six months after that, she had been to another three physicians and a fourth hospital. The information began accumulating rapidly. Because many of the visits were second opinions with physicians who needed to work in concert with each other, we needed to make sure they had the information they needed when they needed it.

We chose a two-tiered strategy. For the first visit to each physician, we brought copies of all of her previous medical records. Second, we created a secure, password-protected Web site that housed all of Emmalea's medical records. We provided each of her physicians with password and Web site information so they could upload their own information and view information from each other. Some physicians were not comfortable uploading information. In those cases, we requested hard copies of the records and uploaded the documents ourselves. Ultimately, it was up to us to keep the site accurate and up-to-date.

A Solution Provided by Your Healthcare System

Many major healthcare organizations today have developed or are developing their own Web-based health records. These Web sites are accessible to patients of the healthcare system and contain all relevant information, including prescriptions, appointments, referrals, and health information/medical records. Cleveland Clinic's "MyChart" Web site (*mychart.clevelandclinic.org*), and Beth Israel Deaconess' "PatientSite" (*www.patientsite.org*) are excellent examples of how efficient and meaningful online medical records can be. These two systems are highly structured, organized, complete, and easy to access.

Hospital owned Web-based health records contain information from the hospital's providers. Documentation about the healthcare you receive elsewhere is not integrated into your overall health record. If you are, however, a long-term patient within the same system, these Web-based products are amazing additions to your healthcare tool set. You should ask your physicians if they, or the hospital where they admit patients, provide an electronic patient record that is available for your use.

Figure 4.3 Cleveland Clinic MyChart Health Records Overview[3]

Health Summary	Includes your current diagnoses as released by your physician. Learn more about your diagnosis by clicking on the underlined diagnosis name.
Medications	View a list of your current medications, request prescription renewals, and learn more about your medications by clicking on the underlined medication name.
Test Results	Click on the "Final Result" option to view the details of your recent tests and read explanatory notes, if added by your physician. Click on the underlined test name to see a description of what the test is and what it means.
Health Reminders	Lists the tests or immunizations recommended for people your age, gender, and, in some cases, diagnoses. Due dates help you decide when to request the tests or procedures. Find out more about a test by clicking on the test's name.
Visit History	Includes a list of your appointments and attending physician. For more information on a particular physician, click on his or her name. Click on "Details" to see more information about a particular visit, such as vital signs, patient instructions, and orders associated with that visit.

A collaborative web-based approach for the future. Members of our firm are located in different geographic areas. We have a virtual office. Sometimes it is challenging to brainstorm or have group discussions. We can accomplish some of this via conference calls. But, we also use intranet-based discussion groups. These discussions allow everyone to see, read, and comment on each other's contribution to a particular topic. Each of us receives automatic alerts through our e-mail when one of the group members has made an addition to an online brainstorming session. We make better decisions because we can continuously view and comment on each other's work.

Someday, perhaps, healthcare will embrace an open, yet individually protected, system to allow all physicians who care for the same patient to engage in electronic communications, similar to an online discussion group. The communication process would be akin to the interactions among the attending physicians, residents, and interns in a typical teaching hospital. But this system would cut across all healthcare organizations and physicians, regardless of which institutions they are affiliated with or where they are located. The ultimate benefit of online patient communications would be the best possible care to you, the patient.

YOUR HEALTHCARE STORY BENEFITS YOU, YOUR FAMILY, AND OTHERS

The impact of your healthcare story will likely go beyond you and your family. Early in my career, I worked in the medical record department managing the cancer registry for George Washington University (GWU) Hospital. A cancer registry maintains a collection of detailed information on every patient treated for a diagnosis of cancer anywhere within a healthcare system. The goal of registries is to gather as much information as possible for research purposes in the hope of discovering improved treatments and cures. Today, cancer registry activities are an even higher priority than they were in the 1980s when I worked in the field.

A large group of physicians, some with renowned accomplishments in cancer treatment and diagnosis, supported the cancer registry at GWU Hospital. We met monthly to review the current database of cancer patients and to discuss results of any studies that we were performing either for the hospital, the medical school, or the American College of Surgeons, the national sponsor for cancer registries at the time. Our team at GWU dedicated a tremendous amount of time and resources to collect and analyze information on cancer patients. Back then, researchers considered cancer patients' records so important that we stamped *CANCER* in 4-inch-high red letters on the front cover of every record. It was a way of ensuring the cancer registry did not miss any useful information. Today tagging is done electronically.

When I first began working in the cancer registry, I marveled at the detailed information we maintained on every patient. Much of that information was from the patient's medical record. Minute details describing the exact circumstances surrounding when, where, and how a patient first discovered a lump or other abnormality that led to a cancer diagnosis sometimes went on for several paragraphs. We scrutinized personal habits, like smoking, and included the age a patient began smoking, how many cigarettes were smoked per day, the time of day they were smoked, the brand of cigarettes, and so on. Family history details were also often lengthy and informative. We sent our quantitative data—of this we were most proud—to the State Department of Health and the federal government's Centers for Disease Control and Prevention (CDC). These agencies combined our data with that of approximately 4,000 other participating hospitals to use in national cancer research initiatives.

The cancer registry followed up on patients at least once a year. If the patient had not been in the hospital within the past 12 months, it was our responsibility to call the patient and ask general questions about how she was doing. This undertaking remains a crucial function in medical research because follow-up information provides cancer survival statistics. For the follow-up, we had a standard script and always explained our purpose in calling. Even then, I was surprised at how willing patients were to divulge private information about themselves and their treatment to strangers over the phone. They seemed eager to provide information that could possibly help themselves and others. Researchers used the information we collected to determine, for example, that early screening for breast cancer and colon cancer can improve a cancer patient's outcome. Cancer registries are just one example of how your health information—your story—is strung together to help other patients throughout the world.

Key Highlights

One of the most important parts of your medical record is the *history and physical.* You can ensure the accuracy of this information by describing your symptoms as specifically as possible. You should provide complete and accurate information about past illnesses, social practices, and family health history. Your health information can have a larger effect on medical advances than you may realize, especially if you have a certain disease, such as cancer or AIDS. Medical research studies include your anonymous health information to determine best treatments and cures.

Key Actions

- Create your personal medical record. Start out brief and focused, adding details as you go.
- Describe your symptoms with detail, accuracy, honesty, and completeness.
- Provide accurate information about past illnesses, lifestyle, and family health history.
- Ask questions if you don't understand something your healthcare provider says.
- Obtain treatment and discharge instructions in writing. If you need more details, ask for them.

Key Take-Away

Always provide detailed, accurate, honest, and complete information to your healthcare practitioners.

Endnotes

---

[1] American Health Information Management Association, *www.ahima.org.*
[2] American Medical Informatics Association, *www.amia.org.*
[3] Cleveland Clinic MyChart site, *mychart.clevelandclinic.org.*

CHAPTER

5

Understanding Who Uses Your Health Information and Why

As a general rule, the most successful man in life is the man who has the best information. —Benjamin Disraeli

I had just earned my bachelor's degree and had little work experience when the director of quality at a local community hospital hired me as her assistant. This was my first hospital job, and I was charged with helping to improve the quality of patient care. My biggest responsibility was to review patient medical records and report results. I had never seen a medical record before or even been inside a hospital.

Alice, the director, and the other women in the department were nurses. I, on the other hand, was a liberal arts graduate with experience teaching high school French. Alice surely did not realize the big job ahead of her when she hired me. On my first day, Alice assigned me to review patient records to determine who had been given antibiotics after surgery. She showed me where the antibiotics were recorded in the record, and then left me to begin my review. It never occurred to me to ask Alice for names of antibiotics. As a kid, I remembered my mother referring to penicillin every so often if my brothers or I needed a prescription to fight an infection. So, I proceeded to review the records with the presumption that penicillin was the only antibiotic.

I reported to Alice later that day that only 12 percent of the patients I reviewed were given antibiotics or, in my translation, penicillin. Surprised by my results, she reviewed my work. By her discovery of my second missed record, where the patient received the antibiotic, Gentamycin, she knew something was awry. Without embarrassing me, she quickly located a book that listed antibiotics. She left me alone with the book and the records to continue my review. I was on my way to becoming a proficient quality reviewer. My exposure to Alice and my nursing co-workers was a positive learning experience for me. My exposure to the hospital's physicians, on the other hand, was not as positive. One of my responsibilities was to report to the physicians the results of the quality assurance studies I performed. The first time I had to report unfavorable results was for one of the "old guard" surgeons, Dr. Friedman.

Using an IBM Selectric typewriter and lots of Wite-Out, I focused on creating elaborate tables and on other artistic qualities of the report. Unfortunately, I didn't think much about the fact that the report showed Dr. Friedman did not order antibiotics for two patients when the study criteria showed he should have. One of the patients who did not receive antibiotics had a severe postoperative infection. Alice had reviewed the information and thought it was clearly a physician's error. However, Dr. Friedman had a defense that had to do with the standard of care. Moreover, Dr. Friedman was wondering who exactly I was to question his authority. "My God, you are not a doctor. You are not even a nurse," he reminded me in front of the entire committee. His voice became louder as he continued to rip apart every piece of information in the report. I was in shock. I could not respond.

Dr. Friedman left the room, slamming the door. I soon found out that this type of reaction would be the norm, not the exception, when delivering unfavorable report results to the physicians. That night at home, I realized that while the encounter with Dr. Friedman frightened me, it also aroused my curiosity. Looking back now, I realize I should have familiarized myself with the medical staff and considered how to anticipate and manage their undesirable reactions before I delivered the report.

Certainly, the physicians on the review committee and my colleagues in the medical records department were all seeking the same goal: high standards and quality patient care. Yet my unfavorable report obviously put Dr. Friedman on the defensive. I began to ask myself how these separate, but integrated groups—the hospital, physicians, and patients— could work together to advance overall healthcare goals. I wanted—I *needed*—to learn more about how the hospital-physician-patient triad worked. This anecdote shows us how the information in each of our medical records—our story—becomes part of the bigger picture. As a patient, you may not consider yourself or your medical record as part of a larger entity. But your medical record provides detailed information that plays an important role in the quality of healthcare.

Two books, *Wikinomics*[1] and *The Wisdom of Crowds,*[2] describe how each of us plays a role in creating intellectual capital for the good of the whole—how collective wisdom shapes society. Likewise, your health information is pieced together with others' health information to tell a bigger story—about treatment and prevention of ailments affecting millions of people, such as cancer, cystic fibrosis, Parkinson's disease, and HIV. Just imagine the possibilities for improving healthcare if we all were to be conscious contributors to our own health story.

WHO USES YOUR HEALTH INFORMATION?

The following list highlights a number of people and organizations who use your healthcare information:

- Your healthcare team
- The legal system
- Your health plan
- Researchers
- Healthcare administrators
- Quality rating companies
- You

Figure 5.1 shows the *typical* top five uses of health information compared to the *ideal* top five uses. In the *typical* top five, your use is not even listed. But, in the ideal list, I rank your use second, following your practitioner's use. I also combined quality and payment, since in the future, insurance companies will likely use quality measures to determine whether to pay for care and how much to pay.

Figure 5.1 Use of Health Information: Typical Versus Ideal

Typical Top Five Uses of Health Information	Ideal Top Five Uses of Health Information
1. Physician diagnosis, treatment, and communication among your healthcare team	1. Physician diagnosis, treatment, and communication among your healthcare team
2. Payment for your care	2. Your own reference and sharing purposes
3. Research	3. Payment for your care and quality-of-care measurement
4. Planning for future patient care	4. Research
5. Quality-of-care measurement	5. Planning for future patient care

Now, let's take an in-depth look at each of the ways your healthcare information is used. These details can help you understand why your providers ask certain questions, what they are writing down, and why. You'll see how important it is for you to ensure your records are accurate and complete.

Your Medical Record: A Communication Tool for Your Healthcare Team

You may have several professionals providing your care. These providers primarily communicate with each other through your medical record. If, for example, a physician admits you to the hospital, even for one day, at least seven healthcare professionals will likely be involved in treating you, and they will each write in your medical record. These clinicians commonly include the emergency room (ER) physician, your primary care physician (PCP), a specialist, three nurses, and a radiologist. The following are examples of the observations and treatment each healthcare provider documents in your medical record:

- **Emergency room physician**. More than 40 percent of patients admitted to the hospital come through the emergency room.[3] If you go to the ER, a physician who specializes in emergency medicine takes a history from you regarding your reason for coming to the emergency room and she performs a physical examination. The ER physician then documents your diagnosis and treatment orders.
- **Primary care physician (PCP).** Your PCP is responsible for coordinating your overall healthcare. She maintains records of any specialists' evaluations that she orders while you are under her treatment. If you are hospitalized, your PCP, also known as your *attending physician,* is generally responsible for coordinating care among any specialists. Your PCP is also usually the physician responsible for documenting orders for your discharge from the hospital.
- **Surgeon.** If you are admitted to the hospital for a surgical procedure, your attending physician may be your surgeon. She documents the reason for your surgery, explains risks of the procedure, and obtains your informed consent. If you have other health problems in addition to the condition for which you are receiving surgery, the surgeon may order evaluations from other specialists. The surgeon also documents the details of the procedure she performs on you.
- **Specialists**. Specialist physicians are also called *consulting physicians.* The consultant is an expert in the area in which you are suspected to have a problem. Examples of specialists include cardiologists, neurologists, endocrinologists, and gastroenterologists. Generally, a specialist physician will evaluate you in response to a request by your PCP.
- **Unit nurses**. In the inpatient hospital setting, nurses provide continuity for your care. Present on all hospital units 24 hours

a day, they regularly monitor your vital signs and implement physician orders, such as medication administration. Nurses provide significant documentation in your record, including times and dosages of medication and observations of your condition.

- **Radiologist.** The radiologist is the physician who reads and interprets your x-rays, MRIs, CT scans, and other types of images. He generally does not provide direct treatment to you. Rather, he is in direct contact with your x-ray film, MRI reading, or CT scan output. The radiologist reads and interprets each of your tests and then documents his impression or diagnosis in a formal report that becomes part of your medical record.
- **Pathologist**. The pathologist is another physician who provides indirect treatment. She works in the laboratory, analyzing tissue or body fluid removed from you during surgery. If the pathologist does not find any abnormalities, she documents a negative report. If she does find some abnormalities, she documents her impression and a suspected or confirmed diagnosis.
- **Therapist**. Like other clinical specialists, therapists evaluate and treat you based on your needs and your doctor's orders. Examples of therapists include physical therapists, respiratory therapists, speech therapists, and occupational therapists. Each of these clinicians documents his evaluation of your condition in a formal report called a *consultation.* In addition, whenever a therapist provides treatment, he documents the details of the treatment in your record.

Everyone on your healthcare team needs to know about *all* of your diagnoses, treatments, and reports completed by the other members of the team and filed on your record. Your medical record is the vital instrument containing all of this healthcare data about you. Figure 5.2 illustrates some of the healthcare providers who create and refer to your medical record.

Figure 5.2 Some Healthcare Providers Who Create and Refer to Your Medical Record

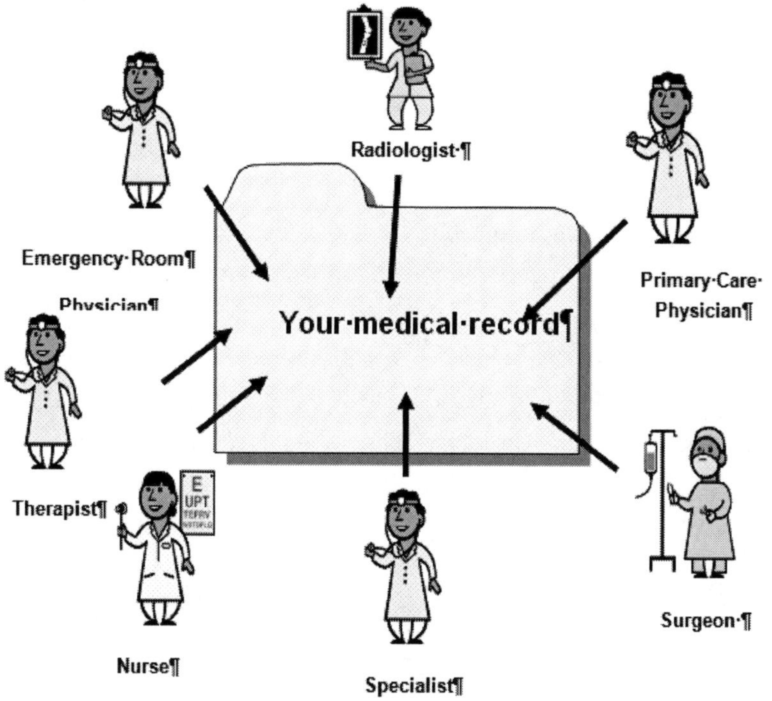

Your Medical Record: Legal Evidence That Care Was Provided to You

Your medical record is a legal document. It is kept in the "normal course of business" and is a "business record." Therefore, your medical record can be used as evidence in any legal inquiry. All entries in your record are supporting evidence of the care provided to you, including when, by whom, and the outcomes of that care. Your record is referenced in any medical malpractice or other related legal actions that involve your care.

Physicians are acutely aware that medical record information may potentially be used "against them," particularly in medical malpractice actions. In fact, this is why many physicians now practice "defensive medicine" in the United States. In other words, doctors may document to reduce their exposure to unfavorable legal actions.[4] Once, during a hospital training session for cardiothoracic surgeons, I learned that the physicians were not documenting heart failure for all of the patients who appeared to meet the clinical criteria for that diagnosis. I explained the importance of clearly and completely documenting every diagnosis, so other healthcare professionals would fully understand the patient's needs and provide proper care. Our discussion continued for quite some time until one surgeon said, "If you want to know the truth, I don't document heart failure on any of my patients who are on or who might need, disability insurance in the future. This diagnosis can cause them to be rejected for disability benefits." It was this physician's belief that insurers could use a patient's prior history of heart failure to deny disability benefits. And, as the surgeon explained, he did not want to be responsible for his patient being rejected for insurance benefits. Other surgeons around the table shook their heads in agreement.

So, it struck me: these surgeons believed that sacrificing accurate documentation was beneficial to the patient. Admirable and caring as this action may seem, it actually could be detrimental to the patient. For example, if other physicians referenced inaccurate records, they might prescribe wrong medications and possibly make the patient's condition worse. Furthermore, if that were to happen, the surgeon who failed to document the heart failure diagnosis might end up with liability issues to address. Obviously, the hospital needed to address this documentation issue with its entire medical staff.

When I reviewed Emmalea's medical records from her first hospitalization following her initial seizure, I noticed that although verbally we had been told her diagnosis was juvenile myoclonic epilepsy (JME), her written diagnosis was seizure disorder, which physicians believe carries much less social stigma. In addition, depending on the state, the difference in documentation could also mean the difference between whether the patient's driver's license is suspended or not.

Your Medical Record: Verification Your Health Plan Needs

Health plans perform regular audits to make sure that what they paid for actually happened. They use your medical record to verify that their payment is justified. You are the one most at risk if the insurer audits your medical record. If the insurance company decides not to pay the healthcare provider or only pays a portion of the bill, the healthcare provider may bill you directly for the balance due. You can help ensure proper insurance payment by providing accurate and detailed information to your physician.

Health plans evaluate your health information in three primary ways to determine payment for your healthcare:

1. **Pre-certification or pre-approval.** Many health plans require your physician or other healthcare provider to submit information about your condition to them so they can approve the care *before* it is provided. This is particularly true in the case of tests like MRIs and CT scans, as well as certain surgeries.
2. **Billing generated.** Your healthcare providers must submit a bill to be paid by your health plan. Your medical record must substantiate all the information on the bill. In essence, the bill should be an abbreviated form of your medical record.
3. **Documented information required.** Health plans reject a high percentage of claims the first time they receive them. They often request additional information about your healthcare services to determine whether they will pay the bill. Some health plans may request your entire medical record for the billed services. Others may request specific documents in your record, such as test results and surgical reports.

Your Medical Record: A Source for Research Studies and Reporting

Many different organizations conduct medical research, including medical schools, hospitals, associations like the American Cancer Society, and foundations. All have similar goals: to understand, treat, and prevent illness, and promote the well being of individuals in our society. Medical records play a big role in helping researchers achieve these goals.

The information in your medical record—each diagnosis, test, treatment, and procedure—has a code. These codes are put into searchable databases, allowing medical researchers to identify individual patient records that may be eligible for research studies.

Medical researchers use health information in two ways. Sometimes patients volunteer for clinical trials and their information is verified with the medical record. Other times, just the patient's medical records are used in the research. From these studies, researchers are able to draw conclusions about treatments that yield improved outcomes.

Your Medical Record: A Tool for Healthcare Planning

Hospital or doctor's office staff use patient records to attempt to identify trends in care and treatment to ensure adequate staffing. For example, if there is an increase in patients who have chest pain without a heart attack, a hospital may add a chest pain clinic to provide specialized care for these patients. This could help avoid using ER beds that heart attack or other acutely ill patients may need.

State and federal government officials also sometimes use medical records to plan for future healthcare needs. Aggregated data helps officials determine where communities need more (or fewer) healthcare organizations and to identify the most urgent healthcare priorities. For example, Medicare may detect an increase in cardiovascular disorders and, therefore, fund a greater number of cardiology residency programs in certain parts of the country.

Your Medical Record: A Tool to Measure Quality

Measuring the quality of medical care is a practice that has grown substantially over the past two decades. Today, hundreds of quality measures exist, and they all use information from medical records. For example, quality reviewers may look at whether a patient with a heart attack received aspirin within one hour of hospital admission or was asked about any family history of heart-related illness. Healthcare organizations, hospital-accrediting groups, and consumer advocate organizations use health information to rate the overall quality of U.S. healthcare. First, reviewers categorize your health information by diagnosis. Next, they consider other information, such as treatment, the numbers and types of other diagnoses, and any complications. Then they compare this information, such as your age and length of hospital stay to determine the quality of healthcare provided. Several different sources of analyzed data for healthcare quality are available. (For more details about measuring quality, see chapter 10.)

Your Medical Record: For Your Own Reference

Your medical record is, or should be, an important reference for you, your family, and your future generations. Today, few people use their own medical records, but with online personal medical records becoming easy to access and use, I hope this trend will be reversed. As I discussed in chapter 4, your goal should be to maintain complete copies of your health information, for your benefit and for the benefit of your family.

Key Highlights

Many people, groups, and organizations use your health information for a variety of reasons. The primary reason for documenting your healthcare in your medical record is to ensure that your healthcare providers continually make appropriate diagnoses and give you the best possible care. Various organizations also use your health information to benefit the healthcare system and society through research, healthcare planning, and measuring healthcare quality.

Key Actions

- Understand the different roles of your healthcare team in regard to documenting in and using your medical record.
- Ask for a copy of your medical record at the end of each healthcare visit, so that you have complete records to refer to as needed.
- Review your record for accuracy and ask questions if you see information you don't understand or that you believe is incorrect.

Key Take-Away

Because your health information is used by many organizations to benefit you as well as to advance medical research, you should take an active role in ensuring your health information is accurate and complete.

Endnotes

[1] Tapscott, Don. *Wikinomics*. The Penguin Group, 2006.
[2] Surowiecki, James. *The Wisdom of Crowds*. Anchor, 2005.
[3] Kozak, L.J.; DeFrances, C.J.; Hall, M.J. *National Hospital Discharge Survey: 2004 Annual Summary with Detailed Diagnosis and Procedure Data.* National Center for Health Statistics. Vital Health Statistics, 13(162). 2006.
[4] Definition of "defensive medicine" from MedicineNet, *www.medicinenet.com*.

CHAPTER

6

Knowing Your Rights: Health Information Privacy and Ownership

I was brought up to believe that the only thing worth doing was to add to the sum of accurate information in the world.
—Margaret Mead

As I walked from my midtown apartment to the Memorial Sloan-Kettering Cancer Center in New York City, I pulled my coat tighter—partially because of the blistering cold, but mostly because of growing concern for my sister-in-law, Vera. She had recently been diagnosed with breast cancer and had her first visit with her physicians at the center scheduled for 9 a.m. Nearly everyone in our large, close family came. We came with newspapers, coffee, or doughnuts. But mostly, we came to offer Vera support during this difficult time.

None of us suspected at 8:45 a.m. that we would still be waiting in the same spot at 10 a.m. with no further progress. At 8:45, the members of Vera's entourage were the only people in the waiting room. By 10, we were just one group among many others. All were there for the same reason, all focused on one member of their group. Finally, at about 10:15, a small woman dressed in white walked to the front of the room and loudly shouted, "Vera Reynolds!" Startled, we jumped up, ruffling papers and spilling coffee. Then, just in case everyone had not clearly heard her name the first time, the woman yelled out again, "Vera Reynolds!"

We assembled into a line and followed the woman to the examining room. That day, as we listened to the doctors and asked a hundred questions, what seemed to us to be the beginning of a long journey, must also have been an emotionally wrenching one for Vera. But she didn't show it then, nor as she went through two surgeries and 16 weeks of chemotherapy. She went back to work a week after her surgery and worked all through chemo. Nearly three years later, she continues to move forward with an excellent prognosis and a positive outlook.

Recently, Vera and I discussed her experiences with breast cancer as I was writing this book. Her stories illustrate some important issues, beginning with that first Memorial Sloan-Kettering Cancer Center visit. I considered her experience in relation to a patient's right to privacy. Our group of eight sat amongst 50 or 60 other patients with their own groups in that waiting room. Although no one likely knew anyone outside of his or her own group, everyone there shared the bond of fighting the common enemy—cancer. Before we left that waiting room, everyone knew Vera's first and last name. Vera suffered no direct harm when the woman in white broadcast her full name. Calling out only her first name could have helped to avoid the situation altogether.

HIPAA AND PATIENT PRIVACY RIGHTS

Patient privacy rights have always been an issue in healthcare. Until the mid-1990s, many hospitals commonly published the names of every patient admitted to the hospital in the local newspaper. The list of hospital admissions at the small community hospital where I worked in rural New Jersey was a daily topic of conversation at the local beauty parlor and coffee shop.

At that time, how much patient information a hospital could give to newspapers, and whether a hospital had rules prohibiting a physician from discussing patient cases in public areas depended on state laws. Some states had clear-cut laws protecting patient privacy rights, while others had none. This patchwork quilt of laws often confused healthcare administrators and practitioners.

In 1996, however, the federal government passed the Health Insurance Portability and Accountability Act (HIPAA), which, among other things, mandated a minimum set of privacy protections for all patients. HIPAA gave you the right to:

- Obtain and inspect a copy of your medical records
- Request a correction of inaccurate health information
- Find out where your health information has been shared for purposes other than care, payment, or healthcare administrative purposes
- Request special restrictions on the use or disclosure of your health information
- Request that your providers share your protected health information with you in a particular way
- See a provider's policy on confidentiality[1]

HIPAA also addressed health information rights: who can access information and what they do with the information. With the growing pharmaceutical industry and the economic strength it began to wield, many patients worried that hospitals would sell their information to pharmaceutical companies for marketing purposes. HIPAA allayed these concerns before they became reality. Certainly, HIPAA improved patient information privacy laws. Whether processes had just gotten lax, or there was a lack of awareness for patient privacy, is unclear. What is clear is that HIPAA provided one uniform law spelling out your rights regarding your health information.

Your Right To Request a Correction or Make an Addendum to Your Medical Record

Of all of your HIPAA rights, your right to modify your record deserves special attention. Perhaps you were not aware of this right, or maybe you feel uncomfortable asking your doctor to change your medical record. It's no different from making sure your driver's license, passport, or credit report is accurate. It is important to take the same approach to health information. The first step in making the request is ensuring you understand the information. However, like the next story illustrates, what you may perceive as incorrect, may be a matter of opinion.

My husband Joe is an attorney who represents many healthcare providers. The patient of one of Joe's physician clients requested a copy of his medical record from the physician. After reviewing his record, the patient asked the physician to delete or change certain information. The particular statement the patient wanted amended was from his history and physical. It said, "Patient is not adequately groomed with evidence of gross neglect. Patient is obese." The patient claimed the information was inaccurate. From a legal perspective, the patient also claimed the information was libelous. Because the statement is the clinician's opinion, the information is not, in fact, libelous. However, when you read the statement, you can probably understand why the patient was upset. The physician should have been more objective in his documentation. Whether a patient is adequately groomed is a judgment call. The physician could have written that the patient met the criteria for obesity given his body mass index (BMI). A correct, objective statement related to the patient's actual BMI would not have been able to be challenged successfully by the patient as inaccurate.

As we all become more familiar with our health information rights, requests for healthcare providers to make changes to the information may become more common. This process is also another way to keep our healthcare providers accountable and in check. (For a sample request form to change or amend your health information, see figure 6.1.)

Figure 6.1 Sample Form: Request for an Addendum or Correction

Request for an Addendum or Correction

Section A: Patient Information [Name, Address, Date of birth]

Section B: What Information Is Incorrect or Incomplete?

Name of the Document	Date of Document	Author of document	Incorrect or Incomplete Information

Section C: Request To Add an Addendum (for Adult Patients)

You have the right to provide ABC Medical Center with a written addendum to your record. If you clearly indicate in writing that you want the addendum to be made part of your medical record, we will attach it to your records and include it whenever we disclose the item or statement you believe to be incorrect or incomplete. To add an addendum to your record, please provide us with a statement in the space below regarding the item you believe to be incorrect or incomplete.

Figure 6.1 Sample Form: Request for an Addendum or Correction (Continued)

Section D: Request to Add a Correction (Amendment) If you believe that the protected health information we have on file about you is incorrect or incomplete, you have the right to ask us to correct the information in your records. To request a correction to your protected health information, please complete this section. Please tell us what changes you would like to make to the information you described in Section B.
Please give a reason why you want this change.
We must tell you within 60 days if we will change your protected health information as you requested, or that we need more time (up to 30 extra days) to decide. We do not have to change your protected information if: 1. We did not create the information, or the person who created the information is unavailable to act on your request to change it (for example, the doctor who originally created the information has died). 2. The information is accurate and complete. 3. You do not have the legal right to access the protected health information you want changed. 4. The protected health information you want changed is not part of the designated record set. This includes your medical records, billing records, and records containing your protected health information that we use to make decisions about you.

Your Right to a Legible Medical Record

Your right to a legible medical record is not explicitly stated in HIPAA. It is implied in your right to "request a correction of inaccurate health information." HIPAA, therefore, gives you the right to an *accurate* medical record. The Oxford English Dictionary (OED) defines *accurate* as "careful, precise, lacking errors, arising from careful effort." The OED defines legible as "handwriting that is clear enough to read."

You have the right to accurate (careful, precise) information in your medical record. *Accurate* is actually a much higher standard than *legible*, which is only "clear enough to read." If your medical record is illegible, you can request that the unreadable information be documented in an accurate manner: careful, precise, and lacking errors. You can make your request using the *Request for an Addendum or Correction* form.

When Your Records Can be Used without Your Consent

One of the primary objectives of HIPAA is to protect your health information from inadvertent or inappropriate disclosure to third parties. However, HIPAA does allow your health information to be disclosed without your consent in special circumstances.

- **Your record can be used for treatment purposes without your consent.** This means that any providers, *within* the organization where your record was created, have the right to review your record to care for you. This use of your record does not require your consent.
- **Your release is not required for payment purposes.** For example, your surgeon sends a bill to your health plan for a hernia repair he performed on you. In processing the bill, the health plan decides it needs more information before it will pay. It wants to review your entire medical record. You will

not be asked to authorize this, or similar, uses of your medical record by health plans.

- **You will not be asked to authorize the use of your medical record for administrative purposes**. For example, the Joint Commission on Accreditation of Healthcare Organizations accreditation team is at the hospital for an inspection. The team requests a group of records to review as part of the accreditation process. You will not be asked to authorize this or similar uses of your record.
- **There are certain uses of your record that are required by law.** For example, if a healthcare provider receives a subpoena for your medical record, she must comply with the request. Your authorization would not be obtained in these situations.

YOU OWN YOUR HEALTH INFORMATION, BUT IT IS YOUR RESPONSIBILITY TO OBTAIN IT

Although HIPAA guarantees you access to your medical records, HIPAA does not clearly spell out ownership rights. You *do* own your health information, but it is generally accepted in the healthcare industry that the provider who collected the information owns the medium on which it is stored. [2] This means that the provider owns the original copy of your health information.

Propped up against the wall in my walk-in closet sits a large radiology film tucked inside a folder. The film contains several MRI images of my pelvis with a stress fracture. The folder is stamped with the following statement: “X-ray films owned by MRI Center.” Although the statement claims I am not the owner of the film, I contend that I am the owner. The premise that we own our health information, but the healthcare provider owns the media on which the information exists is a difficult one to apply. How can you separate the information on that MRI from the film that houses the image? Does the statement of ownership mean that the patient owns words, but not pictures? No authority has ever officially stated this, so the actual owner of that radiology film, for example, remains ambiguous.

The absolute ownership of patient information is not necessarily as confusing as the x-ray film. The bottom line is that you own all health information recorded and maintained on you—and you can request copies of it, which may include x-rays, MRIs, or other data stored on paper, film, or CD. Unfortunately, most patients do not know that they own their information or may not even care to own it. Can you imagine owning something that would potentially give you more insight into yourself or empower you and never knowing about it? The obvious question to be asked is: If I own it, why don't I have it? It is up to you to obtain your information from all of your healthcare providers and to store that information in whatever media you choose, paper or a computer file. Just because you own the information does not mean you automatically receive a copy of it or have access to it. It's your responsibility to initiate the request.

A story about requesting your medical records. My husband Joe serves as the self-appointed guardian for our family's essential information and cherished photographs. As part of this responsibility, he visited the many healthcare providers who cared for Emmalea during her first hospital stay to obtain copies of her medical records. He first went to the hospital's health information management (HIM) department, also known as medical records. He still claims that he was verbally assaulted by the woman behind the sliding glass window. He thought he arrived prepared with the necessary information to obtain a copy of Emmalea's medical record. However, the woman barraged him with questions about his identity, Emmalea's signature on the release form, and the exact dates of care needed in the copy of the record.

Joe produced his driver's license and completed the detailed release forms. He also voiced his concerns to the department director about the process and the time involved. Then he paid $200 for 80 pages of information. But after getting over his initial irritation with the process, he walked away several hours later with a newfound respect for people like HIM professionals who are so passionate about protecting patients' interest in their health information.

Next, Joe went to the other end of the hospital's campus for copies of the MRI, CT scan, and EEG results. There, he had a very different experience. At the radiology department, where he requested the MRI and CT scan copies, the woman behind the sliding glass window was much more obliging. She did not ask for a release form and did not even care who Joe was, let alone ask for his identification. She burned the complete report results onto a disc and handed it over within minutes, no questions asked. Joe, thinking the process was too easy, asked for two additional copies. He had the copies in hand within another few moments. He had a similar experience in the neurology department and walked away with three copies of the report and EEG test on CDs within minutes, without providing any ID or consent form. We've learned that this process of endless interrogation in the medical record department, while clinical departments hand out patient information in an almost whimsical fashion, seems to be common in many healthcare organizations.

Where to Obtain Your Health Information

The health information management (HIM) department typically maintains, stores, and distributes medical records. This is true for hospital inpatient records, but it may vary for outpatient or clinic records. When Joe went to the hospital to collect Emmalea's health information he had to visit three different locations to get all of it. The hospital was fairly sophisticated in its use of technology and even boasted a partially electronic medical record. However, the electronic systems in the neurology and radiology departments were not integrated with the other systems, so we had to piece the information together to obtain a complete medical record for Emmalea. Gathering Emmalea's records was frustrating for Joe, but he also knew how important it was to have a complete record of Emmalea's healthcare.

Depending on the type of care you have received and where, you may need to either visit or make requests to several locations to ensure you have a complete record. Not only is the system of caregiving often fragmented, but the system of record keeping is as well. In almost all instances, you are the only common thread in the system.

Three Types of Health Information: Traditional, Clinical, and Financial

Providers maintain three different types of health information about you: traditional, clinical, and financial. You generally need to request each type of information from a different department or individual in the organization. In Emmalea's case, Joe obtained her traditional record from the HIM department. He obtained her clinical records from the departments of neurology and radiology. For the financial record, we used the explanation of benefits (EOB) statement that we received from our insurance plan. Alternatively, we could have requested Emmalea's financial record from the hospital's business office.

A more detailed description of these three types of records may help you to better understand their contents and their use. The traditional record is what is commonly referred to as your medical record. Kept in the HIM department, it contains a record of your history and physical; notes from physicians and other clinicians; and reports from consultants, surgeons, and others who have treated you. It also includes laboratory test results, nurses' notes, medication records, and physician notes. The clinical record, on the other hand, is the technical media that generally only trained experts can read and interpret. Examples of these records include x-ray films, EEG readings, CT scan screens, echocardiograms, and MRI films. These records are stored in the relevant clinical department, such as neurology, cardiology, or radiology. Finally, the financial record is your bill for services. Your bills are protected just like your medical records because all bills for healthcare services contain clinical information, including your diagnoses and procedures. These records are stored in the healthcare provider's business office.

How to Obtain Your Health Information

Your health information is sensitive and personal. You have legal rights regarding your health information. But beyond that, the protection of your information related to your health is also a moral and ethical obligation for every provider. No one is more aware of the importance of protecting your health information than the healthcare providers who create the information. That's why there are stringent rules about the release of health information. At times it may seem these rules were designed to frustrate you, like in Joe's experience. In reality, the process for requesting and obtaining health information is designed primarily to protect you.

Once you have identified where you need to go to request your health information, you will need to fill out the release of information (ROI) form for that organization. A completed, signed ROI form, is the organization's documentation that you have requested your health information and asked that it be sent to yourself, a family member, your physician, or other provider. In our case, Emmalea needed to sign off on the ROI, indicating that the hospital could release information to her father. Without that form properly completed, the hospital would not have given copies of her records to Joe.

ROI forms are specific to every hospital and physician office, so be sure to obtain a copy of the correct form. (See figure 6.2 for a sample ROI form.) In the hospital setting, you can call the HIM department. HIM departments usually have a team dedicated to managing all requests for medical records. Generally, HIM departments mail or fax the ROI form to you or direct you to a Web site to download and print the form. You might even want to try visiting the hospital Web site before calling the HIM department. A search for "medical record" will likely result in the information you need. Most ROI forms require demographic information and dates of treatment or hospitalization. Hospitals ask the reason for your request. They may waive the copying fee if your reason is for continuing medical care. But it may make a difference whether you want the hospital to send the records to another provider or to you directly.

Most hospitals will charge you, as they did in our case, if the reason for obtaining the information is continued care, but you want the records to be provided to you directly. Many providers do not yet recognize that it really is your responsibility to manage your records. You could explain to the hospital that you are coordinating your own health information among your providers and ask the facility to waive the associated copy fees. By doing so, you are actually relieving the hospital of the future burden of copying your records for potentially several additional providers.

You will also need to document what part of the record you would like to have copied and released. For completeness, it is probably best to check the box on the ROI indicating you want the "complete" record. Healthcare providers are required to give you a choice to designate if you want less than the complete record. If you want to omit certain portions, you may need to document which specific forms or contents you do not want to have copied. Some hospitals provide a list of documents on the form, allowing you to check off the ones you do not want included in your copy.

Patients who have psychiatric, drug and alcohol, or HIV diagnoses have special privacy protections for those conditions. Every consent form must contain a specific statement that requires you to affirmatively state that you would like (or not like) to have psychiatric, drug and alcohol, or HIV information disclosed. If you are obtaining the information for yourself, this is not an issue, but you still need to complete this portion of the form. If you are requesting the records to be sent to another provider or someone else, you may choose not to share this type of information. Keep in mind, though, the more complete your record is, the more likely your future diagnoses, treatment, and care will be coordinated and shared in a way that leads you to your best overall healthcare.

Figure 6.2 Sample Form: Release of Information

Authorization for Use or Disclosure of Health Information

By completing this document, you authorize the disclosure and/or use of your individually identifiable health information, as set forth below, consistent with state and federal law concerning the privacy of your health information.

Use and Disclosure of Health Information

I hereby authorize the use or disclosure of my health information as follows:

Patient name:________________________________

Date of birth:____________________________

Persons/organizations authorized to receive the information:

____

This authorization applies to the following information (select only one of the following):

□ All health information pertaining to any medical history, mental or physical condition, and treatment received EXCEPT:

____

□ Only the following records or types of health information (including any dates):

____

____

I specifically authorize release of the following information:

□ Mental health treatment information

□ HIV test results

□ Alcohol/drug treatment information

A separate authorization is required to authorize the disclosure or use of psychotherapy notes.

Figure 6.2 Sample Form: Release of Information (Continued)

Authorization for Use or Disclosure of Health Information

Purpose

Purpose of requested use or disclosure:
□ Patient care
□ Other:______________________________

Expiration

This authorization expires (not to exceed 24 months):_______________________

Notice of Rights and Other Information

1. I may refuse to sign this authorization.
2. I may revoke this authorization at any time.
3. My revocation will be effective upon receipt.
4. Neither treatment, payment, enrollment, nor eligibility for benefits will be conditions for my providing or refusing to provide this authorization.

Signature

Date:_______________ Time:__________
Signature: ________________________________

If signed by someone other than the patient, state your legal relationship to the patient:

____

Witness:____

Date:_______________________

Frequently Asked Questions for Release of Medical Records

The following are some of the most frequently asked questions and responses regarding requests for information. Actual questions and responses vary, depending on the provider.

Who is authorized to sign for release of my medical record/health information?

- You, the patient
- Anyone who has been granted the power of attorney for you
- A parent, if the patient is younger than age 18
- The parent and minor, if the patient is 12 to 17 years of age and receiving psychiatric, alcohol, or drug treatment services
- Your legal guardian
- The representative of the estate for deceased patients

How much does it cost to obtain a copy of my health information?

- Under HIPAA, providers may charge a "reasonable, cost-based fee" that includes the cost of supplies, labor, and postage.
- There is generally no charge for releasing copies of your health information directly to other healthcare providers.
- You will generally be charged a fee for copies you want released directly to you or someone else who is not a healthcare provider. The amount will be specific to each provider.
- Though it is best to obtain your complete medical record, you can reduce costs by requesting specific information rather than a complete record.

Can my spouse obtain copies of my medical record?

Yes, but only with your written consent. You must sign an ROI form authorizing the provider to release copies of your records to your spouse.

Can the information be faxed to me?

Generally, no. Except in an emergency, most providers will not fax medical records or any health information, due to confidentiality issues. The possibility that an unauthorized individual may have access to the fax machine is the basis of the privacy concern.

How long do providers keep records? Or, how far back can I request information?

Most states require healthcare providers to keep medical records for the statute of limitations period for adults and age of majority (18 in most states) plus the statute of limitations period for minors. The time period varies by state, but generally, is anywhere from 7 to 10 years. Some providers keep information much longer than the mandatory minimum, so check directly with your hospital or physician's office.

Can I request birth certificates from the hospital where I was born?

The hospital where you were born has a record of your birth, but not your birth certificate. You can only obtain your birth certificate from the department of health or department of records in the state where you were born.

You own your health information. As with anything you own, it is up to you how, or if, you take care of your property. Being aware of the value of your property, what you can do with it, and how it can help you, may make a difference in whether you choose to exercise the rights you have to your health information. It's your decision to make.

Key Highlights

Even though your healthcare providers keep the original copies, you own your health information. It is your responsibility to request, obtain, and maintain your medical records for your use. Under HIPAA, you have specific rights regarding privacy of your health information. However, HIPAA does allow release of your information without your consent for treatment, payment, and administrative purposes required by law.

Key Actions

- Be aware of how and where to obtain the various parts of your medical records from all your healthcare providers.
- Know your health information protections provided through the federal legislation known as HIPAA.
- Understand that responsibility comes along with ownership. As with anything you own, it is up to you to take care of your health information and to use it to your greatest advantage.

Key Take-Away

When you exercise your rights regarding your health information, you empower yourself and you are more likely to get the best possible healthcare.

Endnotes

[1] HIPAA is Public Law 104-191, passed by the 104th Congress. The privacy rule is under Title II of HIPAA.

[2] Huffman, Edna K. *Health Information Management, 10th Edition.* Physicians' Record Company, 1994.

STEP

3

BUILD YOUR RELATIONSHIPS

CHAPTER 7

Recognizing Healthcare as a Right, a Privilege and a Responsibility

Character—the willingness to accept responsibility for one's own life—is the source from which self-respect springs. —Joan Didion

St. Joseph Hospital in Lexington, Kentucky is part of the Catholic Health Initiatives (CHI) system. The hospital is located in the center of the largest city in the eastern half of the state. Fiona took her mother, Mary-Margaret, there for continued, unbearable abdominal and chest pain. Mary-Margaret had no insurance, no money for copays, and no primary care physician. When Mary-Margaret arrived at the hospital's emergency room, she was immediately triaged to the top of the list because of her age (62), severity of her pain, and the yellowish hue to her skin. The EKG technician had already begun cardiac testing and the lab assistant had drawn blood when the registration clerk wheeled her portable computer station into the room to begin collecting information from Mary-Margaret.

Fiona held her breath for a moment, but quickly stepped in front of the computer station to intervene. "My mother is not insured and we have no money to pay you," Fiona blurted out. The registration clerk, a woman about Mary-Margaret's age and build, shrugged her shoulders. "Doesn't matter to me," she said. "I just want to know her name and address for her hospital bracelet." Fiona was stunned. She stepped aside.

After the registration clerk left, Fiona watched while the ER physician, Dr. Munoz, carefully examined her mother. She pressed on her stomach in at least a dozen places. Each time Dr. Munoz asked Mary-Margaret to describe the pain she felt on a scale of 1 to 10, with 10 being the worst pain she could imagine. Mary-Margaret obliged.

The greatest pain seemed to be in the central part of her stomach. Dr. Munoz asked Mary-Margaret a long list of questions. When did she first begin having pains? Were they constant or did they come and go? Was she unusually tired? Had she had any recent transfusions? The questions seemed to go on forever. For certain questions, Mary-Margaret gazed at Fiona to respond. She was just too tired to speak and beginning to feel disoriented. Dr. Munoz sensed this and ordered some radiology tests immediately to rule out what she suspected was cancer of the liver.

Ten minutes after Mary-Margaret returned from the radiology department, Dr. Munoz came into her room. She explained to Fiona and Mary-Margaret that the tests pointed to a disorder with Mary-Margaret's liver and possibly her pancreas. Dr. Munoz had already ordered a consultation with Dr. Jamison, an oncologist, to confirm the diagnosis and begin treatment to ease Mary-Margaret's discomfort.

Fiona cleared her throat and spoke directly to Dr. Munoz. "We have no insurance or money. We can't pay for an oncologist." Dr. Munoz explained that she was only concerned with getting Mary-Margaret diagnosed and treated. She would admit Mary-Margaret to the hospital. At some point, Dr. Munoz explained, a social worker would visit Mary-Margaret to discuss financial arrangements. "For right now," she said, "let's focus all of our efforts on getting your mother well again."

Mary-Margaret was diagnosed with primary pancreatic cancer with extension to the liver. She needed major surgery and extensive outpatient chemotherapy. "It felt like St. Joseph's was turning their full resources to us," described Fiona of the experience at St. Joe's. "They provided chemotherapy, a private room, and created a plan for my mother once she was discharged." Fiona further explained that, "By the time my mother was discharged, we owed St. Joseph's nearly a quarter of a million dollars for her care."

The social worker did visit Mary-Margaret and Fiona, but when she saw how weak Mary-Margaret was, she simply said they could worry about the paperwork later. She assured them that she would walk them through the process of applying for Medicaid. And she said that if Mary-Margaret did not qualify for Medicaid, they would work together to find other solutions. If necessary, the social worker said, the hospital would write off the bill.

The social worker's promise, made on behalf of the hospital, let Mary-Margaret rest easy. Given the seriousness of her condition, additional stress may have harmed her health outcome. Mary-Margaret walked out of the hospital and received continued outpatient chemotherapy and physician office visits over the next few years.

Although I have never been a patient in a CHI hospital, I have had the privilege of working with some of the staff in the CHI corporate office and various hospitals. CHI employees embody the culture of the organization: they are kind and will not settle for less than the best results. The organization posts its values, vision, and mission statements (VVMS) on its Web site. CHI's values are reverence, compassion, integrity, and excellence. Its vision is:

> *. . . to protect the vulnerable; encourage participation in the political process; and safeguard the environment. Advocacy for these and other issues of social justice stems from our leadership position as a builder of healthy communities . . . Catholic Health Initiatives advocates for the kind of systemic change that will provide all Americans with affordable healthcare.*[1]

In an ideal world, healthcare for Mary-Margaret and others like her would be a *right*. For Mary-Margaret, she was fortunate to receive care from an organization that feels a responsibility to its patients, regardless of their ability to pay. In a way, CHI gave Mary-Margaret the *privilege* of free healthcare. The hospital completed the Medicaid application on Mary-Margaret's behalf. And in the end, she did qualify for Medicaid, which covered a small percentage of the hospital's costs.

According to Fiona, Mary-Margaret never once felt like a second-class citizen because she did not have insurance or money to pay for her care. Mary-Margaret's story illustrates the inspiring possibilities that exist in our healthcare system. Her story also shows that organizations with the right VVMS and the right people to carry it out can figure out a way to get things done within our complex system.

IS HEALTHCARE A RIGHT OR A PRIVILEGE?

For people to consider healthcare a right, first the government must recognize it as such for *everyone.* Government-sponsored insurance (Medicare and Medicaid) is the only guaranteed health benefit in the United States, and it is only available for certain classes of the population, namely the elderly and the poor. The answer to the question *is healthcare a right or a privilege?* depends on two things: first, who you are, and second, whether you have completed the appropriate paperwork.

Your Right to Health Insurance if You Are over 64 Years Old or Disabled

Medicare is insurance for the elderly, currently defined as anyone over the age of 64, regardless of ability to pay. Medicare also insures disabled individuals and dependents of disabled individuals. The federal government provides the sole financial support for the Medicare program. Of course, we all pay our fair share in taxes and direct Medicare payments that come out of our paychecks. The 43 million Americans, or approximately 15 percent of the population, currently insured with Medicare include those who meet one of the following criteria:

- Individuals over age 64
- Individuals on disability

- Individuals who have renal failure or ESRD (end-stage renal disease) and certain other diseases
- A child of a disabled parent

Your Right to Health Insurance if You Are Economically Needy

Medicaid is an insurance program that is funded by both the federal government and state governments. Medicaid insures three categories of individuals: economically needy, medically needy, and those who have certain diagnoses. Because each state administers Medicaid, the details of each of the 56 programs (including Washington, D.C., and American territories) vary. The federal government requires states to meet minimum requirements. Each state may offer coverage to more individuals and provide additional benefits.

At a minimum, each state Medicaid program must cover the economically needy. The definition of financial need varies from state to state, but is usually one to two times the poverty level. (To find the eligibility requirements for your state, go to *www.govbenefits.gov*. Under "Benefits Quick Search," select "Medicare/Medicaid." Then select your state to get information and a link to its Medicaid program Web site.) Figure 7.1 below shows 2007 U.S. Department of Health and Human Services (HHS) poverty guidelines.

Figure 7.1 2007 U.S. Poverty Guidelines[2]

Number of Persons in Family or Household	48 Contiguous States and Washington, D.C. ($)	Alaska ($)	Hawaii ($)
1	10,210	12,770	11,750
2	13,690	17,120	15,750
3	17,170	21,470	19,750
4	20,650	25,820	23,750
5	24,130	30,170	27,750
6	27,610	34,520	31,750
7	31,090	38,870	35,750
8	34,570	43,220	39,750
For each additional person, add	3,480	4,350	4,000

Your Right to Health Insurance if You Are Medically Needy

In addition to the economically needy, the federal government will also subsidize certain categories of medically needy patients if the state elects to create and manage the program. It is not mandatory for the state to do so. Medicaid programs for the medically needy are currently available in 34 states and the District of Columbia. (See figure 7.2.) Since each program differs, contact your state Medicaid or Medical Assistance office to determine whether you qualify for any of the program's benefits. The people covered under some of these programs include:

- Pregnant women through a 60-day postpartum period
- Children under age 18
- Blind persons
- Children under age 21 who are full-time students
- Caretaker relatives (relatives or legal guardians who live with and take care of children)
- Women with breast or cervical cancer

- Tuberculosis patients
- Individuals in need of long-term care

Figure 7.2 States (as well as the District of Columbia) with Medicaid Programs Covering the Medically Needy (2005)[3]

Arkansas	Kansas	Nebraska	Tennessee
California	Kentucky	New Hampshire	Texas
Connecticut	Louisiana	New Jersey	Utah
Florida	Maine	New York	Vermont
Georgia	Maryland	North Carolina	Virginia
Hawaii	Massachusetts	North Dakota	Washington
Illinois	Michigan	Pennsylvania	Washington, D.C.
Iowa	Minnesota	Puerto Rico	West Virginia
	Montana	Rhode Island	Wisconsin

Your Right to Health Insurance if You Are Under Age 18

Every state also has a State Children's Health Insurance Program (SCHIP). Most states offer this insurance coverage to children in families whose income is at or below 200 percent of the federal poverty level. The SCHIP eligibility criteria is twice the amounts listed in figure 7.1. In the past five to six years, most states have begun to ensure healthcare coverage for all children for healthcare costs through the state's Medicaid program, even if the children's parents are not eligible for Medicaid.

Is Healthcare in the United States a Right or a Privilege?

In 2005, *USA Today* reported that about 100 million people, or one out of every three individuals in the United States, now have government coverage through Medicaid, Medicare, the military, or federal employee health plans. The newspaper also reported that more than 10 million other people are eligible for Medicaid, but they have not enrolled.[4]

Thus, the more specific answer to the question *Is healthcare in the United States a right or a privilege?* is that it is a *right* for over a third of the people in the United States. In contrast, healthcare is a *privilege* for members of the working class who receive healthcare benefits from their employers. The U.S. Census Bureau estimates that approximately 50 percent of Americans received health insurance benefits through their employers in 2005. About 2 percent of Americans purchase their own health insurance.

WHAT YOU NEED TO KNOW ABOUT YOUR RIGHTS AND RESPONSIBILITIES AS A PATIENT

While American healthcare is a *right* for only certain classes of individuals, once you become a patient, regardless of your ability to pay, you do have some guaranteed rights. And, yes, your rights come along with additional responsibilities as well.

Before he left office, President Clinton secured several significant wins for patients in the U.S. health system. On March 26, 1997, President Clinton created the Advisory Commission on Consumer Protection and Quality in the Health Care Industry. He charged this Commission with making recommendations to promote and assure healthcare quality and value and to protect consumers and workers in the healthcare system. As part of that charge, the Commission developed a "Patients' Bill of Rights."[5] The objectives of the bill of rights are to:

- Strengthen consumer confidence by assuring the healthcare system is fair and responsive to consumers' needs
- Reaffirm the importance of a strong relationship between patients and their healthcare professionals
- Reaffirm the critical role consumers play in safeguarding their own health by establishing both rights and responsibilities for all participants in improving health status

Technically, these rights were provided to recipients of Medicare and Medicaid insurance, but healthcare providers apply the rights to *all* patients. Medicare is the gold standard for healthcare. And, because there are also potential legal issues with treating people differently based on their insurance coverage, Medicare rights can be viewed as the minimum requirements. Our system of state versus federal government also allows the states to offer greater protections or greater rights than the federal government outlines. They just cannot offer less protection. Certain states, like California and Vermont, have traditionally offered much greater rights and protections than the minimum the federal government requires.

Patients' Bill of Rights

- **The Right to Information**. Patients have the right to receive accurate, easily understood information to assist them in making informed decisions about their health plans, facilities, and professionals.
- **The Right to Choose.** Patients have the right to a choice of healthcare providers. This choice must be sufficient to ensure access to appropriate high-quality healthcare, including giving women access to qualified specialists such as obstetrician/gynecologists and giving patients with serious medical conditions and chronic illnesses access to specialists.
- **The Right to Access Emergency Services.** Patients have the right to access emergency health services when and where the need arises. Health plans should provide payment when a patient presents himself to any emergency department with acute symptoms or pain—symptoms a "prudent layperson" ascertains may seriously impair a person's health if untreated.
- **The Right to Be a Full Partner in Healthcare Decisions.** Patients have the right to fully participate in all decisions related to their healthcare. Consumers who are unable to fully participate in treatment decisions have the right to have parents, guardians, family members, or other conservators represent them. Additionally, provider contracts should not contain any *gag clauses* that restrict health professionals' ability to discuss and advise patients on medically necessary treatment options.

- **The Right to Care Without Discrimination.** Patients have the right to considerate, respectful care from all members of the healthcare industry under all circumstances. Consistent with policy benefits and legal mandates, healthcare providers may not discriminate against patients in marketing, enrolling, or providing healthcare services based on race, ethnicity, national origin, religion, sex, age, current or anticipated mental or physical disability, sexual orientation, genetic information, or payment source.
- **The Right to Privacy.** Patients have the right to communicate with healthcare providers in confidence and to have the confidentiality of their individually identifiable healthcare information protected. Patients also have the right to review and copy their own medical records and request amendments to their records.
- **The Right to Speedy Complaint Resolution.** Patients have the right to a fair and efficient process for resolving differences with their health plans, healthcare providers, and the institutions that serve them, including a rigorous system of internal review and an independent external review.

Along with the rights Medicare and Medicaid guarantee, they also stipulate that patients must take greater responsibility for maintaining good health.

Hospital Patient Rights and Responsibilities: Turning Policy into Reality

The Patients' Bill of Rights applies to any care received, whether in a one-room clinic or a 1,000-bed hospital. Many hospitals have taken similar language from their state legislation and applied the rights in a way patients can understand. Hospitals' bill-of-rights statements clearly answer the patient's question, "What are you going to do for me?"

You receive a document of patient rights and responsibilities when you enter the hospital. Most hospitals also post one in the lobby. Each hospital has its own version, but the basics are the same. In a review of 25 different hospital documents of patient rights and responsibilities, about 90 percent of the statements were the same. Hospitals commonly list your right to:

- Considerate, discrimination-free, abuse-free and respectful care
- Participate in your care plan
- Care regardless of your source of payment
- Information about your condition communicated so you can understand it
- Refuse treatment and/or decline to participate in experimental research
- Informed decisions
- Have your advance directives followed
- Family notification of your hospital admission
- Assessment and management of pain
- Be free from restraints or seclusion
- Be informed of hospital rules and regulations
- Know the names of your attending physician and anyone else who cares for you
- Know if your hospital is a teaching organization
- Know if any of your healthcare providers are in training
- Request a second opinion or change physicians
- Privacy of your care and your information
- A safe environment
- Prompt and reasonable responses to any request for relevant services
- Express concerns or grievances and have them resolved
- Review your medical record
- Receive a copy of your bill and have it explained to you
- Have a plan for continued treatment at discharge

- Emergency services
- Access to an interpreter, if necessary
- Full information and counseling about the availability of financial resources to pay or help pay for care
- Visitors

The significance of the patient rights and responsibility statement is three-fold. First, the statement is a means of communicating important information to you about what to expect from the hospital. As a patient, you may not even realize that you have some of these rights. For example, you may not realize you have the right to request a change in your attending physician during your hospital stay or to review your medical record. Second, the statement is a document that you can have with you when you are in the hospital. If there is a misunderstanding or you are dissatisfied with your care, identifying a particular right or rights may help to clarify your position to the hospital staff. For example, during my daughter Emmalea's first hospitalization for epilepsy, the resident physician ordered an injection of low molecular weight heparin to prevent blood clotting from bed rest. She had only been in the hospital for six hours when the nurse came to inject the heparin into her stomach. It was an unnecessary drug at the time. I indicated that she did not want the injection and, initially, the nurse argued with me. Then I reminded her that, as a patient, Emmalea had the right to refuse treatment. She apologized and left the room with her syringe full of heparin. Third, should you find yourself in a defensive position with a hospital, you can use the written statement of your rights as evidence of what the hospital promised to provide to you.

Hospitals also expanded upon your *responsibilities* as a patient. The Patients' Bill of Rights, launched by President Clinton, paved the way by stating you should "take greater responsibility for maintaining good health." Most hospital statements outline five or six patient responsibilities. The most common patient responsibilities contained in hospital statements include your responsibility to:

- Provide a copy of your advance directive to the hospital, if you have one
- Provide accurate and complete information about all matters pertaining to your health
- Follow the instructions and orders of your healthcare team
- Communicate if you do not understand something about your care or treatment
- Report any changes in your condition, including pain, to a member of the team
- Respect the rights and property of others
- Follow the rules and regulations of the hospital
- Keep scheduled appointments or cancel in advance
- Make financial arrangements to pay your bills
- Not take medication in the hospital that your attending physician has not prescribed, unless approved and recorded in your chart

Many patient responsibilities involve compliance with the medical plan and treatment. Working with a team of healthcare providers where there is mutual respect and good communication can inspire you to comply with your treatment plan.

Who Monitors That Your Rights Are Being Upheld in the Hospital?

Although most of your interactions in the hospital are with physicians, nurses, and other clinicians, the hospital's management team, led by the CEO, works to uphold your rights.

If you have ever been in the hospital, did you receive a visit from someone on the top management team? And what about the patients with chronic conditions who have frequent admissions? Shouldn't the hospital administrator know these patients by name and by sight? The typical hospital employs approximately 7.5 staff members per hospital bed. The numbers go up as the hospital size goes up. If only 20 percent of the employees are administrative staff, then there are two administrative staff per hospital bed. Hospital managers are available to you. If you ever feel your patient rights have been violated in a hospital, you shouldn't hesitate to bring your complaint to the attention of a hospital manager.

Do you get to talk with the manager *and* the chef? My husband Joe and I frequent a few restaurants in our hometown of Bethlehem, Pennsylvania. For the past decade, we have dined a few times a week at one restaurant in particular, the Apollo Grill. Dyanne and Rod are the husband-wife owner-operators of the business. Dyanne will either greet us upon arrival and chat with us for a few moments or stop by our table at some point during the meal to see how things are. There are never any problems to report.

I have often wondered over the years if the reason for our satisfaction with the meals is the consistency of the cooking and the cooking staff, all of whom Rod, himself a chef, supervises closely. Or is our satisfaction a result of Dyanne's close communication with every customer who comes in the door? Perhaps, knowing the owner cares about customers and what they think makes the food taste just one iota better. Probably, the combination of the two activities makes for a successful business.

Rod is the expert technician in the kitchen. He makes sure the process flows smoothly. Once the food comes into the dining room, Dyanne and her wait staff take over. These two functions work together to create a satisfied customer. Dyanne and Rod have done this type of work most of their professional lives. They have it down to a science, but they also have a passion for it, which is why I guess most of us keep coming back.

It's not that different in a hospital, or at least it shouldn't be. The expert technicians in the hospital are the clinicians. Like Rod, the attending physicians call the shots and manage the patients' care. The physicians need a team of expert clinicians, including nurses, lab technicians, physical therapists, and others, to provide the best possible care. And, like Dyanne, ideally hospital managers would greet patients at the door or in their rooms (when appropriate) to inquire about their satisfaction with the service and, yes, even with the food.

Would you call the CEO? When my father-in-law was in the hospital in 2006, our family saw firsthand the benefit of hospital administrators as active partners in patient healthcare. Suffering from severe chest pain and shortness of breath, my father-in-law went to the ER. He had a pericardial effusion (fluid around his heart). The fluid had accumulated because of an infection and needed to be drained. Although the condition required emergency care and hospitalization, no hospital beds were available, and my father-in-law had to stay in the ER for about 10 hours until a room was open. The ER staff brought him up to the room on the fourth floor. Shortly after, a transport person whisked him away to the radiology department for follow-up x-rays. However, when the transport person returned my father-in-law to his room on the fourth floor, someone else was in his bed.

Not sure what to do, the transporter parked my father-in-law and his portable bed in the hallway. When my husband Joe arrived, there was my father-in-law, in his hospital gown, walking up and down the hallway because he was bored. Joe attempted to resolve the situation with members of the hospital admissions team. Persisting, he tried the patient advocate. Joe realized that he was not getting anywhere and that it was likely that his father would be spending the night in the hallway unless he did something.

It was a Thursday evening. The hospital senior management team was not in the building, though an administrator is always on call for emergencies. Joe got the name of the hospital CEO and called him directly. Within minutes, a transporter moved my father-in-law to an empty bed. About an hour later, at 10 p.m., the hospital CEO dressed in a suit, white shirt, and tie showed up at my father-in-law's room to make sure he was okay. Then, he stayed while Joe and his sister MaryAnn recounted the challenges of the past 14 hours. The CEO listened to them and promised to make improvements. The CEO's visit turned around my father-in-law's opinion of the hospital and his healthcare treatment. He still speaks highly of the hospital.

In its *Strategies for Leadership* publication, the American Hospital Association (AHA) includes an assessment tool for hospital leaders.[6] One question on the assessment is, "Do members of your management team do 'patient rounds' to find out firsthand about patients' and families' hospital experiences and how well your staff is communicating with them?" Hospital management teams have not commonly practiced patient rounds, but such a practice appears to be on the horizon. Still, it may take a while for visits from hospital management to become the norm.

In the meantime, you can kick-start the process by asking to speak with a manager when you are in the hospital. Perhaps the interaction will provide the manager with useful feedback and encouragement to spend 20 minutes a day, or more, visiting you and other patients (when appropriate). This basic practice might improve enforcement of your rights, not to mention quality healthcare and your satisfaction. It may even increase efficiencies . . . so you spend less time in the hospital!

Patient Rights and Responsibilities for Physician Visits

While the general patient statement of rights and responsibilities passed during the Clinton administration applies to all healthcare providers, there are no laws or regulations specific to physician visits like those created for hospital care. Some healthcare organizations that employ physicians, however, have created statements of rights and responsibilities that apply to physician office visits. The lists below identify the more common rights and responsibilities. Additionally, I incorporated some suggestions from Dr. Janet Maurer into this list. She addresses the issues of patient rights and responsibilities in her book, *How to Talk to Your Doctor: The Questions to Ask.*[7] These rights and responsibilities are in addition to the basic rights already discussed in this chapter for Medicare and Medicaid recipients and for hospitalized patients.

As a patient in the doctor's office, you have the *right* to:

- Have your physician explain your diagnosis, as well as tests and treatments, in a way you understand
- Ask your physician to recommend reasonable alternative treatments or medications
- Receive care within a reasonable amount of time when you go to a healthcare facility
- Ask your doctor to notify you of non-office hour coverage, to keep good patient records, and to inform you of services not covered by insurance
- Be informed about the physician's policies regarding patient payment obligations including missed appointments
- Recognize when the physician's knowledge is limited and ask for a second opinion
- Develop a partnership with your doctor in your quest for wellness

As a patient in the doctor's office, you have a *responsibility* to:

- Share information with your doctor about your lifestyle, particularly if it affects your condition or proposed treatment
- Identify goals for each visit to your doctor
- Ask your doctor questions
- Ask your doctor to explain information you do not understand

You can ask your physician or office staff if they have a statement of rights and responsibilities or rules and regulations. If you review it and don't understand something, ask for clarification.

Key Highlights

In the United States, the government provides healthcare to certain citizens, including the poor, the elderly, and children. Your rights as a patient include the ability to access your own medical records, receive information to make an informed decision, and privacy. Your responsibilities include giving your healthcare provider accurate health information, complying with treatment your physician recommends and you agree to, and reporting any changes in your condition to your healthcare provider(s). It's up to you to hold your healthcare providers accountable for respecting your rights and to fulfill your responsibilities as well.

Key Actions

- Do something to contribute to improving healthcare in this country, no matter how small.
- Understand Medicare and Medicaid rights for yourself and for others you may know who are eligible for coverage under one or both of these programs.
- Provide direct feedback about your hospital stay to hospital administrators if you or a family member is hospitalized.
- Know your rights as a patient.
- Know your responsibilities as a patient.

Key Take-Away

Understand and exercise your rights and responsibilities as a confident healthcare consumer.

Endnotes

[1] Catholic Health Initiatives statement of advocacy, *www.catholichealthinit.org.*

[2] *Federal Register*, Vol. 72, No. 15, January 24, 2007, pp. 3147–48.

[3] Centers for Medicare and Medicaid Services, *Medicaid At-a-Glance*, 2005.

[4] Cauchon, Dennis. "Medicaid insures historic number," USA Today. August 1, 2005.

[5] For more information about the Patients' Bill of Rights, visit the Commission Web site: *www.hcqualitycommission.gov.*

[6] American Hospital Association. *Strategies for Leadership: Improving Communications with Patients and Families: A Blueprint for Action.* AHA, 2003.

[7] Maurer, Janet. *How to Talk to Your Doctor: The Questions to Ask.* Simon & Schuster, Inc., 1986.

CHAPTER

8

Communicating with Your Physician: Play an Active Role to Get the Best Results

The most important thing in communication is to hear what isn't being said. —Peter Drucker

I had an abscess of the fourth bicuspid. My general dentist referred me to an endodontist, a dentist who specializes in root canal. Once there, I immediately was ready for the Novocain and drilling to start. To my surprise, the dentist—a young woman in scrubs and sneakers, who looked about 16 years old—had a different plan. She sat down next to me, held out her hand, and with a big, sincere grin, introduced herself as Dr. Kristin Jabbs. She took out a pad of blank, unlined paper and drew a picture of a healthy tooth. Then she drew a tooth with unhealthy inner structure. This was my tooth, she said. Then, she pointed to the different parts of the tooth and explained how she would perform the root canal. She sounded very confident and knowledgeable, just what I expected from a Harvard- and Stanford-educated dentist.

After the picture and explanation, I once again was ready for the drilling to start. She surprised me a second time by continuing her presentation. She wanted to discuss with me my options. I could: (1) do nothing, which, of course, would likely lead to more infection and a worse situation, (2) have the tooth pulled, which would resolve the abscess, but create a void in my gums and require further treatment, or (3) have the root canal, for which she estimated a high likelihood of success. I decided to have the root canal and signed the consent form.

This was my third root canal—but the first time a dentist ever asked me to give informed consent for the procedure. Dr. Jabbs treated me not only like a patient, but also like an intelligent customer. I received excellent healthcare treatment *and* excellent information. Both are necessary for a positive and successful patient experience. Dr. Jabbs also reminded me of something very important—it is my responsibility as a patient to gather as much information about every healthcare procedure as I can and make sure I understand my options before I undergo treatment. Once I have made an informed decision to receive the care, then I should proceed with the care in a proactive, but cautious manner. I hope you will do the same.

This chapter addresses two topics: actions you can take to improve communication with your physician and other healthcare providers; and the content of and requirements for valid, informed consent. If you actively engage in both processes, you are more likely to get the best possible healthcare.

WHAT KIND OF PHYSICIAN-PATIENT RELATIONSHIP WORKS BEST FOR YOU?

Before you determine what type of relationship may work best for you, it is helpful to first define your goals, values, and expectations regarding how you want your physician to interact with you. You can start by re-evaluating your VVMS and then deciding how you want your physician to interact with you.

How Can I Use My VVMS?

Revisit the VVMS that you created in chapter 1 to help you identify what you are looking for in a relationship with your physician. A mutual understanding of your healthcare VVMS between you and your physician is the basis for good communications. Without a common understanding of healthcare goals, you really cannot have effective communication or a meaningful doctor-patient relationship.

About a year ago, I was looking for a new primary care physician. I had heard through some colleagues about a physician in the area who was an MD, but had a holistic approach to medicine. I also heard he focused on diet and nutrition and was a big believer in eating only organic foods. My personal VVMS includes a focus on nutrition and, for me, that means a vegetarian, raw food diet. At my appointment, the physician first asked me about nutrition, which pleased me—until he began to expound upon the importance of meat, poultry, cheese, and eggs in a daily diet. "You need to purchase your food through an organic market, and I can give you some good names," he said. "You cannot be healthy without daily intake of organic animal protein." After the third rendition of this, I stood up, shook his hand, and thanked him for his time. As I was doing so, I checked off in my head, "ask about diet *philosophy* next time."

My experience with this physician is a good example of a philosophical difference between doctors and patients that prevents effective communication. This physician could not understand why anyone would want to be a vegetarian. He was not willing to support any patient who chose that lifestyle. Before you make a first appointment with a physician or other healthcare provider, ask about your specific preferences that might affect the relationship.

How Do I Want My Physician to Interact with Me?

Think about what role you would like your physician to take in making decisions. Researchers have been studying the dynamics between patients and their physicians for decades. Ezekiel J. Emanuel, MD, PhD, and Linda L. Emanuel, MD, PhD, describe four types of patient-physician relationships.[1] They base these relationships on the degree of control that the physician has in the relationship versus the degree of control that you, as the patient, have. The four relationship types are:

- *Paternalism* (the physician has the greatest degree of control)
- *Consumerism* (the patient has the greatest degree of control)
- *Mutuality* (the patient and physician work together)

- *Default* (neither the patient nor the physician is engaged in the relationship, usually meaning the end of the relationship)

Applying your VVMS, what is your ideal relationship type? Does your current physician relationship reflect your VVMS? If not, what do you need to do to achieve your ideal relationship with your physician? On average, a physician and patient discuss six topics during the typical 16-minute physician office visit.[2] Generally, the longest topic takes five minutes. Knowing the limited time you have with your physician, being clear on what you want to address and how you want to make a decision are key to ensuring you have the best possible encounter with your physician. Consider also your physician's basic communication style. Good communication between you and your physician is the cornerstone of your relationship.

A study cited by The American Academy of Ophthalmology (AAO) examines what patients valued most when receiving bad news from their physician.[3] The patients said that it was important to them that their physician:

- Takes time to answer all of their questions
- Is honest about the severity of their conditions
- Provides them ample time to ask all of their questions
- Gives them his or her full attention

The AAO also cites a study that indicates quality is more important than quantity. In the study, patients who were satisfied after a doctor visit overestimated the time the doctor actually spent with them. In contrast, patients who were dissatisfied complained that the doctor seemed in a hurry, even when visits were actually long.[4]

Your Role in Successful Communications with Your Physician

In their book, *Clinical Reasoning in the Health Professions,* Joy Higgs and Mark Jones assert that shared decision making between you and your physician is important for you to consider the outcome a success.[5]

You have the ability to direct or manage the discussion in most situations. Emergency situations—where you may need a relative, friend, medical mentor or other advocate to help you through the process—call for a different strategy. Whatever the situation, it is *your* unique situation—yours to manage in the way that works best for you. See figure 8.1 for a few examples of physician encounters and the different communication needs for each. (See chapter 15 for definitions of the various healthcare facilities listed in figure 8.1.)

Figure 8.1 Different Scenarios, Different Communication Responsibilities

Scenario	Your responsibility
Well Visit—Primary Care Physician	Talk about your values and goals. Identify the six key topics you would like to address with your physician. Provide details of your diet and physical activities.
Sick Visit—Primary Care Physician	Provide detailed information regarding the onset of symptoms, illness, or injury. Note any related information, including diet, activities, and prescription and non-prescription medicine.
Well Visit—Pediatrician	Provide detailed information regarding child's accomplishments and activities since the last visit.
Sick Visit—Pediatrician	Provide detailed information regarding the onset of symptoms, illness, or injury. Note any related information, including medications given prior to visit, diet, activities, sleeping patterns, irritability, crying, rashes, and fevers.
Initial Visit—Specialist	Provide copies of prior records and test results; written record of the types and amounts of medication you take, when you take them, and how long you have been taking them; and records of any events related to your condition (dizzy spells, fainting, seizures, confusion, palpitations). Communicate the details of your symptoms, illness, or injury. If you are experiencing pain, describe the location, time, quality (sharp, dull), and duration of the pain.
Sick Visit—Specialist	Provide detailed information regarding the onset of symptoms, illness, or injury. Note any related information, including diet, activities, and prescription and non-prescription medicine. Also describe any new or different patterns since your last visit regarding habits (sleep, disposition, diet) and your condition.

It is useful to prepare yourself ahead of an initial or follow-up visit with your physician to obtain the greatest benefit from the (on average) 16 minutes you will have together. Given the importance of the interaction, the time you spend preparing for your visit could be the best 15 to 30 minutes you have ever spent. The following are 10 steps you can take before and during your visit to improve communication with your physician:

1. Think about your goals: what do you want to achieve from the visit?
2. Get organized. Create a list of questions you want to ask. Bring relevant medical records.
3. Research your problem to better prepare questions.
4. Decide whether you want your medical mentor to join you.
5. Answer all your physician's questions fully.
6. Tell the physician your goal(s) for the visit.
7. Listen attentively to the physician and maintain eye contact.
8. Repeat instructions or recommendations the physician gives you. Take notes, if necessary.
9. Ask the physician to clarify anything you do not understand.
10. Ask for instructions in writing.

Norman Cousins: Humor and Help for Patient-Physician Communications

Norman Cousins was the famous optimist who healed his own heart disease and chronic autoimmune disorder through laughter and a positive attitude (accompanied by large amounts of vitamin C administered intravenously). Cousins' methods are well documented in his book, *Anatomy of an Illness.*[6] Cousins believed a patient's attitude and willingness to participate in his care along with his physician had an impact on the outcome of his illness. Cousins was asked by the Dean of the Medical School at the University of California, Los Angeles (UCLA) to work on research regarding laughter therapy and the impact of patient attitude on disease outcomes. Cousins also became an important link in patient-physician communications at UCLA.

He worked at UCLA for over a decade. After 10 years in the role, Cousins wrote a second book, *Head First: The Biology of Hope and the Healing Power of the Human Spirit,* which reveals that he played a much bigger role at the medical school than helping with research studies.[7] In particular, he spent a lot of time with patients who had negative or hopeless attitudes about their conditions. Cousins had the time to listen to patients. Patients were responsive to him. They felt good about their time with him and often left their sessions with a more positive perspective and a plan for being more active in their own care. Cousins was well respected by the physicians of the patients he saw. He was often able to identify diet, prescription drug, or other lifestyle issues that should be further investigated by the clinical team. When he passed on this information to the physicians, they acted on it and often produced improved results for the patients.

In *Head First*, Cousins discusses a survey that was conducted at UCLA. The survey asked patients if they had changed doctors in the past five years and, if yes, why. Eighty-five percent of the patients who changed doctors said they did so because of the doctor's communication style or office manner. Cousins says that these patients were "troubled by the insensitivity to their needs, or poor communication techniques, or by lack of respect for the patient's views, or by overemphasis on technology."[8] The results Cousins produced as a "communication intermediary" at UCLA suggest it may be possible for someone in a similar role to provide a positive effect on patient-physician communications.

Clinicians Who Serve as Communication Intermediaries between You and Your Physician

The New York University (NYU) Epilepsy Center uses clinicians who serve as intermediaries for the neurologists, whose time is often limited. Dr. Devinsky, Emmalea's primary neurologist, is available for regular checkups, to discuss medication changes or the need for diagnostic testing, like EEGs or blood tests. He is also available for emergencies and will answer any phone call made directly to him, even if it is not emergent.

At NYU, a team of nurse practitioners (NPs) serve as the backup for the neurologists and, in many cases, are the first string communicators for the patients. There is an ebb and flow of communication needs with epilepsy that centers around seizures, often referred to as "events," by the clinicians at the Epilepsy Center. Often, the time just before and immediately after a seizure is when the patient and/or the patient's family has the greatest need to communicate with their healthcare professional. During these times, it has been helpful for us to have unlimited access to one of the NPs.

The team of clinicians at the Center is well trained and knowledgeable, with direct access to Dr. Devinsky. They are able to devote significant time to listening to my concerns and developing specific strategies to avert a seizure. We call the NPs for prescription refills and questions we have regarding non-acute issues or symptoms. They are always receptive, helpful, and thorough.

In addition to NPs, physician assistants (PAs) can also serve as communication intermediaries between you and your PCP or specialist. Like the nurse practitioner, PAs often work directly with a physician. The PA may be charged with seeing patients for well visits and managing any telephone or e-mail communications.

Before entering into a relationship with a new physician, ask whether the physician employs NPs or PAs. If so, some questions you may want to ask about the NP or PA include:

- What are the NP/PAs' qualifications, credentials, and years of experience?
- How many years of experience has the NP/PA had dealing with my condition?
- How many different patients with my condition has the NP/PA managed?
- What issues will the NP/PA manage instead of the physician?
- When should I contact or call the NP/PA?

Naturopathic doctors can also supplement the patient-physician communication process. NDs focus on finding holistic solutions for the cause of a patient's problem. NDs are specifically skilled at probing for information to identify the cause of your problem. As a result, their communication training is more targeted than many other clinicians. If you choose to be treated by an ND, she can serve as the intermediary between you and your specialists and even between you and your PCP.

Pros and Cons of Using a Clinician as Your Communication Intermediary

There are several pros to working with a clinician like an NP, PA, or ND as a communication intermediary. These clinicians may have more time to spend with you and may be less intimidating than physicians. Additionally, they are probably easier to access than the physician, especially for non-urgent issues. And they can facilitate tasks like prescription renewals efficiently.

There are also cons to interacting with the clinician instead of your physician. These clinicians have limits on the types of conditions or situations they are able to manage for you. Finally, because they do not have the depth of experience and training of a physician, you may not have as much confidence in dealing with them on some issues. Every physician group will have its own unique approach to patient management and communication. It is important for you to determine how to get the best care from the physician of your choice—even if you need to communicate through an assistant or other clinician for your needs.

Communicating Via E-Mail with Your Physician

If you are comfortable communicating via e-mail with your physician, ask if this is an option for needs that arise between visits. More and more physicians are open to communicating via e-mail, especially if the patient initiates the communication.

One of the primary benefits of e-mail communication is that you, as the patient, receive a written, legible record of the information directly from your physician. Questions you may want to ask your physician regarding e-mail communication include:

- Do you communicate via e-mail with patients? May I e-mail you?
- Do you have a written policy regarding e-mail communication?
- Are there topics I should not address via e-mail?
- Is there a charge for e-mail communication? Will insurance cover it?

Communicating on the Telephone with Your Physician

Teleconferencing with physicians has become commonplace in rural or underserved areas of the United States. However, telephone visits with physicians can be useful in other situations as well. Certain chronic conditions, such as epilepsy or migraine headaches that do not require regular physical examinations, are good examples of when telephone consultations may be helpful.

After months of searching for a more natural, alternative treatment for Emmalea's epilepsy, Emmalea and I were relieved to find Dr. Herzog at Harvard Medical Center. He identified the treatment we were looking for. Yet, a 10-hour round trip for each visit was not ideal for us. We were relieved again when he informed us that, since a physical exam was not required for each visit, we could schedule phone conferences for follow-up visits.

This process works well. We prepare our questions ahead of time and take notes during the calls. After each call, Dr. Herzog e-mails the details of decisions and follow-up actions that both he and Emmalea agree to take. The e-mail documentation he provides is not only helpful in clarifying our roles and responsibilities, but also gives us peace of mind that we did not misinterpret anything he said. (If you use telephone conferencing or e-mail for follow-up visits, be sure to check with your health plan about whether it will pay for your doctor's charges.)

Provide Feedback on Physician Communication through Patient Satisfaction Surveys

One way a healthcare provider determines whether you are happy with the care you received is by conducting and analyzing patient satisfaction surveys. If you have ever been a patient in a hospital, you have probably received a survey in the mail. Chances are you did not complete the survey, since generally only about 10 percent of *all* surveys (about healthcare or other topics) are completed. But completing a survey from your physician may help you to understand what your physician values. Furthermore, if your concerns differ from those on the typical healthcare survey, it may be helpful for you to communicate that. Common questions contained on a patient satisfaction survey ask you to rate the:

- Skill and knowledge of the physician
- Likelihood of recommending the provider to friends and family
- Staff's concerns for your privacy
- Physician's effort to include you in decisions about your treatment
- Coordination of your care across different treatment areas
- Time your physician spent with you
- Staff's ability to address your emotional needs
- Friendliness/courtesy of your physician
- Physician's concern for your questions and worries

INFORMED CONSENT: ESSENTIAL COMMUNICATION FOR DECISION MAKING

In 1914, New York Supreme Court Justice Benjamin Cardozo ruled that informed consent for surgery was mandatory because "every human being of adult years and sound mind has a right to determine what shall be done with his own body."[9] Today, your physician must obtain written informed consent from you for any procedure, invasive treatment, or non-routine treatment. (See sample informed consent form in figure 8.2.)

Informed consent acknowledges your basic human right to make decisions according to your concept of what constitutes a good life. Your signature on a consent form is only symbolic. Your actual consent happens during a discussion with your physician. Physicians have a responsibility to inform you of the risks and benefits of surgery or treatment and to do their best to make sure you understand.[10] When your physician explains a procedure or treatment so you can make an informed decision, at a minimum, he should include:

- Your diagnosis or condition
- The nature and purpose of the treatment or procedure
- The risks and benefits of the treatment or procedure
- Other treatments that may be available and their risks and benefits
- The risks and benefits of not receiving the treatment or procedure

The responsibility for informed consent does not rest solely with your physician. You have a duty to be sure that you understand the information your physician has given you. You also have the right to request that your physician review information with you.

Questions you should ask before consenting to a procedure include:

- How serious is my diagnosis?
- Why do I need the operation?
- What happens if I don't have the operation now?
- What kind of anesthesia will I have?
- How long will it take me to recover from the procedure?
- How many times have you performed the procedure?
- What has been your experience in performing the procedure?

- Can you provide me with an illustration or video of exactly what the procedure involves?
- Is there discomfort associated with the treatment you are recommending?
- What methods do you recommend to prevent or relieve the discomfort?
- What are the immediate, short-term, and long-term side effects of the treatment?
- How will treatment, or not having treatment, affect my normal functions and activities?
- How long will the treatment last?
- How much does the treatment cost?
- How long before I can resume my normal activities?

Informed Choice

In his book, *How Doctors Think,* Jerome Groopman, MD talks about how he likes to use the term *informed choice* instead of *informed consent.*[11] When Emmalea visited the neuroendocrinologist at Harvard, he also referred to the process of *informed choice* before describing all possible treatments.

Using the term *choice* allows us, as patients, to understand it is our decision that determines the next step. *Informed consent* sends the message that your healthcare provider is looking for consent—your having a choice appears less clear. The bottom line is that better-informed patients have better outcomes, faster recoveries, and fewer complications.[12] So, it is in both your best interest and your physician's to make the most well-informed decision possible.

An example of "un"- informed consent. About a year ago, I had porcelain veneers designed for my teeth and fit into my mouth by a local, prominent dentist. Our five-minute conversation preceding the start of the procedure was not very informative, but I should have realized the extent of what I was to undergo based on its price tag alone. The dentist asked me if I had any questions. I asked him what, if any, type of problems or complications might I expect. He did not expect any and noted that this was, after all, a cosmetic procedure. I did not receive or sign a consent form.

Given how my teeth look, I rate this dentist's work high, a 10 on a scale of 1 to 10. However, his failure to address a number of issues prior to the procedure knock my rating down to about a 5. These unaddressed issues include the amount of time and Novocain the treatment required and the pain I would experience. As it turned out, I spent 14 hours in the chair and had so much discomfort between the temporary and final settings over three months, I could not chew anything or drink anything hot. And for months after the procedure, I continued to have pain and sporadic gum inflammation.

In retrospect, the list of "I should have's" go on forever. *I should have* asked many more questions pre-procedure. *I should have* shared with him the fact that I have Temporomandibular joint disorder (TMJ), a chronic inflammation of the joint in my lower jaw that could have impacted the outcome of the procedure. *I should have* done more research about possible side effects or complications before I went to the office. I *should have* asked to sign a consent form. Basically, *I should have* asked him all of the questions I've listed for you in this chapter.

Figure 8.2 Sample Form: Informed Consent

Informed Consent: Flexible Sigmoidoscopy

This document provides you, the patient, with written information regarding the risks, benefits, and alternatives of the procedure above. This consent form is a supplement to the discussion you have with your physician about the risks, benefits, and alternatives to the procedure. Please read this document thoroughly. It is important that you fully understand this information. If you have any questions regarding the procedure, ask your physician prior to signing the consent form.

The Procedure: Flexible sigmoidoscopy is an examination of the interior of the left side of the large intestine, where colon cancer is most common. The areas examined are called the descending colon, sigmoid colon, rectum, and anus. In the first part of the examination, the doctor uses a gloved finger to lubricate the anal canal and feel for tumors. In the main part of the examination, the doctor uses a long, flexible, lighted tube (the sigmoidoscope) to look inside the colon.

Benefits. You might receive the following benefits from flexible sigmoidoscopy. The doctors cannot guarantee you will receive any of these benefits. Only you can decide if the benefits are worth the risk.

1. Flexible sigmoidoscopy may reduce your chances of dying from colon cancer because it helps to identify colon cancer and potentially pre-cancerous polyps at an early, curable stage.
2. There can be no guarantee that the procedure will find all cancers or that any cancer found is necessarily curable.

Risks. Before undergoing this procedure, understanding the associated risks is essential. No procedure is completely risk-free. The following side effects are known to occur, but there may also be unforeseen risks not included in this list. Risk of serious complications, such as perforation or significant bleeding, is about 1 in 100,000, with the need for transfusion and the likelihood of death far less common. Nevertheless, it is important that you be aware of the following:

1. You may experience discomfort or pain. Abdominal discomfort lasting after the procedure occurs in about 5 percent of cases.
2. You may develop dizziness or during or after the procedure.

Risks Continued

3. There may be bleeding if the sigmoidoscope scrapes a blood vessel or hemorrhoid, or after a biopsy; this occurs in less than 2 percent of cases.
4. The procedure may create a hole in the wall of the colon, called a perforation. This rare complication may require surgery.
5. Patients who have had flexible sigmoidoscopy, in rare cases, develop infections of the colon, bloodstream, or heart.
6. You may experience allergic reactions to the medicines or instruments used during the procedure.
7. You may require hospitalization resulting from complications of the procedure; this occurs in about 0.6 percent of cases.

Alternatives. The alternatives to this procedure include:

1. Barium enema (colon x-rays)
2. Colonoscopy (examining the entire colon under mild anesthesia)
3. Testing the stool for blood
4. Having no colon examination

If you decide not to have this procedure, there may be associated risks. Discuss these risks with your doctor.

I discussed the above risks, benefits, and alternatives with the patient. The patient had an opportunity to have all questions answered and was given a copy of this information sheet.

Patient questions:

Physician notes:

Physician Signature Date

____________________________ ________________

Patient Signature Date

____________________________ ________________

Using Multiple Means to Ensure You Are Well Informed

There are two formal requirements for informed consent: (1) the physician discusses the treatment or procedure with you, and documents the discussion, and (2) you, the patient, sign a consent form. Additional strategies by you and your physician may be particularly helpful for complex conditions or conditions that have multiple treatment options. First, mid-level practitioners or ancillary staff can help explain the alternatives. Receiving the information from an additional person can be reinforcing and clarifying. Second, if applicable, ask your physician to illustrate the procedure or provide a resource, including DVDs for you to view.

Key Highlights

Actively communicating with your physician is important to ensure you receive the best possible care. Different situations call for different types and modes of communication. Consider communicating with your healthcare providers via e-mail or telephone, if possible. It is important to understand all components of informed consent for any procedure or treatment. Your physician has a responsibility to inform you of the risks and benefits of any treatment. You have a responsibility to make a well-informed choice.

Key Actions

- Build a strong basis for communication with your physicians by making sure they understand and respect your health values.
- Ask whether your physician is willing to communicate with you via e-mail or phone if you prefer this method of communicating.
- Make sure your physician gives you verbal and written information about the risks and benefits of any non-routine procedure or treatment.

- Ask questions about the risks and benefits of a procedure or treatment if you don't understand something.
- Sign an informed consent form *only* if you fully understand the risks and benefits and feel comfortable going forward with the procedure or treatment your doctor recommends.

Key Take-Away

When your doctor recommends a procedure or treatment, he should provide you with complete information, including an informed consent form, and you should be confident that you are making an informed *choice.*

Endnotes

[1] Emanuel, Ezekiel J., MD, PhD, and Emanuel, Linda L., MD, PhD. "Four Models of the Physician-Patient Relationship," *Journal of the American Medical Association,* 267, no. 16 (1992): 2221-28.
[2] Tai-Seale, Ming. *ACSM Health and Fitness Journal,* January/February 2007.
[3] Baile, Walter F. *Conversations in Care,* Chapter 1: "The Importance of Physician-Patient Communication." EMD Pharmaceuticals. (*www.aao.org/practice_mgmt/patient_ed/effective.cfm#talking*)
[4] Korsch, Barbara M.; Gozzi, Ethel K.; and Francis, Vida. "Gaps in doctor-patient communication: I. Doctor-patient interaction and patient satisfaction," *Pediatrics,* 42, no. 5 (1968): 855-71.
[5] Higgs, Joy and Jones, Mark. *Clinical Reasoning in the Health Professions.* Butterworth-Heinemann, 1997.
[6] Cousins, Norman. *Anatomy of an Illness as Perceived by the Patient.* W.W. Norton & Company, 1979.
[7] Cousins, Norman. *Head First: The Biology of Hope and the Healing Power of the Human Spirit.* Penguin Group, USA, 1989.

[8] Cousins, Norman. *Head First: The Biology of Hope and the Healing Power of the Human Spirit.* Penguin Group, USA, 1989.
[9] Schloendorff v. Society of New York Hospital, 211 NY 124, 105 NE 92 (1914).
[10] Bernat, James L. MD, and Lynn M. Peterson, MD, "Patient-Centered Informed Consent in Surgical Practice," *Archives of Surgery,* 141 (2006): 86-92.
[11] Groopman, Jerome, MD. *How Doctors Think.* Houghton Mifflin Company, 2007.
[12] Clancy, Carolyn, MD. Agency for Healthcare Research and Quality, U.S. Department of Health and Human Services.

CHAPTER

9

Getting a Second Opinion: What to Do When Doctors Disagree

Honest disagreement is often a good sign of progress.
—Mahatma Gandhi

Emmalea had her fifth grand mal seizure exactly 365 days after her first. Both days were Fridays. Both days were just after she had returned from a trip. These facts were not the most striking similarities between the two seizures. As we examined each of the seizures more closely, we realized that each one had occurred within three days of the end of her menstrual cycle. Actually, this was not the first time we had wondered about a relationship between the seizures and Emmalea's menstrual cycle. When we previously brought this concern to her primary neurologist, he said we needed much more data before assuming a relationship existed. However, it was never clear how much data we needed. In addition, more data meant one thing to us: more seizures, the very thing we were trying to avoid.

We needed to find a doctor who would help us address the relationship between seizures and the menstrual cycle. Our current neurologists listened sympathetically, but their focus was on treating her seizures with anti-epileptic drugs (AEDs). The endocrinologists were experts in hormones, but they did not treat epilepsy. In fact, they expressed concern about practicing outside their area of expertise. The gynecologist prescribed birth control pills, but would not discuss any relationship between seizures and menstruation.

Just when things seemed hopeless, I found an article on the Internet about seizures related to the menstrual cycle. This article even gave the phenomenon a name: *catamenial epilepsy*. The article referenced a physician from Harvard, Dr. Andrew Herzog, who had been researching the relationship between seizures and menstruation for over a decade. The more I read, the more certain I felt this doctor would have the answer for us, for Emmalea. Here was the key: He is a subspecialist, a neuroendocrinologist. He is an expert on disorders of the nervous system *and* hormones. Certain hormones, such as estrogen, progesterone and testosterone, regulate the menstrual cycle. It took five long months until we were able to see Dr. Herzog. When we did, he pulled together the different pieces of the puzzle into one place for us.

A common criticism of physician specialization is that it can result in an overly narrow perspective in diagnosing the patient and overconfidence in the methods of treatment.[1] This is exactly what happened in Emmalea's case. The primary neurologist initially was not open to considering a hormonal reason for her seizures. However, after our visit with Dr. Herzog, we connected our primary neurologist with him to work together to achieve the same goal: keep Emmalea seizure-free. Emmalea's healthcare team now consists of a primary care physician, a primary neurologist, and a neuroendocrinologist.

THE BEST PROVIDERS WANT YOU TO SEEK A SECOND OPINION

The Yale-New Haven Hospital Web site (*www.ynhh.org*) dedicates a page to describing the process for and value of second opinions.[2] It begins:

Americans today are taking more responsibility for managing their own healthcare. They are becoming more informed about their medical problems and treatment options and playing an active role in every decision with their doctors. Increasingly, consumers are seeking second opinions, showing the strong value Americans place on being in control of their health.

Ideally, all healthcare providers would embrace this statement. It supports the growing responsibility of healthcare consumers as well as respect for individual preferences. The Yale-New Haven Hospital Web site goes on to state:

Because of the increase in medical knowledge and new treatments, it is difficult for any one physician to be aware of all the latest information. One result is patients and their physicians together are seeking second opinions so better and more informed decisions can be made.

This statement sums up the overall reasoning for second opinions. It also shows that the staff at Yale-New Haven are grounded in reality because they understand it is difficult for any one physician to have all of the answers.

Second Opinions: When and How Do You Get One?

Getting a second opinion for any type of major surgery or major treatment plan is a good idea. Sometimes you may want a second opinion because even after your physician addresses your questions and concerns, there may be something about the treatment plan that makes you feel uncomfortable.

Maybe you just do not feel at ease with your physician. Listen to your inner voice. If it is your physician's demeanor, philosophy, or some other personality or competency concern, you probably do not only need a second opinion, you probably need a new physician. Here are some common reasons to get a second opinion:

- Your doctor says you need major surgery
- You question whether surgery is the only option for your condition
- You have a chronic condition that seems to be getting worse, with no explanation
- Your regular doctor cannot diagnose your problem
- You have trouble talking with your current doctor
- Your medical condition is not improving
- Your diagnosis is a life-threatening disease

- You have multiple medical problems
- Your physician recommends getting a second opinion
- You have a newly diagnosed chronic condition that requires long-term medication
- You do not feel comfortable with the treatment plan or with your physician

Once you decide you want a second opinion, it is helpful to do two things. First, discuss your desire with your physician. Unless you plan to sever your relationship with your current physician, it is important to be honest about your intentions, as awkward as you may feel. A confident physician should understand your needs, support you, and possibly even recommend other physicians to see. If you cannot have a positive, productive discussion with your physician regarding second opinions, then you probably need a new physician.

Second, identify physicians who are appropriate candidates for second opinions. Certainly consider suggestions from your current physician. You may want to do your own research as well. You can find another physician in several ways. For example, many city magazines publish a "best doctors" list each year. These lists are usually available on the Internet. If a teaching hospital is nearby, check there for specialists. The American Board of Specialties *(www.abms.org)* is a resource for all medical and surgical specialties. Also ask friends or relatives for their suggestions based on experiences they have had. (Please see chapter 13 for more information on specialists).

Second Opinions: What Are You Really Looking For?

Before getting a second opinion, think about what you want to achieve. One of two things can happen when you get a second opinion. The physician offering the second opinion may agree or disagree with the initial physician's opinion. If the physicians *agree* with each other, you have two choices: (1) do what the physicians recommend, or (2) seek a third, fourth, or even more opinions, depending on your concerns. We saw five physicians before we found one able to treat the *cause* of Emmalea's seizures instead of only prescribing medication (AEDs) to block the seizures. If your second physician *disagrees* with your initial physician, you have three choices: (1) do what your initial physician recommends, (2) do what the second physician recommends, or (3) seek a third opinion, or more if necessary.

Consider what it is you want to know. Are you seeking a confirmatory opinion? Are you looking for a different approach or philosophy? Are you looking for a different physician, one whom you feel more comfortable with? Whatever your reason for seeking a second opinion, determine what it is before you make the appointment. Then, once you meet with another doctor, you may be better able to determine your next steps. Whatever the outcome of a second opinion, goal planning can be worthwhile. You will be better informed and more confident in determining your healthcare plan.

Use figure 9.1 to help you think through and document why you are seeking a second opinion. Read the statements within the figure. Which reasons would you rate as most important in seeking a second opinion? Circle the number to the left of the corresponding statement that best describes how important each reason is to you for seeking a second opinion: (0) no reason, (1) somewhat of a reason, (2) a reason, and (3) a strong reason. Prioritize your actions based on those reasons you rate a 2 or a 3.

Figure 9.1 Why I Want a Second Opinion

				Why I Want a Second Opinion
0	1	2	3	I want to confirm my first physician's recommendation.
0	1	2	3	I want a different approach to my treatment.
0	1	2	3	I want to choose a treatment from several options.
0	1	2	3	I want a different physician.
0	1	2	3	Other:

Once you make your appointment for your second opinion, prepare your questions for the visit. Sample questions to ask the physician include:

- Is the diagnosis certain?
- What are alternative treatments?
- What are the risks associated with the treatment?
- What are the risks if I elect not to have the treatment?
- What are the side effects of the treatment?
- Will the treatment affect my quality of life?
- Why does your opinion differ from or confirm the initial recommendation I received?

Medicine is as much an art as it is a science.[3] When physicians disagree, it is difficult to make a decision. With Emmalea, we eventually found physician specialists who worked well together. But if we hadn't persisted in our search for solutions, Emmalea may not have discovered the cause of her seizures or gotten them under control.

Was it ventricular tachycardia (a heart arrhythmia) or not? One evening in the summer of 2006, my husband Joe complained of lightheadedness and tightness in his chest. Although he had no prior cardiac history and did not have a family history of cardiac problems, given his age (48 years old) and current stress level (high), we went to our local hospital's ER. Within minutes of our arrival, he was in an ER bed, hooked up to an EKG monitor, and having blood drawn. Right away, the healthcare team was able to confirm Joe was not having a heart attack.

What happened next was quite interesting. An ER physician came into the room to interview Joe about his symptoms. As Joe responded to the questions, his blood pressure began to rise. The more frequent the questions, the higher Joe's blood pressure rose. When he answered one final question about describing the chest tightness, the EKG monitor made a long beeping noise and several inverted V's shot up on the EKG screen. As the physician stopped the questions, the EKG showed a more normal reading.

Once Joe had calmed down, the physician asked if he had felt the abnormal heart beat that showed up on the EKG. Reluctantly, Joe nodded yes. Sounding ominous, the physician said Joe had been in ventricular tachycardia, a serious heart arrhythmia. Then, Joe gazed past the ER physician to the television to see his favorite team, the New York Yankees, beating the Boston Red Sox. His blood pressure dropped a little below normal.

A few minutes later, a cardiologist came to see Joe. The cardiologist did not believe Joe had been in ventricular tachycardia. He thought Joe had experienced some premature ventricular contractures (PVCs), a fairly benign and limited irregular heartbeat. He said about 70 percent of adults experience PVCs at some point. Sustained or repeated PVCs, he explained, indicate ventricular tachycardia. The only way to prove Joe had been in ventricular tachycardia was to review his EKG results. But that was not possible.

Apparently, Joe's room was the only one in the ER that had an old EKG machine, which did not have paper to record the readings. So, it was the ER physician's opinion against the cardiologist's opinion. Choosing the safest precaution, we decided to go with the ER physician's diagnosis, given its seriousness, and he admitted Joe for further tests. It turned out, the cardiologist was right (thankfully), and he discharged Joe the next day. Despite the doctors disagreeing, our experience was straightforward. The risk of releasing Joe from the ER that night versus keeping him in the hospital another day made our decision easy. Certainly keeping Joe overnight in the hospital was not overly intrusive for him. But not all situations when doctors disagree are as simple as this one.

Was my pelvis fractured or not? In the summer of 2006, I had improved my speed and increased my weekly running routine from 40 to 50 miles a week. I had been running regularly for almost the past two decades. Following a series of competitions I ran as a member of the New York Road Runners, I began to feel some pulling and slight pain in the back of my right thigh. When the pain did not subside, I scheduled an appointment with an orthopedic surgeon.

The pelvic x-ray the surgeon took was normal. However, because of the symptoms, he suggested an MRI to rule out a stress fracture. When I called the MRI center to get my results, I was relieved to hear that the radiologist's interpretation was a stress *injury* and some edema (swelling) of the muscle. There was no fracture. I was satisfied with this diagnosis until I received a call from the surgeon. He also read the MRI and saw a fracture of the pubic ramus. I decided to go with the radiologist's diagnosis since it was what I wanted to hear. I continued to run. When the pain became so excruciating that I could barely walk, I decided to seek a third opinion.

I knew I wanted a diagnosis and treatment from someone who dealt with stress fractures of this type if, in fact, that was what I had. After researching my third opinion options, I chose a new sports medicine facility in our area. My doctor took me into the physicians' work area to look at the original MRI films I had brought. She put the film up on the lighted viewing board and told me that on film, the blank space in between broken bone shows up as white, while the rest of the film is black. With her pencil, she traced the fracture line on the right hip. The area was clearly white.

The doctor explained that the fracture had resulted from years of micro-trauma to my bones due to running day after day. She said that initially and sometimes up until the bone breaks, runners often do not experience warning signs. She also noted the differences on the film between my right and left hips—no white lines on the left. Though she said, in time, a fracture could happen there too with continued running. I left the office a deflated runner, but a more informed healthcare consumer, on crutches with a 12-week plan for recovery.

This example is another simple case without fatal consequences. However, it illustrates the importance of a second opinion for clarification, as well as to convince a patient who is in denial, that the diagnosis is correct. It also demonstrates how effectively a physician can educate the healthcare consumer by showing—not just talking about—diagnostic tools, such as MRI film.

This practice of illustrating the diagnosis to the patient is becoming more common. For example, many cardiologists show patients the film results of their cardiac catheterization procedures to demonstrate heart vessel blockage. In any visit with your physicians, ask to see an x-ray, a CT scan, MRI film, or other tangible information that may help you understand what is going on in your body.

This example also highlights differences that arise between types of practitioners—in my case, the radiologist, the sports medicine physician, and the orthopedic surgeon. Radiologists provide a diagnosis based primarily upon the test, the x-ray, MRI, or CT scan. The radiologist did not directly interact with me. He did not know I was a runner or how many miles I usually run a day. Because radiologists usually only have part of the picture, your treating physician may discount the accuracy of the radiologist's interpretation as he fuses all of the information and test results together for his final diagnosis.

I had asked the radiologist for a diagnosis. However, he probably should not have provided me with his diagnosis and instead should have advised me to speak with my treating physician. Given my healthcare training, I knew better than to accept the diagnosis of a radiologist over an orthopedic surgeon—but I went with the diagnosis I wanted to believe, delaying necessary treatment.

Are symptoms meaningful or not? With juvenile myoclonic epilepsy (JME), one of the common types of seizures patients initially experience is *myoclonus.* This involves quick, brief jerking motions of the limbs, usually the hands or upper limbs. Emmalea had experienced minor (one or two second) jerks for about one year prior to her first grand mal seizure. As is common with many JME patients, doctors did not diagnose her condition until her first full-blown seizure. When Emmalea began the anti-seizure medication, we asked the doctor if the jerking motions would subside. He told us the jerks might never go away. We left the hospital discouraged, assuming the jerks would be a normal part of her life.

About 15 minutes before Emmalea's next seizure, she experienced several jerks. When we described this to the second neurologist we saw, he said the medication should eliminate the jerks, but if it did not, any jerking while on the medication was probably a warning sign of an impending seizure. He also explained that when the jerks start, Emmalea can take an "emergency pill" (Ativan or Valium) to prevent a full-blown seizure. This neurologist's opinion caused us to substantially modify Emmalea's anti-seizure strategy.

These examples of second opinions or doctors disagreeing are all from the patient's perspective. If you are interested in second opinions from the physician's perspective, several books are available, including *Second Opinions* by Jerome Groopman, MD.[4] Dr. Groopman describes several patient scenarios involving second opinions. Two of the scenarios describe second opinions he sought as a healthcare consumer himself—one for his own back problem and one for his son's intestinal problem. Both offer insight into how a physician manages second opinions for his own or a family member's diagnoses and treatment.

Is a Blind Second Opinion a Good Idea?

A blind second opinion requires the second physician to see you under the same circumstances as the first physician. In other words, the second physician does not have access to the notes and records of the first physician. This process ensures that the first physician's findings and recommendations do not influence the second physician.

In theory, a blind second opinion is the best way to obtain the opinion. In reality, it may not be possible. The second physician may require your previous records. And if your first physician is making the referral, he may speak with the second physician about your condition. One of the disadvantages of a blind second opinion is that doctor number two may not be able to tell you why his opinion is different without knowing the basis of the first doctor's opinion. Some hospitals such as Yale-New Haven Hospital suggest another option—that you provide test results, x-rays, and other information without including the first doctor's written diagnosis and treatment recommendation.

INITIAL CONFLICT AMONG YOUR PHYSICIANS MAY NOT BE A BAD THING

Disagreement between physicians is an inherent part of their training. Residents are taught to question their mentors and attending physicians partly to understand why they are treating or caring for patients in the way they are, and partly to arrive at a better result. Such questioning may result in modifying a patient's treatment regimen. Teaching hospitals often promote their residency programs as one of the biggest advantages for patients. Residents act as a system of checks and balances for physicians. Many physicians probably never outgrow the discipline they acquired as residents to question and make sure they have the right answer for the patient.

If your initial and consulting physicians disagree, try not to be frustrated. Disagreement is not necessarily a negative. Lean on your primary care physician. She can help you to: (1) analyze all the available information, (2) decide if you need another opinion or further information, (3) speak with other physicians who have provided opinions, and (4) coordinate discussion among all the physicians. You may want to participate in the discussion or ask your primary doctor to fill you in.

The good news is that there is an upside to most disagreements between or among physicians. In June 2007, *New York Magazine* asked a panel of anonymous physicians to provide their views regarding second opinions. As one physician put it, "Everybody wins."[5] A disagreement between physicians in many cases can result in better outcomes. Disagreements abound in the medical community. The downside of this for the patient can be confusion and frustration, especially if the disagreements are about a current condition. The upside is that the medical community usually has a plan for the traditional, safe treatment, while they battle out new treatment regimens. This culture of disagreement demonstrates that physicians worldwide are never at rest with disease. They are always looking for a better solution, one that is in the best interest of the patient.

Documented Examples of When Doctors Disagree

Doctors do disagree. In fact, frequently groups of physicians become polarized on certain issues. These examples illustrate some disagreements currently getting attention in the media.

Rheumatoid Arthritis: Surgical Versus Medical Treatment
According to the *Journal of Rheumatology,* hand surgeons and rheumatologists often disagree about whether medication or surgery is indicated to treat rheumatoid arthritis.[6] About 70 percent of rheumatologists consider hand surgeons deficient in their understanding of the medical options available to treat rheumatoid arthritis. A similar percentage of surgeons believe rheumatologists lack knowledge of the surgical options for rheumatoid arthritis. The differing opinions may simply be that surgeons tend to recommend surgery while other physicians tend to recommend non-surgical options first.

Uterine Biopsy: Is It Cancer?
A study at Johns Hopkins University found that pathologists who evaluate uterine biopsies disagree 60 percent of the time about whether the specimens contain cancerous cells.[7] Uterine cancer is the most common cancer of the female reproductive system in the United States. Usually, physicians recommend a hysterectomy for uterine cancer.

Dementia: Which Drug Is Best?
Researchers asked 106 psychiatrists from Australian and New Zealand to identify the drug they preferred to prescribe to patients who have dementia with psychotic symptoms.[8] The researchers found much disagreement among the physicians. The researchers also claimed the physicians relied too much on their intuition. While this may be true, it is also possible the physicians based their choices on experience. In

addition, physicians recommend different medications based upon the differences in patients' medical histories.

Annual Checkups: Are They Necessary?
Most primary care physicians and many medical associations around the globe recommend annual physicals. However, the U.S. Preventive Services Task Force states that a healthy person probably does not need an annual physical.[9] This view suggests that people may decide they don't need checkups at all. Consequently, many may not seek treatment until a late stage of a disorder. If you are an adult, the frequency of preventive physical exams is your decision. Most people agree that babies and children should have a checkup at least annually.

Chemotherapy for Breast Cancer: Is It Necessary?
In a discussion televised on ABC News, oncologists from Dana-Farber Cancer Institute and the Memorial Sloan-Kettering Cancer Center disagreed about backing off on chemotherapy for certain breast cancer patients. There is evidence that new, milder, non-chemotherapy medications can be used to successfully treat breast cancer. Dr. Eric Winer, from Dana-Farber Cancer Institute, explained that oncologists are beginning to back off on chemotherapy in selected patients. On the other hand, Dr. Clifford Hudis, from Memorial Sloan-Kettering Cancer Center, said that he was reluctant to withhold chemotherapy on the basis of what he believes is evolving and incomplete data.[10]

Mammograms: Differences in Interpretation
In a study published in the *New England Journal of Medicine,* 10 radiologists reading the same mammogram films differed in their diagnoses 22 percent of the time.[11] In his book, *How Doctors Think,* Jerome Groopman, MD, discusses the differences in radiologists' interpretation, noting that 15 to 20 percent of the time, radiologists reading the same x-ray differ on their diagnoses.[12] Some differences may be due to productivity requirements. Some radiologists are expected to review 150 films per day. Other differences may be due to human error or subjective interpretations.

What to Do If *Your* Doctors Disagree

If you receive different recommendations from various physicians, the following questions may help you decide whose advice to follow.

- Which physician has the greatest amount of experience regarding my condition?
- How does each physician compare to the other in training and certification?
- Where did each go to medical school?
- Is each physician board certified in the field involving my healthcare needs?
- What are each physician's research accomplishments?
- How many patients does each physician treat?

Key Highlights

Getting a second opinion can be helpful when facing a difficult health situation. Some reasons to consider getting a second opinion include: your doctor says you need major surgery, you feel uncomfortable talking with your doctor, or your doctor recommends you get a second opinion. If you are not happy with your doctor's approach, try to find what you are looking for from another physician. Before visiting a doctor for a second opinion, think about why you want the opinion, what questions you have, and how you will decide which treatment regimen to follow if the first and second doctors disagree.

Key Actions

- Seek a second opinion if your doctor recommends a major procedure, such as surgery, or if you feel uncomfortable or uncertain about anything your doctor says.
- Understand why you want a second opinion. Are you looking for confirmation of the first doctor's diagnosis and recommendation? Are you looking for a different approach?

It's important to think about your reasons and have a clear vision before visiting the second doctor.

- Do some research if your doctors disagree and you're not sure whose advice to follow.

Key Take-Away

It is your right and responsibility as a healthcare consumer to seek out and evaluate second, third, and even more opinions about your healthcare.

Endnotes

[1] Dowie, Jack and Elstein, Arthur. *Professional Judgment: A Reader in Clinical Decision Making.* Cambridge University Press, 1988.
[2] Yale-New Haven Hospital Web site (*www.ynhh.org*)
[3] Azzone, G.F. *Medicine from Art to Science: The Role of Complexity and Evolution.* IOS Press, 1998.
[4] Groopman, Jerome, MD. *Second Opinions: Stories of Intuition and Choice in the Changing World of Medicine.* Penguin, 2000.
[5] Kolker, Robert. "What's up docs? A panel of anonymous physicians coughs up secrets of the trade," *New York Magazine.* June 18, 2007.
[6] Alderman, Amy K.; Ubel, Peter A.; et. al. "Surgical Management of the Rheumatoid Hand: Consensus and Controversy Among Rheumatologists and Hand Surgeons," *Journal of Rheumatology.* 30 (2003):1464–72.
[7] The study was conducted by the Gynecologic Oncology Group, headed by Cornelia Trimble, MD, of the Johns Hopkins Kimmel Cancer Center. Findings were reported in June 2004 at the annual meeting of the American Society of Clinical Oncology. For more information, go to *www.hopkinsmedicine.org/Press_releases/2004/06_02_04.html.*
[8] Greve, Melissa and O'Connor, Daniel. "A survey of Australian and New Zealand old age psychiatrists' preferred medications to treat behavioral and psychological symptoms of dementia (BPSD)," *International Psychogeriatrics.* 17 (2005): 195–205.
[9] U.S. Preventive Services Task Force. *The Guide to Clinical Preventive Services.* International Medical Publishing, 2002.
[10] McKenzie, John. "Doctors Disagree Over Chemo for Breast Cancer," ABC News Web site, May 15, 2006 (*abcnews.go.com/WNT/Story?id=1964721&page=1*).
[11] Elmore, Joann G.; Wells, Carolyn K.; et. al. "Variability in Radiologists' Interpretations of Mammograms," *New England Journal of Medicine.* 331 (1994): 1493–9.
[12] Groopman, Jerome, MD. *How Doctors Think.* Houghton Mifflin Company, 2007.

STEP

4

ASSESS QUALITY

CHAPTER

10

Rating the Quality of Your Healthcare Providers and Health Plan

A product or service is not quality because it is hard to make and costs a lot of money. This is incompetence. Customers pay only for what is of use to them and gives them value. Nothing else constitutes quality. —Peter Drucker

In 2004, at the age of 56, Vera learned she had breast cancer. With a long and strong history of breast cancer in her family, Vera had always been conscientious about getting annual mammograms. In fact, in the year-and-a-half prior to her diagnosis of breast cancer, she had two mammograms. As it turned out, the radiologist had overlooked a spot on one of her previous mammograms. An earlier diagnosis might have required less aggressive intervention or less aggressive chemotherapy. There is really no way of knowing for sure. Fortunately, three years later, Vera remains cancer-free.

When Vera learned of the missed abnormality on her mammogram, she wanted to know if the radiologist had been negligent. She consulted with a physician in Washington, D.C., who had served as an expert witness for breast cancer cases. After reviewing Vera's various mammograms, the radiologist told her that an earlier mammogram showed an abnormality in the same place that the tumor developed. She went on to explain that the abnormality on the film was somewhat ambiguous. "Probably 50 percent of physicians would have read the film as normal," she said, "and the other 50 percent would have identified the abnormality." Then, she ended the conversation with, "I would have found the growth. But, I can tell you that I would not hold one of my staff at fault for missing this abnormality."

Vera felt like she had the wind knocked out of her. She left the office in a daze. As she and her husband Craig began the 250-mile journey back home, she wondered why it was acceptable to have only one physician interpret films when patients' lives are at stake. In contrast, Vera thought about her fourth-grade students who take state-standardized tests each year. Even they have the benefit of their tests being graded twice for quality control purposes—and with much less at stake. Vera's story points to important lessons. First, it should be okay to question test results or ask for a second review. Second, it is important to share your stories so that others may benefit.

THE FIRST STEP IN DEFINING QUALITY: WHAT IS IMPORTANT TO YOU?

The Six Sigma quality process, probably the most renowned quality measurement process in the world, defines quality as *the absence of defects.* A defect is the failure of a product or service to meet customer requirements. In healthcare—which includes both clinical caregivers and insurance companies (or health plans)—the customer, or patient, should define the quality. If you want to receive the highest quality of care, you need to be able to articulate your requirements to your provider. This can be difficult for even the savviest patients. This chapter will help you define your requirements so you can communicate them. The chapter will also help you to use and understand the healthcare quality rating tools available to you as a healthcare consumer.

Although it may be more difficult to see the immediate impact of your feedback in a larger provider group or hospital compared to a small, private practice, your feedback is always important. Do not hesitate to provide it. Healthcare providers have a responsibility to analyze all feedback they receive and act upon it to: (1) make things right with the patient, or (2) develop practices to improve quality and patient satisfaction.

The first step in defining healthcare quality is to define what matters most to you. A good place to start is reviewing the values you created in chapter 1. Keep your top three values in mind as you begin conversations with any healthcare provider. Remember: you are the customer and your requirements define the quality of service. Or if you use the Six Sigma definition, you decide whether the healthcare service you received was defect-free.

Unless you communicate your requirements, the chances that healthcare providers will hit your target greatly diminish. Restate your values. Then think about whether your physician's care upholds your values. Read the table in figure 10.1 for an example of how healthcare providers can apply a set of values. Then complete your own in the blank table in figure 10.2.

Figure 10.1 Example of How Healthcare Providers Can Apply Values

Value	Apply the Value to Healthcare Providers' Services	Measure Healthcare Providers' Services
Collaboration	My physician "over-communicates" with me and works with other colleagues to provide me the best care.	I receive a confirmatory e-mail after each visit. When I have anything other than a simple diagnosis, he recommends a second opinion. He brings residents or fellows (doctors who are in training for a particular medical or surgical specialty) in to co-treat.
Innovation	My physician seeks cutting-edge treatment for my conditions.	He uses complementary and alternative medicine (CAM) and recommends another physician who can provide CAM to me.
Growth	My physician takes a holistic approach to my care.	He questions and provides guidance to me on fitness and nutrition, recommends new approaches, and is open-minded to accepting my choices.

Do It Now!

Fill in your values from chapter 1 and then briefly state how you would like those values to be evident in the care you receive. In the third column, decide how you will know.

Figure 10.2 Your Values and How They are Evident

My Values	How I Apply My Values to My Healthcare Provider's Services	How I Measure Healthcare Provider's Services

Provide Feedback About What You Want and Whether You Get It

The best way to ensure that you get what you want is to communicate your goals. To borrow a phrase from author and leadership consultant, Ken Blanchard, "Feedback is the breakfast of champions." [1]Providing your criteria (your values), and then feedback to your provider as to whether your goals were met is the only way to get what you want.

Many organizations change a product or service in response to customer feedback. This often results in happy customers and a growing business. JetBlue's strategy of listening to customers and limiting its service to certain cities is a good example. The company's recent customer service troubles, which happened when it tried to grow outside of its original vision, also indicate how quality can suffer when you deviate from your original VVMS. Hospitals, physicians, and health plans can learn from the JetBlue experience.

JetBlue: Listening to Customers and Focusing on Certain Cities

During his tenure at JetBlue, and as part of his startup strategy, CEO and Founder David Neeleman asked customers what they did not like about their current airlines. The biggest issues were high prices, inadequate legroom, tasteless snacks, beverage carts banging their elbows, and unfriendly attendants. Before Neeleman started JetBlue, he too, was a frequent flyer and had the same complaints. But he had a clear vision.

Neeleman began to change the industry standards when he gambled that customers would be willing to give up first class and full meals in exchange for features that mattered more to them. He started with a "one-class" offering in mind, providing all passengers with the comfort they wanted. All JetBlue flights, most very economically priced, offer more legroom than other airlines as well as leather seats and live satellite television for all passengers. One of the biggest improvements he made was also the least expensive. Neeleman eliminated beverage carts and replaced them with large, attractive baskets that attendants bring directly to your seat, and passengers may choose from biscotti, signature JetBlue chips, and other tasty snacks. In addition, attendants take drink orders by row and serve them from trays, as in a restaurant.

Like healthcare, the airline industry is an old, staid business, where leaders believe they can't change many practices that bother customers. For other airlines, the cost to change some conditions, like legroom, is prohibitive. For JetBlue, a new company with new planes, modifying the design specifications was part of the plan. With a strong vision and with a focus on customer preferences, in four short years Neeleman took JetBlue from an airline with only two airplanes to one with more than 57 airplanes. The airline strategically serves select cities to ensure continued specialization and attention to customer needs.[2]

For hospitals, a similar situation might be patients not wanting to share a room (and especially not a bathroom) with a stranger. For hospitals that are adding rooms or undergoing new construction, it is possible to build single rooms with private baths. But for existing hospitals, this change is probably cost-prohibitive. Less expensive options that hospitals can take include upgrading food quality and selections. They can even make the schedule more flexible. What if patients could eat at their chosen time instead of on the hospital's schedule? Patients might not only be happier, they might be able to eat and sleep better as well.

To ensure consistent, high-quality service, Neeleman knew early on that JetBlue could not service a massive number of cities. Hospitals can also benefit by specializing to increase quality. Some are clearly the leaders in a specific clinical area. Examples of this specialization include the Joslin Diabetes Center affiliated with Harvard Medical School and Memorial Sloan-Kettering Cancer Center. Most hospitals, though, try to be "all things to all patients." While it is not an easy transition, hospitals that focus on what they are the best at, and can create winning service for their patients, will most likely be the sustainable organizations for the future. Michael Porter, a business strategist from Harvard Business School, discusses healthcare strategy, and the need for hospitals to specialize, in his book *Redefining Healthcare.*[3]

What You Think Matters!

Provide positive, constructive feedback, using whatever method works best for you, to your physician, hospital, or health plan. What you think matters! Here are a few ways to give your input:

- Tell your physician during a visit
- Tell the nurse manager on your hospital unit, or ask to talk with the hospital CEO or other administrator
- Write a letter to your physician, hospital administration, or insurance plan explaining what you found to be good, as well as unpleasant, during your visit
- Fill out a patient satisfaction survey if you get one

Provide Feedback through Surveys about Your Care

New legislation requires providers to survey Medicare and Medicaid beneficiaries. Most health insurers are following suit. All patients with health insurance can expect to see surveys now or in the near future. Medicare collects and publishes survey results for three reasons:

1. To find out how patients feel about their healthcare. (Medicare wants to know how and where the healthcare system can improve.)
2. To give people information that will help them to choose their providers. (Ideally, healthcare providers who receive low ratings will see fewer patients and, eventually, either improve their quality or leave the profession.)
3. To measure quality. (Medicare will begin to reimburse healthcare providers based upon the quality of care they provide. The results of these surveys will determine, in part, whether providers receive a higher or lower payment than what they billed.)

The Consumer Assessment of Healthcare Providers and Systems (CAHPS®) program created the Medicare and Medicaid patient survey. As you read the questions, think about others you might add based on your VVMS. Some of the key questions from the survey are as follows:[4]

- How often did nurses . . .
  - Treat you respectfully and courteously?
  - Listen to you carefully?
  - Explain things in a way you could understand?
- How often did doctors . . .
  - Treat you with courtesy and respect?
  - Listen carefully to you?
  - Explain things in a way you could understand?
- Regarding the hospital environment: How often . . .
  - Were your room and bathroom kept clean?
  - Was the area around your room quiet at night?
- Regarding other concerns:
  - Was your pain controlled?

- Did the hospital staff do everything they could to help you with your pain?
- How often did hospital staff tell you what your medicines were for?
- Did hospital staff describe possible side effects in a way you could understand?
- Did you get information in writing about what symptoms or health problems to look out for after you left the hospital?
- Would you recommend this hospital to your friends and family?

OTHER WAYS TO MEASURE QUALITY

Up to this point, I have been focusing on rating quality based upon your satisfaction with the process of healthcare, the service itself: Were the doctors friendly? Was the bathroom clean? Did your doctor see you in a timely manner? All of these questions concern the *process* of healthcare. However, the *outcome* of the care you receive is another set of criteria for measuring quality.

In the airline industry, the most important outcome is getting customers to their destination on time and safely. JetBlue initially addressed the need for on-time arrivals and departures by using a direct airport-to-airport flight schedule. This strategy gave the airline more control over arrival and departure times, resulting in more on-time flights. As for safety, just before September 11, 2001, JetBlue had already installed steel, bulletproof doors in every cockpit. They were the first airline to comply with new safety regulations.

In healthcare, the outcome measure is improvement in or resolution of your condition. In some cases, where a patient has an acute condition, like pneumonia, and it resolves over a few days with intravenous antibiotics, it is easy to identify that the desired outcome was met. However, in many cases, especially when patients have chronic conditions like hypertension, heart disease, arthritis, and diabetes, it is more difficult to determine whether the desired outcome was achieved.

Some quality measures base a good outcome on whether the patient is still alive. This is the only truly objective outcome by which to measure quality. In truth, the spectrum of outcomes spans a wide range, from a minor improvement of symptoms to complete remission of a condition. To date, no totally flawless methodology for collecting and reporting this information exists. Yet another reason why your feedback about your healthcare experience is important.

Another set of quality measures focuses on how providers do their work. These measures look at the number of different physicians and places you need to go to receive care. They also include a focus on information: whether you have access to your own health information, you understand your medical records, and you have access to information about quality. As you read through the following examples of quality indicators, it may be helpful to rate how important each is to you in defining quality.[5] You may find items to add to your VVMS.

- I have one place to go for healthcare and coordinating the care I need
- All doctors I see have access to my medical records
- I can easily access the information in my medical record
- I have information about the quality of care my doctors or hospital provide
- I have information about the costs of care before I get the care
- Doctors use computerized medical records so my information is available at an appointment
- Doctors and nurses work closely as teams
- Doctors send me reminders to schedule visits for preventive care, including checkups and screening tests

The Physician's View of Quality and Healthcare

Another way to look at quality is through the eyes of the physician. Of course, because of obvious biases, avoid making this your primary way of analyzing quality in healthcare. Still, the physician's perspective is useful. According to *Physicians' Views on Quality of Care,* which reports the results of a survey conducted by The Commonwealth Fund, physicians' most common problems with quality in healthcare all involved health information and lack of coordination of care. Some of the issues identified by physicians include:[6]

- Patient's medical record, test results, or other relevant clinical information were not available at the scheduled visit
- Providers had to repeat tests or procedures because findings were unavailable or inadequate for interpretation
- Patient experienced a problem following hospital discharge because physician did not receive timely information from the hospital
- Patient care was compromised due to conflicting information from different doctors or other health professionals
- Patient had a positive test result that providers did not follow up appropriately
- Patient received the wrong drug, wrong dose, or had a preventable drug interaction

The survey also showed that physicians believe that more time with patients would improve the quality of patient care. The desire for more time with patients is not limited to physicians in the United States. In an article in the *British Medical Journal,* Ian Morrison and Richard Smith describe the phenomenon known as "hamster healthcare," which requires physicians to "spin their wheels" doing more and more with no end in site.[7] Even though the average length of an office visit is only 16 minutes in the United States, some managed care companies have set the goal for office visits at six to eight minutes. Many of the strategies to improve patient care articulated by physicians involve time, communication, and technology. The Commonwealth Fund's *Physician's Views on Quality of Care* report stated that physicians consistently believe the following six activities will improve patient care. As you read them, consider which activities would most improve the care you receive:

- Having more time to spend with patients
- Better patient access to preventive care
- Improved teamwork and communication
- More use of computer technology
- Better information on best physician specialists and centers
- Better treatment guidelines for common conditions

RESOURCES TO ASSESS PROVIDER QUALITY: JCAHO AND OTHERS

Hundreds of Web-based resources are available to healthcare consumers to get information about healthcare provider quality. It can be difficult to find accurate information, and the credibility of many sites is uncertain. So it is best to use sites that are from well-known organizations. The premiere accrediting body for virtually all types of healthcare organizations is the Joint Commission on Accreditation of Healthcare Organizations (JCAHO).[8] Go to the JCAHO Web site (*www.qualitycheck.org*) to find out whether a healthcare organization has JCAHO accreditation. If an organization is accredited, JCAHO indicates whether the organization has received its "gold seal of approval." Additional ratings for services or certain conditions are also available on the site. In general, avoid treatment from providers unless JCAHO has accredited them. Once you determine JCAHO has accredited a particular organization, then use other Web-based rating tools to refine or validate your selections.

When I chose the quality ratings websites for this chapter, I used the following criteria: (1) credibility, usefulness, and meaningfulness of the information, (2) user-friendliness, (3) level of innovative, reliable information, and (4) frequency of use by healthcare consumers. When you rate a new physician or hospital, record the physician or hospital ratings from all Web sites you consult for comparison. If the healthcare provider does not fare well on at least three of the sites, do not use the provider. Continue your search.

Centers for Medicare and Medicaid Services (CMS)

www.hospitalcompare.hhs.gov

Because the Centers for Medicare and Medicaid Services (CMS) measures come from the federal government, they are the gold standard in quality measures.[9] Medicare quality measures are process measures. They measure specific treatments that patients receive for certain diagnoses or symptoms. Both the government and the private healthcare industry consider these treatments to be the best practice. They are likely to result in the best patient outcomes.

The graphs on the Medicare Web site show how well a hospital meets Medicare criteria for a particular diagnosis. (See figure 10.3 for a sample.) In general, avoid using any hospital rated below the top 10 percentile for each measure.

Figure 10.3 Heart Attack Patients Given Aspirin at Arrival (2007)

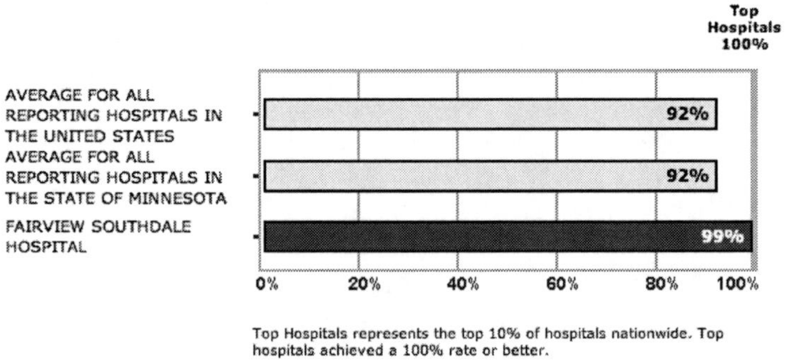

CMS recommends that hospital staff give aspirin to heart attack patients when they arrive at the hospital. The sample graph in figure 10.3 shows that Fairview Southdale Hospital meets the recommended procedure of giving aspirin to heart attack patients at arrival 99 percent of the time. The standards against which the hospital is measured are nationwide (92 percent) and statewide (92 percent).

The top 10 percent of providers meet this standard 100 percent of the time.

This is only one of many measures that organizations use regarding care and treatment in U.S. hospitals. Healthcare rating Web sites derive the information from patients' documented medical records. Without this documentation, it would be impossible to evaluate the quality of healthcare services or help you to make well-informed decisions about where you receive care.

U.S. News & World Report's Best Hospitals

health.usnews.com/sections/health/best-hospitals

Each year, *U.S. News & World Report* publishes America's Best Hospitals.[10] The *U.S. News* approach is a little different from most other quality ratings. It rates hospitals based on 16 different specialties. Most other organizations use diseases, conditions, or surgery as their level of analysis. *U.S. News* uses rigorous criteria for ratings, a three-tiered system that considers a hospital's mortality rates, reputation, and quality indicators. The quality indicators include patient volume, relative availability of nurses, advanced technology, and professional credentialing.

The 16 different specialties that the publication rates include: cancer; digestive disorders; ear, nose, and throat; endocrinology; geriatrics; gynecology; heart and heart surgery; kidney disease; neurology and neurosurgery; orthopedics; pediatrics; respiratory disorders; ophthalmology; psychiatry; rehabilitation; and rheumatology. *U.S. News* generates a list of the top 50 to 100 hospitals nationwide in each of these categories, without regard to the type or size of hospital.

The most impressive list generated from the analysis is the "honor roll," consisting of those hospitals that rank in the top tier for at least six of the 16 specialties. In 2007, of the 5,462 hospitals *U.S. News* analyzed through the *U.S. News* criteria, only 18 made the cut for the honor roll list. Johns Hopkins Hospital has topped the "Honor Roll" list for the past seven years. Other hospitals commonly on the honor roll include Mayo Clinic and Cleveland Clinic. The complete list of honor roll hospitals, along with the top 50 hospitals for each specialty area, are listed each year on the *U.S. News* Web site.

The Leapfrog Group

www.leapfroggroup.org

The Leapfrog Group describes itself as:

. . . a voluntary program created to help save lives and reduce preventable medical mistakes by mobilizing employer purchasing power to initiate breakthrough improvements in the safety of healthcare and by giving consumers information to make more informed hospital choices.

The Business Roundtable, a national association of Fortune 500 CEOs, founded The Leapfrog Group. It is a consortium of major companies and other large private and public healthcare purchasers. The group developed criteria for quality based on scientific evidence, endorsed by the National Quality Forum.[11]

Figure 10.4 shows a sample table that lists all hospitals in a specific geographic region. Among other things, the group rates each hospital on the use of computerized physician order entry (CPOE) and employment of intensive care specialists in the intensive care unit (ICU). Studies show that when hospitals use these types of practices, the result is better patient outcomes. The table also compares the treatment protocols for several high-risk treatments to whether the hospitals adhere to safe practices. (See *www.leapfroggroup.org/cp* for a quick link to your hospital search.) Using the table, you can quickly scan several hospital ratings and determine, based upon the amount of shading in each circle, which hospital fares the best—the greater number and greater percentage of shading in the circles, the higher the rating for the hospital. The comparison in figure 10.4 indicates the hospital to pick is Lehigh Valley Hospital in Allentown, PA.

Figure 10.4 Sample: A Leapfrog Comparison (2007)

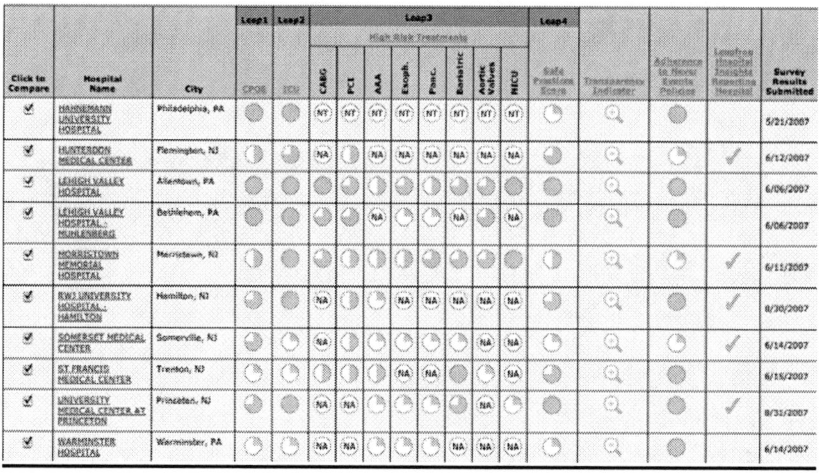

HealthGrades

www.healthgrades.com

HealthGrades estimates that three million individuals research hospitals, doctors, and nursing homes each month on its Web site. This consumer-focused site rates the quality of care at nearly every hospital in the country for 32 different procedures, a process that involves the analysis of 40 million records. The site also contains cost information on procedures to help consumers make sound decisions.

HealthGrades compares hospitals in the same geographic region, using a five-star system. (See figure 10.5 for an example.) It bases its ratings on outcomes: whether the patient had any complications while hospitalized and whether the hospital discharged the patient. One star means the hospital is below expected measures, three stars means the hospital measures are as expected, and five stars means the hospital measures are better than expected. In figure 10.5 you can see that the two hospitals with the highest ratings are hospitals that specialize in orthopedic procedures.

Figure 10.5 2007 HealthGrades Ratings of Hospitals' Performance of Total Knee Replacement (Using Data from 2003–2005)[12]

★★★★★ Best ★★★ As Expected ★ Poor

Current Ratings	Previous Ratings	America's 50 Best Hospitals	Clinical Excellence-DHA	Patient Safety-DHA	Specialty Excellence	Quality Reports

Hospital's Name	Major Complications
✚ = view details	2007 Ratings **Total Knee Replacement**
High Volume Hospitals	
✚ Hospital For Joint Diseases Orthopaedic Institute New York, NY	★★★★★
✚ Hospital For Special Surgery New York, NY	★★★★★
✚ Beth Israel Medical Center* New York, NY	★★★
✚ Cabrini Medical Center New York, NY	★★★
✚ Lenox Hill Hospital New York, NY	★★★
✚ Mount Sinai Hospital New York, NY	★★★
✚ St Luke's Roosevelt Hospital New York, NY	★★★
✚ New York Presbyterian-Columbia* New York, NY	★
✚ New York-Presbyterian/Weill Cornell* New York, NY	★

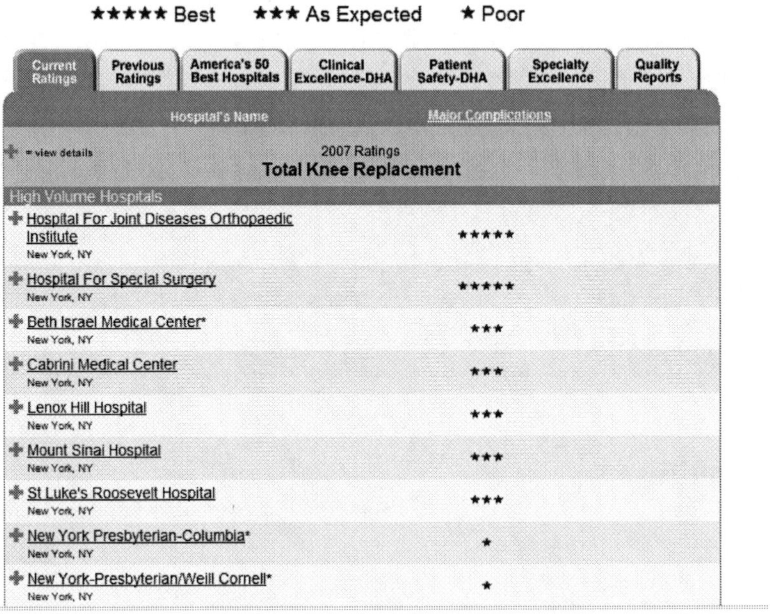

Vimo

www.vimo.com

Vimo provides resources that allow you to take charge of your healthcare spending. It compares pricing information for every procedure by the hospital.[13] Since most pricing information is not shared openly by the provider with patients, this is a novel idea in healthcare. As we begin to assume more of a burden for increased deductibles and hospital and doctor fees, cost will become an even more important component of quality.

An innovator in the field, Vimo shows consumers exactly what each hospital charges for a particular surgery. It also identifies how often a hospital performs a certain surgery compared to the hospital that does this type of surgery the most in the nation. The more often a surgery is performed, the greater the likelihood of a successful outcome.[14]

The pricing information includes a list price as well as a negotiated price for each surgery. The negotiated price is what insurance companies pay. In some cases, the insurance company pays as little as 30 percent of the provider's charge. The norm is about 50 to 60 percent. Vimo provides national averages and information for individual hospitals. In the example in figure 10.6 from the Vimo Web site, a knee replacement search shows information for all hospitals, for the hospital that charges the least, and for the hospital that performs the surgery the most.

Figure 10.6 Vimo Report on Knee Replacement (2007)

National Statistics for Knee Replacement

Number of cases for this procedure group:	485,849
Number of hospitals reporting cases for this procedure group:	3,527
Average list price for this procedure group:	$41,400
Average negotiated price:	$13,000
Average length of stay:	5 days

Least Expensive Hospital in America for Knee Replacement

Hospital Metropolitan Tito Mattei Street 128 Km 1.0 Yauco, Puerto Rico 698

Cases per year:	30
List price	$4,400
Negotiated price:	$4,400

Hospital Where Knee Replacement Is Most Commonly Performed
Hospital for Special Surgery 535 East 70th Street New York, NY 10021

Cases per year:	2742
List price	$49,800
Negotiated price:	$22,000

The Commonwealth Fund

www.cmwf.org

The Commonwealth Fund is a private foundation that promotes better access, improved quality, and greater efficiency in healthcare, particularly for society's most vulnerable people. Results of *all* of The Commonwealth-funded studies are available to consumers free of charge. The surveys and publications produced from this organization every year are too numerous to count.

The Commonwealth Fund defines quality as care that is: (1) right or correct care for the patient's condition, (2) coordinated across providers, and (3) patient-centered. In its 2007 study on quality of care, *Aiming Higher: Results from a State Scorecard on Health System Performance,* the Fund rated healthcare quality by state.[15] Based on its criteria, The Commonwealth Fund identified the following as the top 15 states, in order, for healthcare quality: Rhode Island, Maine, Massachusetts, Connecticut, Iowa, New Hampshire, Vermont, Wisconsin, Nebraska, South Dakota, Michigan, Minnesota, Montana, Pennsylvania, and Delaware. And the Fund rated the following as the bottom 15 states: Georgia, Kentucky, Idaho, Arkansas, New Mexico, Louisiana, Oklahoma, Mississippi, Florida, Texas, Arizona, Utah, Alaska, California, and Nevada.

RESOURCES TO ASSESS THE QUALITY OF HEALTH PLANS

When provided with any additional information, almost two-thirds of healthcare consumers change their minds about health insurance choices.[16] In fact, the more information healthcare consumers review, the more likely they are to change what is important to them. In addition, the more experience people have with the healthcare system, the more qualities they identify as important. For these reasons, it is important for you to be as familiar with health plan information as possible.

Quality Reports on Health Plans, Generally: CAHPS®

Consumer Assessment of Healthcare Providers and Systems (CAHPS®) has the most comprehensive reporting system available for informing the public of health plan quality. (See its Web site at *www.cahps.ahrq.gov.*) The quality ratings include all categories of health plans: private, Medicare, and Medicaid. CAHPS® collects the data from healthcare consumers directly. The 2006 report collected data in 2004 and 2005 from 126,985 respondents for commercial health plans, 93,379 respondents for Medicaid programs, and 97,955 respondents for Medicare.[17] (See figure 10.7.)

While the data is helpful and interesting, it is also limited. The biggest pitfall is that the survey is not specific by plan. It groups all commercial insurers together. Likewise, even though each state administers Medicaid, CAHPS® provides only overall results. And although Medicare recipients may receive health plan administration through one of several managed care plans or fee-for-service plans, CAHPS® also groups all Medicare results together. The reason for grouping the data together is that the number of respondents in any one plan is too small to be of any significance.

CAHPS® survey responses are shown below. Time is a common concern for patients in all types of plans. The survey shows significant problems in the areas of delay in seeing a physician, time spent with physicians, and getting care quickly. When comparing overall ratings for plans, primary care physicians, and specialists, for private insurers and Medicaid recipients, the rating of a 9 or 10 only occurred about 55 percent of the time, but was 69 percent for Medicare.

Figure 10.7 2006 CAHPS® Survey Responses

Question	Best Rating	Medicare (%)	Medicaid (%)	Commercial Insurer(%)
Getting needed care	Not a problem	84	67	76
Delays in care waiting for health plan approval	Not a problem	80	57	68
Getting care quickly	Always	58	45	46
How often were you taken to the exam room within 15 minutes of your appointment?	Always	28	21	20
Doctors communicate well	Always	69	62	61
Doctor spent enough time	Always	62	54	52
Courteous and helpful office staff	Always	79	67	66
Customer service	Not a problem	65	69	64
How much of a problem was it to find health plan information?	Not a problem	55	69	56
How much of a problem was it to find help by calling the health plan?	Not a problem	65	65	65
How much of a problem did you have with paperwork from the health plan?	Not a problem	75	72	72
Overall rating of primary care physician	9 or 10	68	59	54
Overall rating of specialists	9 or 10	68	59	58
Overall rating of health plan	9 or 10	69	55	55

National Committee on Quality Assurance (NCQA)

The National Committee on Quality Assurance (NCQA) is a nonprofit organization that has been dedicated to improving healthcare quality since 1990. NCQA's Web site states:[18]

Every year for the past five years, these [health plan] numbers [of clinical quality] have improved; healthcare protocols have been refined, doctors have learned new ways to practice, and patients have become more engaged in their care. Those improvements in quality care translate into lives saved, illnesses avoided and costs reduced.

This is just one example of NCQA's laser-sharp focus on accrediting health plans. On the Web site, under the "report cards" tab, you can search to see how your health plan compares with others. If NCQA does not accredit your plan, find out why. Most credible, quality plans with an HMO, PPO, or POS offering, participate in the NCQA process. Accredited health plans must comply with more than 60 standards and report their performance in more than 40 areas to earn NCQA accreditation.

NCQA derives its criteria from the Healthcare Effectiveness Data and Information Set (HEDIS) measures. More than 90 percent of U.S. health plans use HEDIS to measure performance. Using HEDIS allows NCQA to compare quality across all health plans. HEDIS measures important diagnostic information including:

- Asthma medication use
- Continued beta-blocker treatment after a heart attack
- Controlling high blood pressure
- Comprehensive diabetes care
- Breast cancer screening
- Antidepressant medication management
- Childhood and adolescent immunization status
- Advising smokers to quit

NCQA assesses each plan on five specific areas: access and service, qualified providers, staying healthy, living with illness, and overall accreditation. As with CAHPS®, the plan assessment is also connected into the providers of care. The reason for including information about physicians on the NCQA assessment is that there is really no way for you to assess whether you feel you are improving without including the provider in the equation. Once you get to the Report Cards home page (from *www.ncqa.org*), you enter the state and type of health plan you are interested in reviewing. A report similar to the one in figure 10.8 will be returned to you. For accredited health plans, each category is rated anywhere from one to four stars. One star = provisional accreditation, 2 stars = accredited, 3 stars = commendable, and 4 stars = excellent.

Figure 10.8 Sample: NCQA Report

Plan	Access & Service	Qualified Providers	Staying Healthy	Getting Better	Living with Illness	Overall Accreditation	Quality Plus Distinction
Aetna Health Inc. (Ohio)	★★★★	★★★★	★★★★	★★★★	★★★★	EXCELLENT	
Anthem Health Plans Kentucky, Inc.	★★★★	★★★★	★★★★	★★★★	★★★★	EXCELLENT	
CIGNA HealthCare of Ohio, Inc.	★★★★	★★★★	★★★	★★★	★★★★	EXCELLENT	

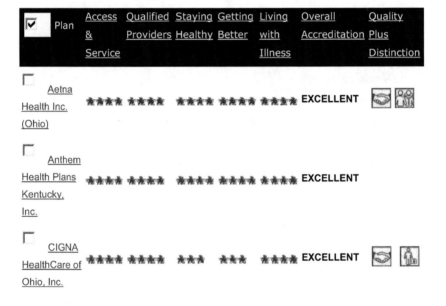

Quality Reports on Specific Health Insurers: *U.S. News* Best Health Plans

Each year, *U.S. News & World Report,* in collaboration with NCQA, publishes the Best Health Plans. The list recognizes the top ten commercial and top five Medicare and Medicaid plans in the United

States. On its Web site, *U.S. News* states that, "Picking the right health plan is like looking at houses whose windows are blackened and whose doors lack knobs: you can't tell what they're like inside."

In 2006, NCQA examined 684 plans for the Best Health Plans list. (See *www.health.usnews.com/healthplans.*)[19] Plans that commonly top the honor roll include Harvard Pilgrim Care, Tufts Associated HMOs, and Blue Cross and Blue Shield of Massachusetts. In addition, there were 158 plans that did not report data and, therefore, NCQA could not rate them. They are listed on the *U.S. News* Web site after the ranked health plans. If your plan is one that did not report data, ask the plan administrator why.

Key Highlights

There are multiple ways of defining healthcare quality. It is important to define quality care for yourself before you use the many resources available to evaluate healthcare services and plans. Defining quality care for yourself allows you to follow your own values when choosing your resources. Once you determine what you value most in your healthcare experience, think about how your provider and health plan meet those values, and how you can measure whether they continue to meet your requirements. Many resources are available to check the quality of providers and health plans in your area.

Key Actions

- Define what quality healthcare is to you, using your values from chapter 1.
- Think about how your providers and health plan can meet your expectations for quality.
- Identify how you can measure whether your provider and health plan meet your expectations.
- Communicate with your physician and other providers about your expectations.
- Give providers and health plans feedback about their services.

- Check quality resources to determine whether a current or prospective healthcare provider or health plan meets quality standards.

Key Take-Away

Give your healthcare providers feedback about their care and use your quality rating resources to guide your decisions.

Endnotes

---

[1] Blanchard, Kenneth, Hershey, Paul, Johnson, Dewey, (2007) Management of Organizational Behavior: Utilizing Human Resources, Prentice Hall, New York

[2] Wynbrandt, James, (2006) Flying High: How JetBlue Founder and CEO David Neeleman Beats the Competition... Even in the World's Most Turbulent Industry. James Wiley and Son Publishers.

[3] Porter, Michael E. and Olmstead Teisberg, Elizabeth. *Redefining Healthcare: Creating Value-Based Competition on Results.* Harvard Business School Publishing, 2006.

[4] Consumer Assessment of Healthcare Providers and Systems (CAHPS®) Hospital Survey (*www.cahps.ahrq.gov*).

[5] Harris Interactive, Inc. *Commonwealth Fund Survey of Public Views of the U.S. Healthcare System, 2006.*

[6] Audet, A.J.; Doty, M.M.; Shamasdin, J.; and Schoenbaum, S.C. Physicians' Views on Quality of Care: Findings from the Commonwealth Fund National Survey of Physicians and Quality of Care. The Commonwealth Fund, May 2005.

[7] Morrison, Ian, and Smith, Richard. "Hamster healthcare," *British Medical Journal.* 321 (December 2000): 1541–2.

[8] Joint Commission on Accreditation of Healthcare Organizations, *www.jcaho.org.* JCAHO Web site (*www.qualitycheck.org*)

[9] Centers for Medicare and Medicaid Services, *www.hospitalcompare.hhs.gov*

[10] U.S. News & World Report America's Best Hospitals, *www.usnews.com.*

[11] The National Quality Forum (NQF) is a not-for-profit membership organization created to develop and implement a national strategy for health care quality measurement and reporting. For more information, go to *www.qualityforum.org.*

[12] HealthGrades' data source is the Centers for Medicare and Medicaid Services. The data is from the years 2003–2005. Web site image is used with permission from HealthGrades.

[13] Vimo www.vimo.com.

[14] The Commonwealth Fund. Harris Interactive Harvard 2000 "International Health Policy Survey of Physicians." New York.

[15] Cantor, J.C.; Schoen, C.; Belloff, D.; How, S. K. H.; and McCarthy, D. *Aiming Higher: Results from a State Scorecard on Health System Performance.* The Commonwealth Fund Commission on a High Performance Health System, June 2007.

[16] Lubalin, James S.; and Harris-Kojetin, Lauren. "What Do Consumers Want and Need to Know in Making Healthcare Choices?" *Medical Care Research and Review.* 56, no. 1 (1999): 67-102.
[17] National CAHPS® Benchmarking Database. *2006 CAHPS® Health Plan Survey Chartbook.* U.S. Agency for Healthcare Research and Quality, September 2006.
[18] National Committee on Quality Assurance, *www.ncqa.org*. Web site image used with permission from NCQAA.
[19] NCQA *www.health.usnews.com/healthplans.*

CHAPTER

11

Impacting Healthcare Quality: Medical Research and the Medicalization of Life

The needs of society determine its ethics. —Maya Angelou

"We painted estrogen on the brains of monkeys and watched them have seizures," Dr. Herzog explained to us during our first visit with him about Emmalea's epilepsy. I watched Emmalea's eyes widen in shock at this idea. Dr. Herzog's ground-breaking research found a link between estrogen (which provokes seizures) and progesterone (which inhibits seizures) and seizure activity.

Medical researchers must constantly ensure their work is ethical. The research Dr. Herzog described to us used animals, not humans. Animal research has its own set of issues. Dr. Herzog's treatment for Emmalea, based on his research, involves rubbing natural progesterone cream (made from wild yams) on her skin for eight days of each month. In our case, we are thankful for those monkeys who gave their time, and possibly even their lives, to provide a new and effective treatment for women who have seizure disorders.

Medical ethics are important, attention-getting, and in some cases, urgent issues. In this chapter, I focus specifically on three medical ethics topics and how they affect healthcare quality. I address the overall importance of medical research, the difference between medical research and the practice of medicine, and the "medicalization of life."Medical research is used to identify methods for improving outcomes in healthcare. When we improve outcomes, we improve quality. Therefore, medical research results in improvement of healthcare quality. Dr. Herzog's work in seizure control is a good example of a direct link between research and improved patient quality of life.

The difference between what qualifies as *research* and what qualifies as the *practice* of medicine is not always easy to discern. Information on this topic may help you appreciate your rights if you ever have the option to participate in a medical research study. It is important to understand if your treatment is, in fact, considered to be research. If it is, you have many protections as a study participant. You also will likely not have to pay for the care you receive as part of the research study. In some cases, you may even be paid for your participation.

The medicalization of life is society's growing trend to classify more and more of *life* problems as *medical* problems. For example, there are some claims of an increasing trend to medicate undesired personality traits, as opposed to accepting these differences as normal variations. Depending on how you define quality in healthcare, you may want to decrease or increase medicalization as it applies to you.

The President's Council on Bioethics agenda provides good examples of current medical research and medicalization issues. Even pop culture addresses some of the more interesting research topics on the agenda such as memory boosting and suppression (the topic of the movie *Eternal Sunshine of the Spotless Mind*) and life extension (the topic of the movie *Cocoon*). Some examples of medical research on the agenda are cloning and genetics. An example of medicalization on the agenda is the use of mood control drugs in adults. For a complete list of the agenda items, see *www.bioethics.gov*.[1]

MEDICAL RESEARCH: PATIENT BENEFITS AND PROTECTIONS

Medical research is highly regulated today. However, this was not always the case. Beginning in the early 1930s, a group of approximately 400 illiterate African-American sharecroppers who were infected with syphilis participated in a study. The research was conducted through the public health system in Tuskegee, Alabama without obtaining these men's informed consent. As an incentive to participate, researchers offered these workers various amenities, such as meals, free medical treatment, and burial insurance. In 1972, the truth about the Tuskegee Study was revealed to the public.[2]

Although penicillin had become the standard treatment for syphilis, the study officials denied penicillin to some participants to observe the effects of the advanced stages of syphilis on the human body. This dehumanizing experiment resulted in a series of hearings and regulations, and, eventually, the creation of the National Commission for the Protection of Human Subjects in Research. The commission continuously reviews and updates the guidelines, which research organizations in the United States today follow closely.

The Relevance of the Nuremberg Code

In 1946 the Nuremberg trials first addressed issues of voluntary and informed consent in medical research, when 23 Nazi physicians were tried for crimes committed against prisoners of war. These crimes included exposure of humans to temperature extremes, mutilating surgery, and deliberate infection with a variety of lethal pathogens.[3] One of the outcomes of the trials was the Nuremberg Code, a set of principles that address the rights of a human as the subject of research. The code also addresses the qualifications required of researchers and the standards researchers must observe. The following is a summary of the Nuremberg Code principles for human experimentation:[4]

1. The voluntary consent of the human subject in medical experiments is essential
2. The duty and responsibility for consent rests with the researcher
3. The experiment should yield results for the good of society
4. The experiment should be based on the results of animal experimentation
5. The experiment should be conducted to avoid all unnecessary physical and mental suffering and injury

6. Proper preparations should protect the experimental subject against even remote possibilities of injury, disability, or death
7. Only scientifically qualified persons should conduct the experiment
8. The human subject should be at liberty to end the experiment
9. The scientist in charge must be prepared to terminate the experiment at any stage, if continuing the experiment is likely to result in injury, disability, or death to the experimental subject

Is It Medical Research or Is It Treatment?

In 2006, the Hospital of the University of Pennsylvania (HUP) granted me permission to conduct my doctoral dissertation research with the hospital's internal medicine residents. Carried out with Ian Diener, MD, the research did not involve patient treatment, but rather residents' education. But because human beings were involved in the research, we had to obtain approval from the university's Institutional Review Board (IRB). As part of the approval process, the IRB required that Dr. Diener and I take the university's research ethics course.

The research ethics course was a Web-based set of eight modules. Each addressed a different issue related to possible ethical violations in healthcare research. Some of the hypothetical scenarios required us to identify the difference between patients who formally enroll as participants in a research study versus those who receive a new treatment approach to a particular condition. In one hypothetical case example, a physician treated a patient for a chronic cardiac condition, with little to no improvement over several years. The physician found much literature showing possible advantages of varying both drug dosage amounts and frequency for the patient's chronic cardiac condition. In addition, the literature addressed adding certain vitamin and mineral supplements. Here, the physician was considering two possible techniques: changing the dose and frequency of the drug, and adding nutritional supplements.

In terms of the ethics course, the question was whether to consider this treatment experimental, thus deeming it a form of research. If yes, then the physician would need to inform the patient that this was experimental treatment and research, and the physician would need to go through the IRB just as he would with any other research study. If no, then the physician could go ahead and treat the patient as he would in the normal course of care.

The ethical dilemma here is clear. Let's assume the physician is certain that this new approach will help to improve his patient's chronic condition. He has watched her suffer for over a decade and now has a solution that could, at the very least, improve her quality of life. Such a decision is difficult for physicians to make unless they have clear guidelines on how to determine whether a treatment is experimental in nature or not.

On one hand, the physician believes that the patient can only improve with this new approach. On the other hand, deviation in medical research criteria can become a slippery slope, and potentially, lead to another Tuskegee disaster. In this case, the answer to the question was within the physician's clinical judgment. It was his choice whether to modify the current dose and frequency of the drug and use mineral supplements. He could proceed with the treatment as long as he obtained valid informed consent from the patient. Life decisions, however, are not always as easy to answer as the hypothetical questions presented in a classroom exercise.

Why Nuremberg Was Not Enough: More on the Difference Between Research and Treatment

In the 1960s, newspapers reported stories of researchers in New York injecting elderly, indigent people with live cancer cells, without their consent, to learn more about the human immune system. As a result, a Harvard University physician created a lengthy report that shocked Americans more. The report publicized the fact that such questionable practices were happening in many of America's premier research institutions.[5]

Consequently, the World Medical Association created necessary guidelines that were broader in scope than the Nuremberg

Code. These guidelines, called the *Declaration of Helsinki*, focus on the difference between treatment and research, especially for physicians who are conducting research *and* treating patients. Sometimes the line can blur, and the declaration seeks to provide some clear guidance for physicians. These more specific regulations have created a more ethical environment in medical research. Some key provisions from the Declaration of Helsinki are the following: [6]

- Some research populations are vulnerable and need special protection. The particular needs of the economically and medically disadvantaged must be recognized.
- Special attention is also required for those for whom the research is combined with care.
- When obtaining informed consent for the research project, the physician should be particularly cautious if the subject is in a *dependent relationship* with the physician or may consent under duress. In that case, a well-informed physician who is not engaged in the investigation and who is independent of the relationship should obtain the informed consent.
- The physician may combine medical research with medical care, only to the extent that the research is justified by its potential prophylactic, diagnostic, or therapeutic value. When medical research is combined with medical care, additional standards apply to protect the patients who are research subjects.

Another provision of the Declaration of Helsinki guides physicians who, like the example in the research ethics course I took, seek to treat a patient with a condition that has no effective treatment. This provision defers to the physician's judgment as long as the physician obtains informed consent from the patient. The relevant sections state:[7]

- In treating a patient, where proven prophylactic, diagnostic, and therapeutic methods do not exist or have been ineffective, the physician, with informed consent from the patient, must be free to use unproven or new prophylactic, diagnostic, and therapeutic measures, if in the physician's judgment it offers hope of saving life, re-establishing health, or alleviating suffering.

- Where possible, these measures should be made the object of research, designed to evaluate their safety and efficacy. In all cases, new information should be recorded and, where appropriate, published.

Being part of a research study is a clearly defined situation. Treatment by your physician with a new technique that, in his judgment, is likely to provide an improved result is less clear. Even if your treatment classifies as medical practice as opposed to an experimental treatment defined as part of a research study, it is still your responsibility to be aware of your rights as a patient. Namely, you need to be aware of your right to provide informed consent before you agree to such treatment. The lack of distinction between research and treatment is partly because they often occur together. In addition, departures from standard treatment practices are often called *experimental*, but the terms *experimental* and *research* are not carefully defined. Other considerations in determining the difference between research and medical practice also merit examination. (See figure 11.1.)

Figure 11.1 Additional Considerations in Determining the Difference Between Research and Medical Practice[8]

Concept	Practice of Medicine	Research
Who is involved?	Individual patient	Groups of participants
What is being done?	Enhancing the well-being of the patient	Testing a research hypothesis
What is the outcome?	Reasonable expectation of success	Unknown until the research is complete
What is the purpose?	To provide diagnosis, treatment, or therapy to the patient	To contribute knowledge about the condition being studied

Informed Consent for Research

Providers must follow specific requirements of informed consent for research purposes. (Chapter 9 covers informed consent for general treatment purposes.) There is widespread agreement that informed consent for research must contain three basic elements: (1) the physician researcher must provide information to the patient, (2) the patient participant must understand the information, and (3) the patient must voluntarily participate in the study.

There are several additional guidelines for obtaining informed consent for research purposes. These include:

1. The consent must contain a statement that the participant can ask questions and withdraw from the experiment at any time.
2. The researcher must reveal information about the study that "a reasonable volunteer" would wish to know to make a decision.
3. A special problem arises when informing participants of some aspect of the research that may affect the validity of the study. Here, it is sufficient to let the participant know that some features of the research will not be revealed until the research is over.
4. Researchers must present information to participants in an organized manner, giving participants sufficient time to review and consider all of the issues.
5. Researchers must present information using language participants can understand. Researchers cannot offer participants excessive or improper "rewards," as this would influence participants' ability to participate voluntarily.
6. Researchers in a position of authority, or who have commanding influence, over a potential participant should not ask the person to be in a study. This also can influence their ability to participate voluntarily. This can apply to patients asked by their regular doctor to participate in one of her studies. In these cases, outside physicians should be asked to obtain informed consent from the patient-participants.

The physician in charge of a research study is known as a principle investigator (PI). If you have the option of participating in a research study, it is the PI's responsibility to inform you of the risks, benefits, and other details. However, it is also your responsibility to understand the risks and benefits of participating in any research. Ask if there is a control group in the study. Participants in the experimental group receive the treatment that the study is testing. Participants in the control group do not receive the treatment that the study is testing. Instead, control group members receive a placebo.

A control group is a necessary part of almost any scientifically valid study. Because random assignment is also part of a scientifically valid study, you can not ask to be assigned to a specific group. However, if there is a control group, you can ask the PI if, after the study is concluded you can be informed as to whether you were in the control or treatment group. Furthermore, if you were assigned to the control group and the research proved successful, you will want to ask if you can receive the treatment free of charge for the same length of time of the study. According to informed consent guidelines, the PI should reveal all information about the study that a "reasonable volunteer" would want to know to make a decision. The control group inquiry is a reasonable question for you to ask. In addition, the guidelines state that problems could arise when informing participants of some aspect of the research that may affect the validity of the study. In these cases, the PI can let you know that some features of the research will not be revealed until the research is over. Here is your opportunity to inquire as to any post-study benefits you can receive if, in fact, you were assigned to the control group.

Control group dilemmas can occur in any experiment. I faced an ethical dilemma in the research study I conducted with the internal medicine residents at the University of Pennsylvania Hospital. I was specifically testing the impact that different educational training programs have on the quality of the residents' documentation in patient medical records. The study design called for dividing the 90 medicine residents who participated in the program into three groups. Two groups participated in different training programs and received feedback and practice to improve their documentation. One group, the control group, received no training. It was necessary for some of the residents to have no training so I could analyze if there was a difference between some intervention and no intervention.

However, as an educator, I could not justify only providing training to two-thirds of the residents. With the assistance of Barry Fuchs, MD, the PI from the University of Pennsylvania, I designed the study so that once we completed the training and data collection, I provided the same education to the residents in the control group. I walked away from the research with a clear conscience. I had done the right thing. It may not always be this easy. But, as a possible study participant, knowing what the parameters are and what decisions you have the right to make can help you better navigate through the research process.

THE MEDICALIZATION OF LIFE

The phrase, *medicalization of life* refers to "society's growing trend to classify more and more *life* problems as *medical* problems" and treating those problems with pharmaceutical or surgical intervention.[9] There is a spectrum of medicalization issues that includes those a physician may treat with prescription medication and surgery to those that are cosmetic in nature. Many advertisements describe how to treat problems like restless leg syndrome, sexual dysfunction, and insomnia with a prescription drug and physician visit. These are examples of the medicalization of life today that 20 years ago we did not even have a medical diagnosis for. At the extreme, medicalization involves treating natural life consequences, such as minor body image issues, being slightly overweight, or experiencing hair loss as diseases that must be eradicated.[10]

Medicalization involves asking questions, such as:

- When does a deviation from normal need medical intervention?

- Does every episode of depression or attention deficit require a medical intervention?
- What are appropriate alternative treatments?

On one end of the medicalization spectrum, an individual may be experiencing anxiety or depression. To the extent that any condition interferes with a person's ability to function effectively on a day-to-day basis, it is important to treat it. Physicians have professional judgment parameters in applying clinical criteria. If you choose to seek medical intervention for such a condition, your physician may recommend treatment with prescription drugs. You make the decision.

At the other end of the medicalization spectrum are conditions like wrinkles, hair loss or yellow, crooked teeth. If you have any of these conditions, you need to discern for yourself whether you need, want, or can afford medical or surgical intervention for problems like these. Whether you choose to seek medical intervention for a natural consequence of living may not be as important as how you do it. We count on our physicians to act ethically and in our best interests when making decision about when and if to treat a symptom, a condition or a "common life consequence." It is also your responsibility to use your VVMS to drive your decisions.[11]

In his book, *Listening to Prozac: A Psychiatrist Explores Antidepressant Drugs and the Remaking of the Self,* Peter Kramer, MD, refers to one component of the "medicalization" of mental health as "cosmetic psychopharmacology." In particular, he addresses the ability of Prozac to alter patients' personalities. Even when a patient is no longer depressed, he could use Prozac to sustain the personality change. Dr. Kramer describes the phenomenon as patients becoming "better than well. . . . patients acquiring extra energy and becoming socially attractive, through the continued use of Prozac when they may no longer have needed it to treat depression."[12]

Medicalization speaks to an issue of fear—fear that society continues to "lower the bar" in defining what is a disease in need of medical treatment. The following are some common conditions that may be life consequences and may receive treatment as medical diagnoses:

- Menopause
- Mood disorder
- Dyslexia
- Attention deficit hyperactivity disorder (ADHD)
- Hair loss
- Insomnia
- Obesity
- Restless leg syndrome
- Acne
- Sleep disorder
- Wrinkles
- Depression
- Yellow teeth
- Anxiety
- Headaches
- Sexual dysfunction
- Everyday unhappiness

Medical Ethics and Pharmaceutical Companies

Medicalization has grown partly because of changes in the way pharmaceutical companies interact with patients. Prior to the mid-1990s, pharmaceutical companies interacted with patients only indirectly, through patients' physicians. Today, we are all flooded with information about new treatments for existing conditions, as well as conditions we never considered treating before.

On the positive side, ads provide information that may help us become better-informed consumers. On the negative side, some of the ads extend the definition of *sick*. Therefore, it is important to view ads with a critical eye, keeping in mind your personal VVMS. If you follow your core values and use trusted physicians who practice ethically, information overload is likely to be more manageable.

The pharmaceutical (pharma) industry interacts with both patients and healthcare providers. Pharma interacts with you through numerous clinical trial research studies. The same research regulations and laws apply to pharma firms as to academic medical centers. Because of the size of the industry, pharma firms wield enormous power. The firms are constantly looking for ways to impact the decision making of physicians. The pressure for a physician to prescribe a certain drug can be significant. This pressure can in turn, impact you.

In his book, *How Doctors Think,* Dr. Jerome Groopman describes some of the challenges his colleagues have faced when they refused to succumb to the pressures of some pharmaceutical salespeople.[13] Federal law now prohibits pharmaceutical companies from providing gifts, such as expensive trips or meals, to physicians as a sales incentive. Yet companies find ways around these laws. For example, they may classify trips as educational opportunities for doctors by arranging for guest speakers and special training events.

Direct-to-consumer marketing is another market pressure doctors face. The pharmaceutical commercials directed to you, the healthcare consumer, are generally very effective. As a result, many patients pressure physicians today to prescribe certain medications, such as Viagra, Lipitor, or Ambien. While switching a drug brand is not likely to be harmful, it is important that physicians are free to use their own judgment in sifting through all the choices they have in prescribing a drug..

Generic Versus Brand Drugs: Pros and Cons

Pharmacies regularly substitute generic forms of brand medications, unless the physician states on the prescription that the patient must use the brand drug. This is generally a good practice. At the very least, generic drugs help contain costs for everyone involved.

Using generic drugs can affect the quality of care in some cases. This came to our attention when Emmalea saw one of the neurologists at New York-Presbyterian Medical Center, Carl Bazil, who has both an MD and a PhD in pharmacology. Well-versed in FDA regulations for generic drugs, he addresses this issue in his book, *Living Well with Epilepsy and Other Seizure Disorders: An Expert Explains What You Really Need to Know.*[14]

Emmalea's Pennsylvania-based neurologist prescribed Zonegran, 100 mg per day, to control her seizures. When Dr. Bazil asked to examine the bottle, he pointed out to us that the label said *Zonisimide*, which is the generic version of Zonegran. Generic drugs, he informed us, are permitted a "20 percent deviation in strength either way." We looked at him dumbfounded until he applied his comment specifically to us. "Mrs. Russo," he said, "this means that a 100 mg capsule of Zonisimide, the generic drug, could actually contain as little as 80 mg or as much as 120 mg of the drug and still be within the FDA's criteria."

Such a difference in dose might not hamper treatment for many conditions, but for others, like epilepsy, precision in the amount of drug being released daily is key. Dr. Bazil went on to explain that the first prescription might contain 80 mg of the drug. If this did not control Emmalea's seizures, a neurologist would likely double her dosage. Depending on the pharmacy and its current vendor, the next dosage could be as high as 120 mg per pill. The likelihood was uncertain. But, it was at least theoretically possible, then, that Emmalea could go from 80 mg per day to 240 mg per day of the drug because of the dosing parameters for generic drugs. She could be tripling her dosage, even though she was only taking twice as many pills.

In a perfect world, for certain conditions *where exact precision in dosage* is even more critical, the pharmaceutical firms and pharmacies would have access to this information, and their computer systems would not allow them to fill prescriptions for specific conditions with a generic drug. Certainly, doctors have the option to indicate *no generic* on any prescription they write. In fact, even if there is no medical reason for not using a generic, you can request that your pharmacy fill the prescription with the brand drug. If you do, you will probably have to pay a higher rate for the drug. Be aware of issues that may adversely affect you and act accordingly.

Trust Yourself

You can take several actions to avoid the medicalization of your life. First, be aware of messages in the media. Do not blindly assume that a symptom you may have, which an ad presents as a condition, merits treatment with a prescription drug. Second, develop a trusting relationship with your physician, especially your primary care physician. Having the ability to discuss your questions and concerns with him will decrease the likelihood of becoming a victim of medicalization. Third, use your own logic and intuition. Ask yourself whether your quality of life will be significantly better if you take a drug, for example, to stop your leg from shaking now and then when you are falling asleep. And fourth, remember your VVMS from chapter 1. If you are deviating from those goals by pursuing treatment for a common life consequence, you may want to rethink your decision.

Key Highlights

There is a difference between medical research and medical treatment. It is your physician's responsibility to communicate the differences to you and obtain the proper consents. Medical research is a highly regulated activity that seeks (after many years of problems) to protect research participants and to determine healthcare treatment specifications. "Medicalization" is defining an increasing number of life's problems as medical problems. Use your own VVMS and input from your primary care practitioner to determine if, and when, you want to use the healthcare system to address a natural consequence of living.

Key Actions

- Understand that there is a difference between medical treatment and research.

- Approach any opportunity to participate in medical research in an informed manner.
- Use your VVMS to determine if you want to use medical care to address a natural consequence of life.

Key Take-Away

Measure the great opportunities that exist in medical research, as well as medicalization issues, against your own values statements.

Endnotes

---

[1] The President's Council on Bioethics (*www.bioethics.gov*).
[2] Centers for Disease Control and Prevention (CDC), *www.cdc.gov/tuskegee/timeline.htm.*
[3] National Institutes of Health. *Guidelines for the Conduct of Research Involving Human Subjects at the National Institutes of Health.* (2004): 15.
[4] Reprinted from *Trials of War Criminals before the Nuremberg Military Tribunals under Control Council Law.* 2, no. 10 (Washington, D.C.: U.S. Government Printing Office, 1949): 181–2.
[5] Wood, Anne; Grady, Christine; and Emanuel, Ezekiel J., MD. "The Crisis in Human Participants Research: Identifying the Problems and Proposing Solutions." Posted at *www.bioethics.gov/background/emanuelpaper.html.*
[6] World Medical Association, *www.wma.net/e/policy/b3.htm.*
[7] Ibid.
[8] National Institutes of Health, *www.nih.gov.*
[9] Smith, Richard, MD, speaking at the World Association of General Practitioners, as quoted in *Medical Post,* Toronto. 39, no. 39 (Oct. 29, 2003): 50.
[10] Menke, J.M. "The Medicalization of Health," *Dynamic Chiropractics.* 24, no. 19 (2006).
[11] Welch, Gilbert; Schwartz, Lisa; and Woloshin, Stephen. "What's making us sick is an epidemic of diagnoses," *New York Times.* January 2, 2007.
[12] Kramer, Peter D., MD. *Listening to Prozac: A Psychiatrist Explores Antidepressant Drugs and the Remaking of the Self.* Penguin Group, 1997.
[13] Groopman, Jerome, MD. *How Doctors Think.* Houghton Mifflin Company, 2007.
[14] Bazil, Carl. *Living Well with Epilepsy and Other Seizure Disorders: An Expert Explains What You Really Need to Know.* Harper Resource, 2004.

STEP

5

UNDERSTAND THE PEOPLE

CHAPTER

12

The Making of a Doctor: Understanding Physician Training May Help You Understand Your Physicians

Everyone has a doctor in him or her; we just have to help it in its work. —Hippocrates

In 1986, at about 4 p.m. on a Saturday, I arrived at the hospital to give birth to Emmalea. Joe and I had decided to use the Lamaze method of natural childbirth, and as we entered the hospital doors, we felt confident in this decision. Though I had previously requested Dr. Chaudry, my obstetrician, to write an order for anesthesia (just in case), we felt it was best to learn natural techniques for both my comfort and for the well-being of the baby. Once my labor really kicked in, though, our two Lamaze sessions went right out the window. The pain was excruciating! After what seemed like my thousandth attempt at the "hee-hee-hoo" breathing technique that we had learned to get me through contractions, I begged for drugs. Thankfully, the nursing staff quickly complied.

At 4:55 p.m., one of the nurses turned me onto my left side and within a few minutes, the epidural anesthesia was flowing. I was still lying on my left side when, 10 minutes later, I could feel more anesthesia being shot into my catheter. As the hour progressed, still lying on my left side, the pain remained. Dr. Chaudry's order allowed another dose at 7 p.m., which I promptly received. Then I heard the nurse telling the anesthesiologist that I had already received two doses, not only the initial one. Apparently, the change of shift occurred at 5 p.m., and the first anesthesiologist was probably writing his note in my record at the same time the second anesthesiologist was giving me his dose. It was not until after he gave me the anesthesia at 7 p.m. that the second anesthesiologist realized I had received an extra dose. I overheard the anesthesiologist and nurse as they agreed that the extra dose of epidural was not a big deal. *Not a big deal to them*, I thought. I was still in a massive amount of pain and wondering what the purpose of the epidural anesthesia was at this point.

Soon, the nurses announced that the baby was crowning. I had not seen Dr. Chaudry yet that day and was starting to worry that he might not be there to deliver the baby. However, just in time, Dr. Chaudry came gliding in. The next scene was like a symphony, perfectly orchestrated. Dr. Chaudry took charge of the room like the seasoned professional he was. In a matter of minutes, the baby popped out into his hands, he handed her over to the nurses for Apgar scoring, and the next thing I knew he was gone again.

The moment Dr. Chaudry left was the same moment I realized I was a mother. Emmalea Christine Russo was born on September 20, 1986, at 7:20 p.m. Just as many women say, the pain is worth it once you see your child. The only problem was I should not have experienced the kind of pain I did, especially since I received additional doses of anesthesia. Still, at that moment, it didn't matter. All I could see was my beautiful baby girl.

Several hours after the delivery, however, my left leg and foot were still numb. When I mentioned this to the floor nurse, she furrowed her brow and replied, "It almost sounds like they didn't turn you over!" *Turn me over!* "What does that mean?" I anxiously asked. She then carefully explained the process to me. Usually, she said, when an anesthesiologist administers an epidural, the nurses turn the patient onto one side so the anesthesiologist can access her spinal canal. Once the anesthesia is flowing, the team waits a little bit before turning the patient over onto her other side. This way the anesthesia makes its way to *both* sides of the body.

Hearing this explanation was a revelation. I quickly confirmed that no one had turned me over to my other side. She shook her head as she looked at me and said, "Poor thing, you must have been in a lot of pain on your right side." Now things were starting to make sense. "Don't worry," she said, patting me gently on the shoulder. "By tomorrow, you'll be fine."

Later that day, when the doctor discharged Em and me, my left leg was still numb. I assumed the situation would continue to get better over time. When the numbness continued, I called Dr. Chaudry, who again reassured me that everything would be fine. As the water ran over my face in the shower the following morning, I attempted to pick up the soap and realized I had no control of the muscles in my hand. I made my way out of the shower and when I looked in the mirror, I was horrified to see that the left side of my face was drooping, like someone who had just had a stroke. My mind raced with panic: how could I have had a stroke at my young age? Just as these thoughts entered my mind, I realized that I could not have possibly had a stroke. I was thinking clearly and was not confused. My mind flashed instantly to the epidural and I went out to tell Joe. As soon as I tried to speak, I realized that I had no control over my tongue and couldn't form words.

At the ER, after a lot of poking and prodding, the official diagnosis documented on my chart was "neurological event related to epidural anesthesia leaking into the subdural space, probably due to excessive dosage." Slowly, over the course of the next 24 hours, my normal functioning returned. However, I continued to suffer from some residuals of the epidural, like occasional numbness in my leg for years, but the symptoms were not debilitating.

I felt the anesthesiologists' care in my case was suboptimal. I imagine if we had contacted the hospital's risk management staff, they probably would have offered us a settlement. Yet here is the issue: although I had a complaint with the hospital and the anesthesiologists, I had a good relationship with my obstetrician, Dr. Chaudry, who delivered Emmalea. Even though he was not present when I received the anesthesia, legal practices would have required me to cite everyone involved in the case, including Dr. Chaudry. I was not willing to do that.

Many books and journal articles state that the best way for physicians to avoid medical malpractice claims is to develop and maintain good communications and relationships with their patients. My story with Dr. Chaudry is a good example of just this. But when, exactly, do physicians learn and develop the skills to be good communicators, necessary to be effective physicians? Undergraduate and graduate business programs have majors where students study for three to five years to perfect communication skills. Do we expect physicians to sandwich this skill in between gross pathology and human genetics? What if a physician is not a good communicator? Should she only become a type of specialist who doesn't practice direct patient contact, such as a pathologist performing autopsies or studying blood samples, or a radiologist interpreting x-rays?

THE MAKING OF A DOCTOR

After completing their bachelor's degree, physicians have at least seven more years of formal education. Four years are in medical school, and at least three in a residency program. For many physicians, residency can be five, six, or—for specialties like neurosurgery—up to nine years long. Physicians must complete all the training and education on a full-time basis. No other professional training has the time requirements of the physician. And, it is probably safe to say, there is probably no other profession with the depth and breadth of knowledge requirements either.

Who Becomes a Doctor?

Medical schools make the first cut in deciding who becomes a doctor. About 15,500 new physicians graduate from 125 medical schools and 27 osteopathic medical schools in the United States each year. Medical schools generally only accept college graduates with strong academic records (usually at least a 3.5 GPA). They are looking for people who are willing to take the time and effort to make a serious contribution.[1] That contribution can be in a volunteer program, an academic pursuit, research, or even sport. Applicants have to show that they are willing and capable of working hard enough to accomplish an important goal.

In addition to academic records and standardized test scores, medical schools also assess every applicant's personal statement. The following are brief excerpts of medical school student essays.[2] The first is from an applicant who worked on his grandfather's farm in Hungary and organized financing for the first private hospital in Estonia:

Genetics and biochemistry represent the future of medicine and the area in which someone with ambition, a desire to work for the public good, and the necessary technical background could make the most significant contribution. Motivation, independence, maturity, precisely those qualities my experiences in Eastern Europe instilled, will be essential to a fruitful career. I can imagine none potentially more fulfilling, nor a more worthy aim for my life's work, than connecting the worlds of medical science and international public health.

The second essay comes from a survivor of anorexia who became an emergency medical technician and a medical volunteer in Honduras. She was also an HIV test counselor:

I decided that I wanted to be a doctor sometime after my four months of incarceration in Columbia Presbyterian Children's Hospital in the winter of 1986–87, as I struggled with anorexia nervosa. Through the maturation process that marked my recovery, I slowly came to realize that my pediatrician had saved my life—despite my valiant efforts to the contrary. Out of our individual stubborn wills was born a kind of mutual respect, and he is one of the people who make up my small collection of heroes . . . Speaking with patients, doctors, and community members has opened my eyes to some of the difficulties involved with healthcare provision, and I hope I have given some inspiration or comfort in exchange for the knowledge I have received. I want these lessons in openness and compassion to shape my understanding of medicine and allow me to become the type of doctor I admire.

Expectations of Medical School Students

After completing a bachelor's degree, future physicians have at least seven additional years of formal education. Four of those years are in medical school. There are general standards that are required for accreditation by the Liaison Committee on Medical Education (LCME). Each medical school develops its own unique curriculum. The LCME ensures that every program meets the basic competency requirements for medical school education.[3]

Some curricula, like the following example from Johns Hopkins School of Medicine, contain more electives and one-on-one planning. Other programs limit electives and have less of an individualized approach. Most medical schools publish their curricula on their Web sites.

Instruction Leading to the MD Degree, Johns Hopkins School of Medicine

The *first year* primarily centers on normal human structure and function.[4] Required courses include:

- Molecules and Cells (integrated coverage of biochemistry, cell biology, genetics, cell physiology)
- Anatomy
- Immunology
- Neuroscience
- Introduction to Behavioral Science
- Epidemiology
- Organ Systems

Principles of developmental biology are incorporated into the anatomy, neuroscience, and organ systems courses. The year also includes a course, *Patient, Physician, and Society*, involving ethics, history of medicine, cultural arts, physician-patient relationships, and the role of physicians in prevention and research. It also includes

Introduction to Medicine, in which students spend time working with a community-based private practice physician.

Second-year students study the causes and effects of diseases in pathology and human pathophysiology. They also learn about the action of drugs in pharmacology. All of these courses are taught in an integrated fashion as organ systems. In addition, students are introduced to the elements of history taking, physical examination, and clinical medicine in the clinical skills course. The patient, physician, and society course continues for the four years of the curriculum.

In the *third and fourth years*, each student follows an educational program adapted to his or her particular interest and needs. With the advice of a faculty advisor, students schedule a course sequence in these nine academic quarters that meet the following requirements:

- Medicine (9 weeks)
- Surgery (9 weeks)
- Pediatrics/Neonatology (9 weeks)
- Psychiatry (4 weeks)
- Neurology (4 weeks)
- Ophthalmology (1 week)
- Obstetrics/Gynecology (9 weeks)
- Emergency Medicine (4.5 weeks)
- Ambulatory Medicine (4.5 weeks)
- Electives (30 weeks)

Hot Topics in Medical School

In addition to the LCME accreditation requirements, the American Association of Medical Colleges (AAMC) has developed a list of "Hot Topics" in medical schools.[5] The AAMC recognizes these topics as important for a successful residency experience. As you read the topics, it may be helpful to determine which areas of training you consider essential. You may also want to ask your physician if he had training in these areas.

Many medical schools are beginning to require some time be spent on each of the topics during the medical school student's career. At least half of all medical schools require their students to take coursework in each of these hot topic areas:

- Alternative and Complementary Medicine
- Communication Skills
- End-of-Life Care
- Family and Domestic Violence
- Healthcare Finance, Quality Improvement, and Systems
- Human Development and Life Cycle
- Medical Ethics
- Medical Genetics
- Medical Socioeconomics
- Nutrition
- Pain Management
- Patient Health Education
- Prevention and Health Maintenance and Counseling for Health-Risk Reduction
- Substance Abuse
- Chemoprevention Methods
- Disease Screening Tests and Health Surveillance Strategies

In addition to classroom and laboratory classes, medical schools require students to spend time in hospitals. Third- and fourth-year medical school students rotate through different medical and surgical specialties in the hospitals affiliated with their medical schools. This practical experience prepares students for their upcoming residency.

COMPETENCIES FOR ENTRY INTO RESIDENCY

After students graduate from medical school, the AAMC asks the graduates to rate themselves on three specific skills in preparation for residency. The assessments address graduates' communication, patient care, and patient advocacy. As you review these competencies, identify the ones most important to you based on your VVMS. You might even want to use this criteria to refine your VVMS. You can use this information to compile interview questions for new physicians.

How Well Can Medical School Graduates Communicate?

The communication skills that the AAMC asks graduates to rate themselves on include their ability to:

- Discuss a prescription with a patient
- Provide safe sex counseling to patients whose sexual orientation differs from their own
- Discuss treatment options with a woman who has late-stage breast cancer
- Initiate discussion of do-not-resuscitate (DNR) orders with a patient or family member
- Negotiate with a patient who requests unnecessary tests
- Assess the health practices of a patient using alternative therapies
- Use a computer-based clinical record-keeping program
- Use various forms of telemedicine
- Use a computerized clinic scheduling system
- Use a PDA (personal digital assistant) for clinical purposes

How Prepared Are Medical School Graduates to Treat Patients?

The list of assessments for which medical school graduates rate their level of preparedness before starting their residencies includes 56 patient care and medical management and policy topics. This list illustrates the wide range of topics that physicians need to understand after they complete medical school. In order to successfully complete their residency, they must master these skills. You can find the complete list of 56 topics at *www.aamc.org*. The following list is a sample of these topics:

- Care of healthy and sick older adults
- Delivering services to the underserved
- Care of hospitalized patients
- Diagnosis and management of disease
- Teamwork with health professionals
- Ethical decision making
- Physical rehabilitation
- Health promotion and disease prevention
- Women's health
- Interpretation of clinical data and lab reports
- Culturally appropriate care for diverse populations
- Continuity of care

How Prepared Are Medical School Graduates to Advocate for Patients?

One final area where the AAMC asks medical school graduates to assess themselves is in their level of commitment to do the following:

- Advocate at all times for the interest of one's patients over one's own interests
- Advocate for access to healthcare for members of traditionally underserved populations
- Engage in lifelong learning to stay abreast of relevant scientific advances
- Avoid conflicts of interest inherent in financial and organizational arrangements for the practice of medicine
- Practice compassionate treatment and respect patients' privacy and dignity

- Value, honesty, and integrity in all professional interactions including interactions with patient's families and colleagues
- Engage in ethical decision making
- Be aware of and manage major ethical dilemmas in medicine that arise at the beginning and end of life
- Be aware of and manage the major ethical dilemmas in medicine that arise from the rapid expansion of knowledge in genetics
- Recognize and accept limitations in knowledge and clinical skills and commit to continuously improve knowledge and skills

Expectations of Medical Residents

Any medical school graduate who wants to practice medicine and become a licensed physician must generally complete at least four years of residency in a U.S. teaching hospital. A few general medicine residencies, like family practice, are three-year programs.

Despite the fact that medical residents are technically still finishing their education, interns (first-year residents) and residents are employees of the hospital. They earn a minimal salary, which Medicare and the federal government subsidize. However, the hospital manages their day-to-day instruction. (For information about types of hospitals where medical school graduates can complete their residency requirements, see chapter 16.)

The Accreditation Council for Graduate Medical Education (ACGME) governs residency education and training requirements.[6] The ACGME competencies for resident training are in six basic areas:

1. Patient care
2. Medical knowledge
3. Practice-based learning and improvement
4. Interpersonal and communication skills
5. Professionalism
6. Healthcare system-based practice

In the area of interpersonal and communication skills, residents are required to develop certain skills before they complete their residency. As you review these competencies, you will probably agree that all are essential for a physician to be effective at treating and caring for patients. For successful completion of the program, the resident must be able to:

- Communicate effectively with patients, families, and the public, as appropriate, across a broad range of socioeconomic and cultural backgrounds
- Communicate effectively with physicians, other health professionals, and health-related agencies
- Work effectively as a member or leader of a healthcare team or other professional group
- Act in a consultative role to other physicians and health professionals
- Maintain comprehensive, timely, and legible medical records

In the area of professionalism, residents must also develop certain abilities. They must demonstrate:

- Compassion, integrity, and respect for others
- Responsiveness to patient needs that supersedes self-interest
- Respect for patient privacy and autonomy
- Accountability to patients, society, and the medical profession
- Sensitivity and responsiveness to a diverse patient population

Residency programs have standardized measures for evaluating residents' medical knowledge and expertise. You may wonder how residents are evaluated in their ability to demonstrate their professional responsibilities such as compassion, respect, and sensitivity. If you have a specific interest in how, for example, the teaching hospital where you might receive care in the future applies these ACGME requirements, check the hospital Web site. Every residency program is required by the ACGME to have one designated coordinator of the program. He will be able to provide you with all the information you need about the residency program. For more information about residents and teaching hospitals, see chapter 16.

PROFESSIONAL EDUCATION REQUIREMENTS OF A DOCTOR

Once a physician completes residency, she still has many continuing education obligations. These requirements ensure the physician is in good standing to practice medicine and are addressed below.

Physician Licensure Requirements

Each state governs physician licensing requirements. The states generally require the physician to:[7]

1. Be of good moral character
2. Be at least 21 years of age
3. Meet education requirements, including graduating from an accredited U.S. or foreign medical school
4. Successfully complete a minimum of four years of residency in a hospital residency program accredited by the ACGME
5. Meet examination and experience requirements
6. Be a U.S. citizen or an alien lawfully admitted to permanent residence in the United States

State licensure is a minimum requirement for every doctor to have the right to practice medicine within that state.

Board Certification Requirements

Board certification goes above the minimum requirements of licensure. While licensure is required to practice medicine and regulated by the state where the physician practices, board certification is optional for most specialties. Certification, whether in a specialty or subspecialty, involves rigorous testing and evaluation by peer physicians. The official board of the medical specialty regulates board certification for each specialty. For example, family practice physicians take their board certification exams through the American Board of Family Practice Medicine. Physicians, healthcare institutions, insurers, and patients recognize certification as the gold standard for assessing a physician's knowledge, experience, and skills for providing quality care in a certain specialty.

Check the American Board of Medical Specialties (ABMS) Web site (*www.abms.org*) to determine whether your physician is board certified.[8]

Continuing Education of a Doctor

Physicians must comply with continuing medical education (CME) requirements to maintain their state license. These requirements vary from state to state, but support the ever-changing climate of the medical world. Medical practices have changed so much and, hopefully, will continue to change, improve, and evolve for many years to come. In addition to state CME requirements, physicians who are board certified have fairly rigorous annual continuing education requirements in order to maintain their certification. Most hospitals also require certain continued education for their physicians in order to maintain status as a physician who can admit patients to the hospital.

Where and When Do Physicians Learn to Document?

As I've previously discussed, physicians must document the care they provide to you in your medical records. Yet only one component of clinical documentation—taking medical histories—is included in the medical school curriculum. ACGME requires that residents must be able to maintain comprehensive, timely, and legible medical records.

However, unless a medical school has an elective on documentation requirements or the hospital residency program contains special training in documentation, it appears that physicians' knowledge of documentation needs to be intuitive or picked up as on-the-job training. My research with clinical documentation practices and residency programs confirms this notion. For nearly 20 years, my colleagues and I have conducted many training sessions on clinical documentation. In a research study, in cooperation with the University of Pennsylvania, we measured the need for and results of clinical documentation training. Before training, we measured 91 physicians' documentation skills by administering a pre-test. The average score was 67 percent. After several hours of training and about two weeks of practicing the skills, the average score rose to 95 percent. In comments collected during the study, most residents felt they received basic information regarding documentation practices during medical school, but were not thoroughly taught the six key concepts of clinical documentation: (1) legibility (2) completeness (3) reliability (4) accuracy (5) preciseness (6) timeliness.

After their training, residents commented that they wished they had received similar training and feedback on their documentation practices in both medical school and earlier in their residency. When we asked residency program directors why they did not train residents on documentation practices, they replied that there simply was not enough time.

As a patient, you can hold your physician accountable for good documentation. One way to do this is to request your records from your physician each time you have a visit. Just knowing that you are going to read your medical record may influence your physician to document more legibly, timely, and completely.

Key Highlights

To get a proper perspective on your physician, it may be helpful to understand the expectations placed on him. Becoming a physician requires at least seven years of formal education after receiving a bachelor's degree. This includes successful completion of medical school and a residency program. Beyond that, there are continuing education requirements to maintain state licensure and board certification.

Key Actions

- Understand all the expectations that are placed on physicians but, at the same time, make sure you have a physician who meets the values you have for your own healthcare.
- Make your physician accountable for good documentation in your medical record.

Key Take-Away

Your knowledge of the extensive education and training requirements of your physician may help you understand your physicians better and collaborate with them to receive the best possible healthcare.

Endnotes

[1] From StudentDoc, *www.studentdoc.com/medical-school-requirements.html.*
[2] Student essays are from the Web site *www.bestpremed.com.*
[3] Liaison Committee on Medical Education, *www.lcme.org.*

[4] Johns Hopkins School of Medicine, *www.hopkinsmedicine.org.*
[5] American Association of Medical Colleges, *www.aamc.org.*
[6] Accreditation Council for Graduate Medical Education, *www.acgme.org.*
[7] For information about state licensing requirements, go to *www.docboard.org/docfinder.html.*

CHAPTER

13

Understanding Medical and Surgical Specialists and Other Providers

In a democracy, dissent is an act of faith. Like medicine, the test of its value is not in its taste, but in its effects. —J. William Fulbright

In August 1986, Joe had just passed the bar and was starting a clerkship with the Honorable Rufus King of the Superior Court in Washington, D.C. The judge and his wife, Karen, invited us to dinner at an Italian restaurant on Dupont Circle. I was eight months pregnant and had already gained 45 pounds. Other than the weight gain and moving a little slower because of it, I was feeling very energetic and having what my obstetrician, Dr. Chaudry, referred to as an "uneventful" pregnancy. Wearing one of my final-stage maternity dresses and my last pair of stretched-out black leather flat shoes, I braved the 98-degree heat to take the subway to DuPont Circle. At dinner, we enjoyed a light-hearted conversation, mostly about our baby on the way and the Kings' recent adoption of a baby boy. The evening ended as uneventfully as it began. We thanked the Kings and hopped on the subway to home.

At 3 a.m. acute pain in the upper portion of my stomach woke me. The pain and the location were familiar. I had been carrying around a pile of stones and sludge (like mud) in my gallbladder since I was in college. Back then, the doctor said that since the contents were sludge and two or three rather large stones, there was no chance of clogging any of the ducts, so surgery was not required. He told me to stay away from fatty and creamy foods as much as possible, foods like the huge plate of tortellini alfredo I had eaten earlier that evening.

The pain had always been bad whenever I had a gallbladder attack, but with the baby crowding everything, it was unbearable. Because we were in an HMO, the hospital we needed to use was about 25 miles away. At about 4 a.m., we landed at the ER, which luckily for us, was not busy. As soon as the nurses saw my belly, the shouts began, "She's in labor!" I kept shouting back, "This is not labor. This is a gallbladder attack!" My words did not matter to them. All of the circumstantial evidence pointed to the fact that I was in labor. Within minutes, I was in the labor room hooked up to a fetal monitor.

Fortunately, my obstetrician, Dr. Chaudry, was in the hospital, having just delivered a set of twins. By the time he arrived at my room, everyone knew I was not in labor, but I was still in excruciating pain. Joe explained my history with gallstones and gallbladder attacks to Dr. Chaudry. To ease the pain, he gave me Demerol through an intravenous line. The pain was gone in minutes.

I then had an ultrasound. The radiologist confirmed the diagnosis of gallstones. Although the episode appeared to be over, as a precaution, Dr. Chaudry sent me to a surgeon. Just for some added assurance, he said. Although I do not remember the surgeon's name, I do remember his brusque manner. I was sitting on the cold metal table in the traditional paper gown, still feeling some of the anxiety from the previous night's events. He walked in the door, flipped open my chart and without even looking up at me, said, "This gallbladder needs to come out and the sooner the better. I would like to schedule the surgery for tomorrow." That was it, no exam, no discussion.

Did he even notice, I wondered, that I was pregnant? My head spun as I thought about the concept of surgery the next day. I managed to eek out, "What about the baby?" His matter of fact response was, "Well, we'll just take the baby." I do not recall if he said anything more after those first few words. "We'll take the baby," just kept going through my head. He said the words like removing the baby was a routine operation, like removing a gallstone or an appendix.

I jumped off the table and began changing into my clothes right in front of him. "I am not having surgery," I said, "This baby is not ready to be born." Without additional comment he replied, "That's your decision. I'll note that on your record." I immediately went to Dr. Chaudry's office, where he apologized for the surgeon's behavior. He mentioned that the surgeon was not a member of the HMO. That, however, did not explain the surgeon's lack of compassion for my situation. Dr. Chaudry suggested I visit another specialist, a gastroenterologist, later that same day.

As soon as I walked through the gastroenterologist's door, I could tell the experience would be different. The office staff was warm and friendly. The doctor was relaxed, offering me a warm handshake and steady eye contact. During the exam, he talked to me the entire time, explaining what he was doing and why and encouraging me to ask questions if I had any. After the exam, he asked me to meet him in his office.

He showed me the films of my gallbladder and explained what was going on. It was the same story I had heard seven years ago. Like the physician then, and for all of the same reasons, he also believed that surgery was not necessary. The gastroenterologist did give me some detailed instructions, and he recommended a strict diet with no fatty foods, nuts, or seeds, which I promised to follow. Then he shook my hand and wished me well. Emmalea was born five weeks later. I still have my gallbladder. I have never had another gallbladder attack.

This kind of story happens in healthcare frequently. The same patient. The same problem. Two different doctors. Two different approaches. Yet my experience was about more than just doctors disagreeing. Here were two different practitioners, each practicing his specific trade. Surgeons operate. Gastroenterologists explore.

I am oversimplifying and generalizing the issues. However, the point is that the physicians' opinions differed because each was practicing his own specialty. Dr. Chaudry followed a conservative path in having a surgeon evaluate me first. He wanted to make sure he obtained adequate consultation, so that even if I elected not to have surgery and later had a complication due to my gallbladder, Dr.

Chaudry would have done his job. Dr. Chaudry was my primary care physician in this case. He coordinated the process. The two consultants presented me with choices. In the end, I decided.

WHAT IS SPECIAL ABOUT SPECIALISTS?

Unlike the primary care physicians (PCPs) addressed in chapter 2, specialists complete additional training in a specific medical or surgical area, such as cardiology or gastroenterology. Most primary care physicians spend three to four years in residency. The training of a specialist can last from one additional year of residency (for example, radiologists or neurologists) to as many as nine additional years (for certain neurosurgical subspecialties).

According to the Accreditation Council for Graduate Medical Education (ACGME), the term *fellow* is used by some sponsoring institutions and in some specialties to designate participants in subspecialty graduate medical education (GME) programs.[1] The exact number of years of training for fellows depends on the subspecialty, the focus, and the hospital where the resident or fellow is training. In most of the specialties described below, I include a range of years for training.

Sixty percent of the 15,000 doctors who graduate from medical school each year practice in a medical or surgical specialty.[2] Today, the American Board of Medical Specialties (ABMS) lists on its Web site (*www.abms.org*) 37 specialties and 109 subspecialties. These include only those specialties that require an exam for board certification. There are three broad categories of specialties and subspecialties: medical, surgical, and medical-surgical (physicians who do both).

Understanding the different specialties should help you make more informed decisions about your healthcare. Additionally, understanding specialists' education and training, such as knowing how a cardiothoracic surgeon *becomes* a cardiothoracic surgeon, may also be helpful in guiding your decision making. The American Medical Association (AMA) publication, *Physician Characteristics and Distribution in the U.S.,* contains statistics of physicians in specialties with at least 20,000 members.[3]

Specialty	Number of physicians
Obstetrics	35,800
Psychiatry	35,124
Anesthesiology	34,795
General Surgery	30,452
Emergency Medicine	24,393
Diagnostic Radiology	22,037
Orthopedic Surgery	20,974
Cardiology	20,494

Which specialist is the right specialist?

Most specialties are easily distinguished from each other, but the differences between certain specialties may blur. In others, there is clear overlap. When Emmalea had her first seizure, we did not have to ask. We knew that her specialist would be a neurologist. When her seizures were not controlled with AEDs alone, we began searching for options outside of the specialty of neurology. Dr. Herzog provided us with the solution. He is both a neurologist and an endocrinologist. Emmalea needed Dr. Herzog's expertise and razor sharp focus on "menstrual cycle-related seizures" to be seizure-free. In your own searching, you may need to look beyond the obvious specialty to find the answer. Your PCP, your medical mentor, or even your primary specialist can advise you. In our case, Emmalea's primary neurologist helped us find her neuroendocrinologist.

Overlap in specialties exists when different specialists do the same thing, or at least to a non-clinician, appear to do the same thing. For example, both orthopedic surgeons and neurosurgeons perform surgery to repair herniated discs in the back. In most cases, however, neurosurgeons only operate when the herniated disc is in the cervical spine (closer to the brain) or when it involves some portion of the lining around the spinal cord. Orthopedic surgeons repair any type of herniated disc.

There are other areas of overlap in specialties. Anesthesiologists, physiatrists, and neurologists can all be certified in pain management medicine. Family practice physicians, internal medicine and orthopedic surgeons can all be certified in sports management. Dermatologists and allergists both treat immune disorders. Neurosurgeons, vascular surgeons, and vascular radiologists can all perform vascular surgery. Orthopedic surgeons and podiatrists both perform surgery on the foot and lower leg. Some of the differences in the services these different specialists can provide are obvious, others are more subtle. To get the best result, involve your PCP in decision making whenever you need or think you may need a specialist.

Do I Need a Referral to See a Specialist?

It depends. In the past, health plans had significant limitations on when you could visit a specialist without being referred by their PCP. In fact, HMO's even called their PCPs "gatekeepers" to signify the role they played in limiting your access to physicians besides the PCP. When Congress passed HIPAA in 1997, the legislation provided you with the right to choose your PCP. Your health plan is no longer permitted to choose your PCP on your behalf. As a result of this legislation, many health plans have also become more flexible with patient self-referrals to specialists.

So, the answer to the question *Do I need a referral to see a specialist?* is it depends on your health plan and the specialist. First, if your health plan allows patient self-referrals to specialists, then you know your plan will pay for your visit. If you are planning to self-refer, you should research your plan's policy. If you cannot get a copy of the policy in writing, obtain verbal confirmation over the telephone from your contact at the plan regarding the plan's stance on patient self-referrals.

Second, although your plan may allow you to schedule the visit directly with a specialist, the specialist may have a different policy. If you know the specific physician whom you would like to make an appointment with, you can call her office to inquire about her policies. Today, the majority of specialists will usually see you without a referral from another physician.

However, if you are self-referring, you should be aware of the potential disadvantages. Most specialists give priority to patients who are referred by a colleague. It is important to keep in mind that any specialists you see, even if you self-refer, will want to send a report of your visit to your PCP. Many specialists will refuse to schedule an appointment with you unless you provide them with a name of a PCP. Their reasons for this are partly to protect or limit their own legal responsibility for your care and partly to ensure you get the highest quality care. Ideally, you should partner with your PCP on all medical issues, including care from specialists, to get the best possible care for yourself.

MEDICAL SPECIALTIES

The ABMS lists 95 medical specialties and subspecialties. Subspecialties are limited areas of medical practice within a specialty. For example, pediatrics is a specialty and pediatric cardiology is a subspecialty. Pediatrics has 21 subspecialties and internal medicine has 18.

Some of the more common medical specialties and subspecialties are listed below, along with explanations about the training and types of conditions these specialists treat. This is only a partial listing of specialties.[4]

Cardiology

Cardiology is a subspecialty of internal medicine. A cardiologist is an internist who specializes in diseases of the heart and blood vessels and manages complex cardiac conditions, such as heart attacks and life-threatening, abnormal heart rhythms. Other conditions that cardiologists treat include heart failure, angina, and chest pain. One procedure a cardiologist performs is cardiac catheterization, which is performed to diagnose problems with the heart vessels. Heart blockages are being treated more and more with less invasive or non-surgical techniques. Cardiologists perform these procedures, including the placement of stents or balloon angioplasties, to open the coronary arteries. They may also place pacemakers or defibrillators to control heart rhythms.

Cardiology training after residency is usually three to four years of fellowship. Board certification in cardiology is by the American Board of Internal Medicine.[5]

Gastroenterology

Gastroenterologists diagnose and treat diseases of the digestive organs, including the stomach, bowels, liver, and gallbladder. This specialist treats conditions such as abdominal pain, ulcers, diarrhea, cancer, and jaundice, and performs complex diagnostic and therapeutic procedures using endoscopes to visualize internal organs for procedures like colonoscopies.

Training beyond residency is usually three years of fellowship. Board certification is available through the American Board of Internal Medicine.

Other Internal Medicine Subspecialties

There are several other medical subspecialties with board certification through the American Board of Internal Medicine. Training post-residency for these specialties is generally two to four years of fellowship. Some of the more common subspecialties are listed below.

- **Endocrinologists** treat metabolic and hormonal disorders. Most endocrinologists focus on treatment for patients with diabetes. They may also treat patients suffering from obesity and morbid obesity.
- **Infectious disease physicians** treat patients with HIV/AIDS, staph infections, and other communicable diseases.
- **Nephrologists** treat patients with kidney failure and other kidney diseases.

- **Pulmonary medicine physicians** treat patients with tuberculosis, respiratory failure, lung cancer, and chronic lung diseases.
- **Medical oncologists** treat patients with all types of cancers and may be involved in supervising their chemotherapy.
- **Hematologists** treat patients with blood disorders including anemia, hemophilia, and sickle-cell disease.
- **Rheumatologists** treat patients with autoimmune connective tissue disorders like rheumatoid arthritis, lupus, scleroderma, and gout.

Emergency Medicine

The emergency physician treats a diversified population of adult and pediatric patients who are acutely ill or injured. Common conditions that an emergency physician may treat include fractures, head trauma, chest pain, heart failure, asthma attacks, and seizures.

The American Board of Emergency Medicine offers certification in five emergency subspecialties. These are hospice and palliative care, medical toxicology, pediatric emergency medicine, sports medicine, and undersea and hyperbaric medicine. Hyperbaric medicine is the delivery of pressurized oxygen to the body. Physicians use it to treat decompression sickness, a condition in which deep-sea divers develop nitrogen bubbles in their bloodstream from coming to the surface of the water too quickly. Hyperbaric medicine is now also used to treat conditions like carbon monoxide poisoning, difficult wounds, crushing injuries, brain abscesses, burns, and anemia due to sudden blood loss.[6] These conditions are likely to be encountered in emergency situations, hence the emergency certification.

Allergy and Immunology

Allergists treat disorders involving the immune system like asthma, anaphylaxis (severe allergic reaction), eczema, and adverse reactions to drugs, foods, and insect stings as well as immune deficiency diseases.

Training beyond residency is generally two years of fellowship. Board certification is offered through the American Board of Allergy and Immunology.[7]

Medical Genetics

Medical geneticists are trained in diagnostic and therapeutic procedures for patients with genetically linked diseases. These specialists use modern cytogenetic, radiologic, and biochemical testing to assist in specialized genetic counseling. This physician implements needed therapeutic interventions and provides prevention through prenatal diagnosis. A medical geneticist also plans and coordinates screening programs for various genetic disorders.

Training beyond residency is two to four years of fellowship. The American Board of Medical Genetics offers different subspecialty certifications in biochemical genetics, cytogenetics, clinical genetics, molecular genetics, and molecular genetic pathology.[8]

Pediatric Subspecialties

Pediatrics is addressed as a primary care specialty in chapter 2. However, the American Board of Pediatrics offers certification in 21 different subspecialties. I highlight some of the more common pediatric subspecialties in this chapter to provide you with an idea of the depth of pediatric medicine overall. Subspecialties in pediatrics include: child abuse pediatrics, neonatal-perinatal medicine, neuro-developmental disabilities, pediatric cardiology, nephrology, transplant hepatology, and sleep medicine.

Training after residency is generally one to three years of fellowship.[9] For a complete listing of all pediatric subspecialties see *www.abms.org.*

Physical Medicine and Rehabilitation

Physical medicine and rehabilitation physicians, usually called physiatrists, diagnose and treat patients with physical disabilities.

These disabilities may be musculoskeletal, like neck and back pain or sports injuries, or other painful conditions, such as carpal tunnel syndrome. The disabilities may also result from neurological trauma or disease such as spinal cord injury, head injury, or stroke. The primary goal of the physiatrist is to restore physical, psychological, social, and vocational function. A physiatrist may use electromyography to supplement the standard history, physical, x-ray, and laboratory examinations. The physiatrist is an expert in therapeutic exercise, prosthetics (artificial limbs), orthotics, and mechanical and electrical devices.

Training after residency is generally one to three years of fellowship. Board certification is through the American Board of Physical Medicine and Rehabilitation. The board also offers board certification in hospice and palliative medicine, pain medicine, neuromuscular medicine, pediatric rehabilitation medicine, spinal cord injury, and sports medicine.[10]

Neurology

A neurologist specializes in the diagnosis and treatment of all types of disease or impaired function of the brain, spinal cord, peripheral nerves, muscles, and autonomic nervous system, as well as the blood vessels that relate to these structures. Neurologists treat conditions such as epilepsy, strokes, multiple sclerosis, Parkinson's disease, migraines, and brain tumors.

Training beyond residency is generally one to two years of fellowship. Certification is through the American Board of Psychiatry and Neurology. Other board certifications offered include clinical neurophysiology, neurodevelopmental disabilities, neuromuscular medicine, pain medicine, and sleep medicine.[11]

Psychiatry

A psychiatrist specializes in the prevention, diagnosis, and treatment of mental, addictive, and emotional disorders such as schizophrenia and other psychotic disorders, mood disorders, anxiety disorders, substance-related disorders, sexual- and gender-identity disorders, and adjustment disorders.

Training beyond residency is generally one to three years of fellowship. Board certification is through the American Board of Psychiatry and Neurology. Additional certifications available are forensic psychiatry, geriatric psychiatry, and psychosomatic medicine.[12]

A Story of Multiple Specialists. Christine took on the role of medical mentor to her husband Jay early in their relationship. When he was 12 years old, Jay learned he had juvenile diabetes. This meant, among other things, that he would be dependent on insulin injections for the rest of his life. Early in their marriage, Jay spent some time in the hospital with a foot ulcer, a retinal disorder, and possible kidney damage, all complications of his diabetes.

Christine sat next to his bed every minute. She watched the nephrologist come to treat Jay's kidney problem, the ophthalmologist to treat his retinal problem, and the endocrinologist to follow his skin ulcer and blood sugar levels. She watched order after order as more medicine was issued and became concerned that the number of drugs Jay would be taking was too much.

When Christine tried to speak to the physicians as they came and went, each really knew only about the problem he was treating. At some point, Christine asked, "Who's looking at the whole picture here?" The response was "your primary care physician." The problem was that the endocrinologist had admitted Jay for the ulcer, and his primary care physician did not even know Jay was in the hospital.

It struck Christine that nobody was making that call for Jay—it was Jay's and her responsibility to notify Jay's primary care physician. Since that day, the physician has been on Christine's speed dial and involved in every aspect of Jay's care. Jay's primary care physician keeps his records. He is the one who evaluates all the treatments and medications ordered by Jay's specialists. Through their partnership, Jay's overall health has improved.

SURGICAL SPECIALTIES

The ABMS lists 28 surgical specialties and subspecialties on its Web site. Anesthesiology, while not technically a surgical specialty, is included in this list because anesthesiologists primarily prepare patients for surgery and monitor them during and after surgery. The most common surgical specialties and subspecialties, along with a brief description of the necessary training and types of conditions these physicians treat are provided below.

Anesthesiology

Anesthesiologists administer anesthesia for pain relief generally and during surgery. Prior to surgery, the anesthesiologist assesses the risk of anesthesia based on the patient's general health and any chronic conditions. The anesthesiologist uses the risk assessment to administer the appropriate type and amount of the drug. Then he monitors the patient in great detail during and after surgery to ensure appropriate response to the anesthesia.

In my training of physicians on clinical documentation, I have found anesthesiologists to be a group of physicians most receptive to learning and applying new information. Anesthesiologists are detail oriented, as their specialty requires. They have a different view of the patient than any other physician on the treatment team.

Training post-residency is usually two years of fellowship. Board certification is through the American Board of Anesthesiology. The board also offers certification in critical care, hospice and palliative care, and pain medicine management.[13]

General Surgery

A general surgeon may manage surgical conditions in the following areas: gastrointestinal tract; abdomen; breast, skin, and soft tissue; endocrine system; head and neck surgery; pediatric surgery; surgical critical care; surgical oncology; trauma and burns; and vascular surgery.

I have found general surgeons to be especially focused and exceptionally quick thinkers. It is often difficult to get their attention long enough to attend a full program because they are so busy. But, when I have gotten their attention, general surgeons have been some of the most intense participants during the training process. This intensity and focus is probably reflective of their need to move from a gastrointestinal to a pancreatic to a breast surgery perhaps all in one day, and do an excellent job on each.

Training post-residency is two to three years of fellowship. Board certification is through the American Board of Surgery. Additional certifications offered by the board include hospice and palliative medicine, vascular surgery, surgery of the hand, and surgical critical care.[14]

Thoracic Surgery

A thoracic surgeon provides the operative care of patients with pathologic conditions in the chest. This includes surgery for coronary artery disease, lung cancer, and abnormalities of the heart valves. Thoracic surgeons, sometimes also referred to as cardiothoracic surgeons, are under some of the greatest scrutiny by the public. Quality ratings, Medicare, and even local newspapers report on mortality ratings for coronary artery bypass surgery more frequently than any other surgery. Surgeons who do the greatest number of coronary surgeries have the best quality ratings and the best outcomes. Training post-residency is generally three to four years of fellowship. Certification is through the American Board of Thoracic Surgery.[15]

Colorectal Surgery

A colon and rectal surgeon is trained to diagnose and treat various diseases of the intestinal tract, colon, rectum, anal canal, and perianal area by medical and surgical means. This specialist also deals with other organs and tissues (such as the liver, urinary, and female reproductive system) involved with primary intestinal disease.

Training post-residency is generally two years of fellowship. Certification is through the American Board of Colon and Rectal Surgery.[16]

Vascular surgery

Vascular surgeons operate on arteries and veins and provide conservative therapies for diseases of the peripheral vascular systems. For further clarification, cardiothoracic surgeons operate on the heart and neurosurgeons operate on the brain. With the introduction of minimally invasive techniques, the numbers and types of surgeries performed by vascular surgeons have grown considerably. Vascular surgeons remove clots in the veins or arteries. They also re-attach the ends of arteries or veins.

Common types of conditions they treat conclude varicose veins, aneurysms, thrombosis, and embolisms. Training after residency is five to six years of fellowship.[17]

Neurosurgery

Neurosurgeons treat patients with disorders of the brain, meninges, skull, and cranial and spinal nerves. They also treat disorders of the pituitary gland and the spinal cord.

In chapter 1, I described my encounter with one of the chiefs of neurosurgery at Johns Hopkins Hospital. This surgeon was extremely reflective and deliberate. He was very attentive during our discussion. He was also very structured in his interaction and did not end the conversation until he was able to tie up any loose ends regarding his responsibilities to the hospital's compliance program moving forward. He is exactly the type of individual I would want to have working on my brain.

Training post-residency is generally four to five years of fellowship. Board certification is through the American Board of Neurosurgery.[18]

Orthopedic Surgery

Orthopedic surgeons generally perform surgery on patients with trauma and with arthritic joints. Examples of trauma surgery include repairs of fractures, torn ligaments, herniated discs, and dislocations. Surgery for joints involves replacement or repair of joints like the hips, knees, and shoulders.

In training programs I have conducted, these surgeons are quick, to the point, and somewhat impatient. They are focused on knowing the end result immediately and pushing forward to get there no matter what. If this disposition is indicative of most orthopedic surgeons, it probably allows them to repair as many fractures, joints, crushed vertebrae, and other injuries, as flawlessly as possible.

Training post-residency is two to three years of fellowship. Additional certifications offered by the American Board of Orthopaedic Surgery include sports medicine and surgery of the hand.[19]

Otolaryngology

An otolaryngologist diagnoses and provides medical and surgical therapy for disorders or injuries of the ears, nose, sinuses, throat, face and jaw. Head and neck oncology, facial plastic and reconstructive surgery, and the treatment of disorders of hearing and voice are fundamental areas of expertise for this specialist.

Training post-residency is three to four years of fellowship. Board certification is offered by the American Board of Otolaryngology.[20]

Plastic Surgery

A plastic surgeon deals with the repair, reconstruction, or replacement of physical defects or cosmetic enhancement of the skin, musculoskeletal system, face, hands, extremities, and breast. Elective cosmetic surgery is an essential component of plastic surgery.

Training is two to three years post-residency. Subspecialty certifications in plastic surgery within the head and neck and surgery of the hand are offered by the American Board of Plastic Surgery.[21]

Urology

Urologists manage conditions of the genitourinary system and surrounding structures including the adrenal gland. Common conditions treated by urologists include prostate cancer, kidney and bladder disorders, and sexual dysfunction. One year of additional training post-residency is usually required. Certification is available through the American Board of Urology.[22]

SPECIALISTS WHO PROVIDE BOTH MEDICAL AND SURGICAL SERVICES

The ABMS Web site lists 14 different specialties for physicians who provide medical and surgical assessment, care, and treatment. The most common of these specialties are obstetrics-gynecology, (OB/GYN), dermatology and ophthalmology. All three of these specialties require two to three years of post-residency training, and they offer board certification.

- **OB/GYN physicians** serve as the primary care physician for women during their pregnancies. These physicians also perform surgeries, such as a caesarean-section (c-section) during delivery. The OB/GYN physician also performs surgery on the female reproductive system, the most common procedure being a hysterectomy, or removal of the uterus. Other board certifications offered by the American Board of Obstetrics and Gynecology include gynecologic oncology, maternal and fetal medicine, and reproductive endocrinology/infertility.[23]
- **Dermatologists** often treat skin cancer, acne, allergy rashes, eczema, wrinkles, warts, and nail infections.[24]

- **Ophthalmologists** often treat glaucoma, diabetic retinopathy, and cataracts.[25]

DIAGNOSTIC SPECIALTIES: RADIOLOGISTS AND PATHOLOGISTS

The ABMS Web site lists 23 different specialties and subspecialties in diagnostic medicine categories. The difference between these diagnostic specialists and other specialists is that diagnostic physicians are more likely to interact with information, fluids, or tissue taken *from* the patient, as opposed to interacting *with* the actual patient. Examples of diagnostic physicians include radiologists[26] and nuclear medicine physicians,[27] whose primary interaction is with films or computer images of the inside of the body, and pathologists,[28] whose primary interaction is with body fluids, tissues, cells, and organs taken during lab testing or surgery.

Diagnostic physicians work with primary care physicians or other specialists to provide a diagnosis based on collected specimens. The greatest number of subspecialties is in pathology, which has 10 subspecialties, including forensic pathology, molecular genetic pathology, and blood banking and transfusion medicine.

OTHER CLINICIANS

Besides physicians many other trained clinicians provide healthcare services. For example, your physician may write an order for physical therapy for you. Then the physical therapist designs a plan for you. Some examples of other clinicians are listed below.

Mid-Level Practitioners: Nurse Practitioners and Physician Assistants

The mid-level practitioner is a licensed healthcare provider who provides a certain level of care to patients. Often, this care is a higher level than what a registered nurse can provide, but less than what a physician provides, hence the designation "mid-level practitioner."

Physician assistants or nurse practitioners are examples of mid-level practitioners.

Mid-level practitioners include certified registered nurse practitioners (CRNPs), nurse midwives, and nurse anesthetists. These professionals are all registered nurses, most with bachelor's degrees or equivalent, and additional training for the certification. Physician assistants graduate from a five- to six-year program. All mid-level practitioners are licensed within the state where they practice.

If permitted by the state where they practice, nurse midwives often treat patients independently. Most other mid-level practitioners work under the direct supervision of a physician. Exceptions are for those practitioners who work in rural areas with a shortage of PCPs. In these locations, federal law allows mid-level practitioners to treat patients for certain conditions without the oversight of a physician.

Nurses

Nurses are, in many ways, the eyes and ears of the physician. Registered Nurses (RNs) are the nursing professionals you are probably most familiar with. Today 2.4 million registered nurses comprise the largest group of healthcare professionals. These individuals have completed either an associates or bachelors (BSN) degree in nursing or have earned a nursing diploma from a school of nursing. RNs must pass a national licensing examination, known as the NCLEX-RN. Nurses may be licensed in more than one state, either by examination or by the endorsement of a license issued by another State. Currently 18 states participate in the Nurse Licensure Compact Agreement, which allows nurses to practice in member states without recertifying. All states require periodic renewal of licenses, which may involve continuing education.

Licensed practical nurses (LPNs) or Licensed Vocational Nurses (LVNs) complete training lasting about 1 year from one of the 1,200 state-approved programs, mostly in vocational or technical schools. All states require LPNs to pass a licensing examination, known as the NCLEX-PN, after completing a state-approved practical nursing program.[29]

Therapists and Other Clinicians

Other clinicians or therapists on your treatment team may include audiologists, occupational therapists, physical therapists, respiratory therapists, speech therapists, nutritionists, lab technicians, radiology technicians, and pharmacists. They all have formal education requirements. In addition, all clinicians and therapists are, at a minimum, licensed by the state where they provide care. Most have continuing education requirements.

Emergency Medical Technicians (EMTs)

In many ways, EMTs are the unsung heroes of healthcare. They are the individuals who respond to some of the worst healthcare problems including trauma, fire, motor vehicle accidents, and heart attacks. Their job "description" involves keeping the patient stabilized until they arrive at the nearest hospital emergency room. However, in reality, they also need to manage the patient's significant others during some of the most heartbreaking and shocking moments for those individuals. I know. I was one of those people.

Emmalea had her second big (grand mal) seizure while she was a passenger in her cousin Valerie's car. Luckily, Emmalea was in her seatbelt and Valerie was able to pull off of the highway and flag down a state policeman. I happened to be traveling on the same highway in the opposite direction. When I received the call from Valerie, I went immediately to the location. My heart pounding in my chest, I saw the ambulance, pulled my car onto the highway median and ran across the opposite northbound lanes. The doors to the ambulance were already shut. I jumped onto the back bumper of the ambulance and held tightly to the door handles, assuming I guess, that they would allow me to stay in that position until we arrived at the hospital. I was banging on the ambulance windows, trying to get

Emmalea's attention. Imagine her own shock to have just regained consciousness from a major seizure, a surreal experience from her own descriptions, and see her mother pounding on the ambulance windows. It was the EMTs who came around to the back of the vehicle and very calmly and politely escorted me to the passenger's seat of the vehicle.

What is even more amazing about many of these individuals is that they may actually be serving, as in our case, as unpaid volunteers with the rescue squad. Other EMTs may be employed by commercial ambulance services or by the hospital's emergency department or intensive care units. The National Registry of Emergency Medical Technicians (NREMT) sets voluntary standards and examines and certifies EMT candidates in 46 states. Individual states set their own standards of certification or licensure. The U.S. Department of Transportation recognizes four levels of EMTs: basic, two levels of intermediate EMTs, and paramedics. Paramedics may administer drugs orally and intravenously, interpret electrocardiograms (EKGs), perform endotracheal intubations, and use monitors and other complex equipment. Emergency treatment for more complicated problems is carried out under the direction of medical doctors by radio preceding or during transport.[30]

MENTAL HEALTH PROFESSIONALS

Many of the individuals I interviewed while researching this book talked about the difficulties they encountered when they or a family member needed a mental health professional. More than 60 percent were searching for a counselor or a therapist for counseling, not a psychiatrist. Only about 50 percent got the help they sought.

Of those who did get help, several tried two or three different therapists before they found a professional they liked. Some people talked about the stigma around seeking mental health counseling. Others talked about the fear preventing them from getting started with a therapist. You may not have considered or sought the services of a mental health professional. If you do find a need, take time to find the therapist who is best matched to your needs.

Mental health therapists have a wide range of educational backgrounds, depending on the state in which they are licensed. Non-physician mental health professionals in some states may have little, or no, formal education, while in other states a minimum of a bachelor's or master's degree is required. Determine whether level of education matters to you and what qualifications you prefer in choosing a mental health professional. Mental health practitioners include psychiatrists (addressed above in the section on specialists), psychologists, social workers, and mental health counselors.

Locating a Mental Health Professional: Personal Recommendations Help

When our family needed the assistance of mental health professionals, I was fortunate to be able to rely on the advice of my cousin Kathy, an experienced therapist. When we spoke about our specific needs, she asked me questions about preferences in terms of gender and age, two issues often related to people's comfort levels when working with a mental health therapist. Kathy also asked me whether we would prefer a therapist in private practice or in a group practice. She also wanted to know whether we were looking for individual or group therapy, since certain therapists specialize in one or the other. Finally, Kathy asked about the general types of issues we wanted to address. Often, therapists specialize in certain areas, like substance abuse or post-traumatic stress disorder. These inquiries were all good questions, and they may be helpful questions for you to think about as well.

After receiving a list of recommendations from Kathy, we found some detailed information about each of them on the Internet. This helped us narrow down the group. Then, we made some calls and spoke with each person over the phone to make a final decision. In each case, our decisions regarding mental health professionals were good ones. Each selection resulted in a positive, lasting relationship.

If you do not have a close friend or relative who can provide some initial referrals, your primary care physician should be able to help you. Ask for more than one referral so you can explore who might be the best fit for you. If you think you may need medication, discuss your concerns with your primary care physician. Your primary doctor may refer you to a psychiatrist.

DENTISTRY

Dentists are an integral part of your healthcare team. Modern dental hygiene has influenced many other medical advances. Dentists may be the first to spot certain diseases, such as throat and mouth cancers. For example, my colleague's dentist, not her physician, discovered her thyroid cancer. Additionally, general infections in the mouth can affect your overall health. It is likely your dentist will help you first with these problems.

All dentists attend dental school for four years after earning their bachelor's degree. Depending on their specialty, dentists earn either a DMD (Doctor of Dental Medicine) or DDS (Doctor of Dental Surgery) degree. Then, they may spend anywhere from one to five additional years in residency. All dentists are licensed by the state where they practice. Board certification is available for general dentistry and dental specialties through their respective boards.

- **Dentists** restore, replace, and extract teeth. These dentists also correct misaligned teeth and provide oral health instruction. After dental school, they spend one to two years in residency.[31]
- **Endodontists** focus their treatment on the dental nerves and pulp and perform surgeries like root canal.[32]
- **Oral and maxillofacial surgeons** focus on injuries and defects of the neck, head, and jaw. They treat conditions like temporomandibular joint disorder (TMJ) and oral cancer. Oral surgeons spend four years in surgical residency after dental school.[33]
- **Orthodontists** address problems related to irregular dental development and missing teeth, problems needing braces. They spend three years in residency after dental school.[34]

- **Periodontists** treat gum disease and problems related to the supporting bones. They also spend three years in residency after dental school.[35]

Key Highlights

Different types of physician specialists work from unique perspectives directly related to the extensive training within their specialties. Understanding the training and focus of each specialist helps you make the most informed decisions for your healthcare needs. At different points in your life, your healthcare team may also include other clinicians, mental health professionals, and dental specialists. You can use your knowledge of the different healthcare professionals and how they can help you to build the best possible healthcare team.

Key Actions

- Familiarize yourself with the different medical, surgical, and medical-surgical specialties.
- Use mid-level practitioners for minor, non-emergent complaints, if you feel comfortable with their level of training.
- Identify a personal or healthcare contact who can refer a mental health professional, if you or a family member needs therapy.
- Include dental health professionals on your healthcare team and obtain your dental records.

Key Take-Away

Your physicians' background and training influences how they assess your needs and treat you. Knowing all of the different specialists and other healthcare providers who may be able to help you and selecting the right one make you a more empowered and knowledgeable healthcare consumer.

Endnotes

[1] Accreditation Council for Graduate Medical Education, *www.acgme.org.*
[2] Gorman, Christine. "Is healthcare too specialized?" *Time Magazine,* September 14, 1992.
[3] American Medical Association. *Physician Characteristics and Distribution in the U.S., 2007 Edition.*
[4] The complete listing of specialties with board certification along with significant detail about the profession can be found at the ABMS Web site at *www.abms.org/Who_We_Help/Consumers/specialties.aspx.*
[5] American Board of Internal Medicine, *www.abim.org.*

[6] *Morrison, Daniel S., MDR, and Kirkby, Duncan, Ph.D. "Hyperbaric Medicine: What Works and What Does Not?" Posted on* Quackwatch.com *on July 18, 2001.*
[7] American Board of Allergy and Immunology, *www.abai.org.*
[8] American Board of Medical Genetics, *www.abmg.org.*
[9] American Board of Pediatrics, *www.abp.org.*
[10] American Board of Physical Medicine and Rehabilitation, *www.abpmr.org.*
[11] American Board of Psychiatry and Neurology, *www.abpn.com.*
[12] Ibid.
[13] American Board of Anesthesiology, *www.theaba.org.*
[14] American Board of Surgery, *www.absurgery.org.*
[15] American Board of Thoracic Surgery, *www.abts.org.*
[16] American Board of Colon and Rectal Surgery, *www.abcrs.org.*
[17] US Department of Labor, Occupational Outlook Handbook, at *www.bls.gov/oco/ocos101.htm*
[18] American Board of Neurological Surgery, *www.abns.org.*
[19] American Board of Orthopaedic Surgery, *www.abos.org.*
[20] American Board of Otolaryngology, *www.aboto.org.*
[21] American Board of Plastic Surgery, *www.abplsurg.org.*
[22] American Board of Urology, *www.abu.org.*
[23] American Board of Obstetrics and Gynecology, *www.abog.org.*
[24] American Board of Dermatology, *www.abderm.org.*
[25] American Board of Ophthalmology, *www.abop.org.*
[26] American Board of Radiology, *www.theabr.org.*
[27] American Board of Nuclear Medicine, *www.abnw.snm.org.*
[28] American Board of Pathology, *www.abpath.org.*
[29] US Department of Labor, Occupational Outlook Handbook, at *www.bls.gov/oco/ocos101.htm*
[30] US Department of Labor, Occupational Outlook Handbook, at *www.bls.gov/oco/ocos101.htm*
[31] American Board of General Dentistry, *www.abgd.org.*
[32] American Board of Endodontics, *www.aae.org/certboard.*
[33] American Board of Oral and Maxillofacial Surgery, *www.aboms.org.*
[34] American Board of Orthodontics, *www.americanboardortho.com*
[35] American Board of Periodontology, *www.period.org/amboard.*

CHAPTER

14

Complementary, Alternative, and Naturopathic Medicine

The natural healing force within each one of us is the greatest force in getting well. — Hippocrates

When Em and I first met Arnold, the owner of a raw food café in Lansdale, Pennsylvania, he didn't say a word to us. Instead, he crouched down slightly to gaze at Emmalea's face. Em cast me a sidelong glance and arched her eyebrow, but I could only shrug. I was just as confused as she was. Then, with a quick look to Em as though asking permission, he took her hands in his. He gently examined them, running his fingers against her nails before standing tall, his arms crossed against his chest. Finally, he said, "I think you have a neurological problem. Probably seizures." Our jaws dropped. My stunned eyes met Emmalea's, and I knew we were thinking along the same lines: Dr. Herzog's description of animal research was nothing compared to this. What was the source of Arnold's knowledge? He explained to us that the dark circles under Em's eyes and the whitish flecks on her fingernails led him to the diagnosis. We hadn't come to Arnold's for medical advice, and we certainly didn't come for a diagnosis. However, we left with an entirely new perspective. What we got from Arnold was not only an astonishing diagnosis from someone who wasn't a health professional, but a thought-provoking lesson in the advantages of a raw food diet, which is really more a way of life, than a diet.

I had read initially about the raw food philosophy in Natalia Rose's books, *Raw Food: Life Force Energy* and *The Raw Food Detox Diet.*[1] In her books, she also provides a listing of raw food resources. Arnold's Way was listed under the resources in Pennsylvania. So we decided to check it out. Both Natalia and Arnold described the same benefits of a raw food diet. The lifestyle involves eating only or primarily "living foods" like fresh organic fruits and vegetables, sprouted grains, germinated nuts, vegetable juices, and cooking nothing above 110 degrees. Foods in their natural states are very easy for the body to digest. As a result, your body can focus on keeping itself as healthy as possible instead of trying to figure out how to process the unending stream of foreign substances that we typically take into our bodies. This is a very simple explanation of the raw food diet. I have included a list of Raw Food resources in an appendix at the end of the book, if you are interested in learning more.

When I first read about the raw food lifestyle, I was intrigued by the prospect of how it might help anyone with a health condition, including epilepsy. Most of the resources talked about how raw food diets have helped individuals with cancer, diabetes, hypertension and other chronic conditions. At the very least, it appeared to be worth investigating.

As Arnold was finishing his lecture to us on the basics of a raw food diet, he began to list out foods that needed to be eliminated from our diets. His list included sugar, wheat, dairy and, of course, anything cooked above 110 degrees. That list accounted for about 70 percent of our current diets. One last thing he said that was extremely important for Em was that she avoid eating soy products. Em and I were a little unsure about this last statement. At the time, Emmalea was a vegan, meaning that she eliminated not only animal products, but also dairy products from her diet. Because of this, soy had been her primary source of protein for the past two years. Eliminating soy, in addition to his other list of foods, from her diet would mean changing about 95 percent of the foods she consumed regularly. As we left, we thanked Arnold and decided to take *most* of his advice.

About a month later, during our visit with Dr. Herzog at Harvard, we heard the word "soy" again. During that visit, he explained that estrogen is a seizure-provoking drug. Soy products, Dr. Herzog explained, contain phytoestrogens – chemicals that mimic the action of estrogens. He stressed the importance of avoiding these types of foods and urged Emmalea to immediately cut them out of her diet. From that day forward, Em officially gave up soy products. In addition, she began using Dr. Herzog's natural progesterone cream every month, to balance what he believed was a deficiency in progesterone production. Since these additions to her treatment regimen, she has had the longest seizure-free stretch yet.

Because we didn't change just one intervention at a time, we may never know the exact reason for her seizure control. Within a one month time period, Emmalea modified her diet by giving up soy and including some components of a raw lifestyle, began using natural progesterone, and changed her AED from Lamictal to Keppra, due to a bad reaction to the original medication. However, all evidence points to the fact that the complementary use of progesterone and diet changes along with her AEDs produced the success that drugs alone could not.

Depending on your philosophy and health needs, complementary and alternative medicine (CAM) may or may not be an option for you. As you read this chapter about CAM, use your VVMS from chapter 1 as a guide to decide for yourself whether CAM may be beneficial to you and how best to incorporate it into your overall health plan.

WHAT IS CAM? (COMPLEMENTARY AND ALTERNATIVE MEDICINE)

CAM is a group of diverse medical and healthcare systems, practices, and products that are not presently considered conventional medicine. Conventional medicine (sometimes also referred to as *allopathic medicine*) is medicine as practiced by holders of MD (medical doctor) or DO (doctor of osteopathy) degrees and by their allied health professionals, such as physical therapists and registered nurses.

Healthcare providers use complementary medicine *with* conventional medicine. For example, they may use aromatherapy to help lessen a patient's discomfort following surgery. In comparison, CAM providers use alternative medicine *in place of* conventional medicine. An example of an alternative therapy is using a special diet to treat cancer instead of surgery, radiation, or chemotherapy.

As scientists prove through more clinical trials that CAM therapies are safe and effective, more providers are likely to adopt them into conventional healthcare. As new approaches to healthcare emerge, the list of CAM therapies changes as well. Some examples of current mainstream treatments that began as CAM approaches include using fish oil to treat heart disease, depression, bipolar disorder, and arthritis; glucosamine to treat arthritis; probiotics (good bacteria) to treat irritable bowel syndrome; and acupuncture for headache pain.

The National Center for Complementary and Alternative Medicine (NCCAM) is the federal government's lead agency for scientific research on CAM. It began receiving funding in 1992 and, in 1993, moved within the National Institutes of Health (NIH). However, it has only been operating near its current funding level since 2002. NCCAM's mission is to explore complementary and alternative healing practices in the context of rigorous science, train CAM researchers, and disseminate authoritative information to the public and professionals. NIH's recognition gives CAM much needed credibility to grow. NIH acknowledges that CAM is always evolving. NCCAM's Web site (*www.nccam.nih.gov*) contains many extensive resources if you are interested in exploring CAM further.[2]

MAINSTREAM MDS WITH A CAM APPROACH

Many physicians take a CAM approach to diagnosing and treating patients, using both CAM and conventional medicine. The physicians discussed in this section are all leaders in complementary medicine.

These physicians are well known for their publications, radio shows, or other public promotion of CAM.

One way to find traditional physicians with a CAM approach is to look for members of state naturopathic associations who have both an MD and an ND. Alternatively, look for MD members of naturopathic associations in your area. For example, see the California Naturopathic Medical Association Web site at *www.calnd.org.* It shows that about one-third of their advisory board members are MDs. An MD who is affiliated with a naturopathic association is going to be familiar with and advocate CAM practices. When you select a physician, discuss your needs to make sure you find the right one for you. You can learn more about some successful approaches to CAM from the publications and teachings of the physicians described below.

Ronald L. Hoffman, MD

I started listening to Dr. Hoffman's *Health Talk* radio show long before I ever heard the phrase *complementary and alternative medicine* or the acronym CAM. His depth of knowledge and the way he applies it simply and logically to each patient's concerns has won him much success. He is one of the few physicians willing to give advice over the radio to countless patients each year. A pioneer in CAM, he summarized the most common concerns of patients in his 1997 book, *Intelligent Medicine: A Guide to Optimizing Health and Preventing Illness for the Baby-Boomer Generation.* This book was billed as "featuring the best of alternative and mainstream approaches."[3]

After taking a four-year hiatus following college, Hoffman decided to study medicine. He previously had run with the Beat poets in New York City, so he had a lot of catching up to do. He earned his MD degree from Albert Einstein School of Medicine and kept his focus on CAM. In his 2006 book, *How to Talk with Your Doctor: A Guide for Patients and Their Physicians Who Want to Reconcile and Use the Best of Conventional and Alternative Medicine,* Hoffman cites these advantages of a CAM approach:[4]

- Patient-centered care

- Lower toxicity and fewer side effects
- Emphasizes the doctor-patient relationship
- Engenders hope
- Focuses on prevention
- Addresses concerns ignored by mainstream medicine
- Makes the patient an active participant in care (most important of all)

In his books, Dr. Hoffman considers the best approaches to certain conditions: conventional or alternative treatment, or a combination of both. Dr. Hoffman believes that conventional treatment is the best approach to certain problems like heart attacks and trauma. However, he believes alternative medicine is the best approach for conditions like back pain, chronic fatigue, irritable bowel syndrome, mild infections, and obesity. For conditions like osteoporosis, hypertension, headaches, diabetes, and anxiety/depression, Dr. Hoffman has found that the use of both alternative and conventional approaches is best.[5]

Mehmet C. Oz, MD

Although he has many medical accomplishments, Dr. Oz's most significant contribution to the healthcare world is his persistent determination to educate patients to take responsibility for understanding their bodies and taking better care of themselves. In addition to patient responsibility, Dr. Oz focuses on basic nutrition and self-management. While the concept of patient responsibility is not limited to CAM practitioners, he has inspired tens of millions of Americans in a very short time. A regular guest on the *Oprah Winfrey Show,* he is likely to reach millions more.

In one of his first books, *Healing from the Heart: A Leading Surgeon Combines Eastern and Western Traditions to Create the Medicine of the Future,* he discusses his willingness to explore complementary approaches to traditional medicine with his patients.[6] But his first big splash into the American conscious came with the publication of *YOU: The Owners Manual: An Insider's Guide to the Body that Will Make You Healthier and Younger,* which he co-authored with Michael Roizen, MD.[7] The book is a must-read.

If you prefer, watch Dr. Oz talk you through and demonstrate heart bypass surgery, digestive disorders, or any other number of problematic health conditions on *Discovery Health.* You can also order DVDs from the Discovery Health Web site (*health.discovery.com*). Dr. Oz and Dr. Roizen also have written *YOU: On a Diet: The Owner's Manual for Waist Management,* and *YOU: The Smart Patient: An Insiders Handbook for Getting the Best Treatment.* Most recently, the two physicians have collaborated on an inspiring audio book, *YOU: On a Walk.*

Andrew Weil, MD

Dr. Weil, a Harvard Medical School graduate, is probably most famous for his series of books on integrative medicine with a focus on healing. In one of his first books, *Spontaneous Healing: How to Discover and Embrace Your Body's Natural Ability to Maintain and Heal Itself,* he explores different case studies of patients told they had no hope of recovery, but somehow, with no intervention, survived and thrived.[8] These spontaneously healed patients often had some belief system, practices, or other approaches that influenced their ability to thrive in the face of what appeared to be a fatal diagnosis. Dr. Weil describes his desire to see NIH's complementary medicine services evolve to focus on the overall concept of healing.

Dr. Weil's books, CDs, and Internet resources are probably the best available on natural healing. He has compiled an excellent history and overview of homeopathic medicine. In most of the alternative treatment he describes, he uses himself as an example. He describes in detail his gastrointestinal problem that mainstream physicians treated unsuccessfully. When he visited an MD trained in homeopathic medicine, his cure using a homeopathic tincture was successful. In his description, Dr. Weil does not pretend to understand the mechanism that cured him, just that it happened. His books explore numerous facets of CAM through research, personal, and professional methods.

Christiane Northrup, MD

Dr. Christiane Northrup, an author and former practicing OB/GYN physician, is known for her empowering approach to women's health and wellness. She believes that, "Once you engage your own inner wisdom, you can change or improve your habits of thought, your emotions, and your behaviors and create a more positive and joyful life experience right away," and, "This process, when engaged in regularly, heals both your present and your future." Dr. Northrup is a leading proponent of medicine and healing that acknowledges the unity of the mind and body, as well as the powerful role of the human spirit in creating health. She has written several health resource books since 1994 including, *Women's Bodies, Women's Wisdom, The Wisdom of Menopause: Creating Physical and Emotional Health and Healing During the Change* and *Mother-Daughter Wisdom: Understanding the Crucial Link Between Mothers, Daughters, and Health.* Dr. Northrup is dedicated to helping women learn how to create health in their lives.[9]

Dean Ornish, MD

Dr. Ornish is one of the first mainstream physicians to contemplate and act on a holistic hunch he had about a traditional clinical belief. He challenged the premise taught in medical schools that once a patient developed hardening of the arteries of the heart, it is reversible only with surgery. Dr. Ornish challenged this notion not only through individual patient case studies, but he also proved it through a formalized clinical trial research study. He showed in his study that CAM practices could not only stop the progression of coronary artery disease, but also reverse it through meditation, a low-fat vegetarian diet, smoking cessation, and regular exercise. His study, published in 1990, is one of the few clinical research trials using CAM methods.

Michael F. Roizen, MD

When I first saw Dr. Roizen on the *Oprah Winfrey Show* in 2004, he was promoting his best selling book, *Real Age: Are You as Young as You Can Be?*[10] I was so impressed with the clear, logical concepts in the book I bought several copies for my friends and relatives. Dr. Roizen uses several questions about medical history, financial and social stressors, eating habits (a lot about this topic), and other important areas to calculate whether your *real* age is higher or lower than your *chronological* age. You can assess your real age on his Web site at *www.realage.com* and receive a real age plan when finished.

Dr. Roizen takes a holistic approach to treating patients, and as co-author of the *You* series of books with Dr. Oz, he focuses on getting patients to take responsibility for their actions and treatment plans. Reaching tens of millions through his books, he has made significant strides in inspiring people to look at all possible contributors to health problems and to take action towards improvement.

Orrin Devinsky, MD

Dr. Devinsky, director of the New York University's Epilepsy Center, is the physician who was the first to provide effective treatment to Emmalea. He also is one of the editors of the book, *Complementary and Alternative Therapies for Epilepsy,* which profiles, among other things, Dr. Herzog's ground-breaking treatment of seizures using natural progesterone and details other possible therapies for epilepsy.[11] Emmalea uses progesterone as a complementary therapy to traditional anti-epileptic drugs.

Dr. Devinsky's willingness to break out of the mainstream mold and edit this book has made an incredible difference in Emmalea's life, and I am sure, in the lives of others who have epilepsy. After a first read of the book, I identified a list of seven CAM strategies for epilepsy. These included antioxidants (in the form of foods like sweet potatoes and carrots), 400 IU (International Units) of vitamin E daily, 50 to 150 milligrams of vitamin B-6 daily, zinc, copper, and magnesium supplements, and melatonin. While Dr. Devinsky does not endorse any of these treatments as singular solutions, he provides information for patients to make well-informed decisions.

Joel Fuhrman, MD

Fasting and Eating for Health: A Medical Doctor's Program for Conquering Disease, the title of Dr. Fuhrman's 1995 book, tells you a little something about his philosophy.[12] However, once you read the book, you realize he is speaking from experience. His father was cured of chronic arthritis after an almost month-long fast where he existed on nothing but water. After several physicians could do nothing for him, Dr. Fuhrman was able to cure his own chronic musculoskeletal condition with a 46-day water fast. This experience spurred him to leave professional figure skating (he was a member of the U.S. Olympic team) and enter medical school. He graduated from the University of Pennsylvania Medical School and currently practices in New Jersey.

In his new book, *Eat to Live: The Revolutionary Formula for Fast and Sustained Weight Loss*, Fuhrman helps readers learn to eat "right."[13] The front cover of the book quotes Dr. Mehmet Oz: "A medical breakthrough. If you give this diet your complete commitment, there is no question in my mind that it will work for you."

SIX PRINCIPLES OF NATUROPATHIC MEDICINE

Naturopathy is a school of medical philosophy and practice that focuses on improving health and treating disease chiefly by assisting the body's intrinsic ability to recuperate from illness and injury. According to the Association of Accredited Naturopathic Medical Colleges (www.aanmc.org), naturopathic doctors practice the following six principles:

1. **First do no harm.** The process of healing includes the manifestations of symptoms, so any therapy that interferes with this natural healing process by masking symptoms is considered suppressive and should be avoided.
2. **The healing power of nature.** The healing power of nature has two aspects: first, that the body has the ability to heal itself and it is the naturopathic doctor's role to facilitate this natural process; and second, that nature heals. Following this principle includes getting enough sleep, exercising, proper nutrition, and, if needed, additional "earth food," such as herbs or algae (a living organism). Plants can gently move the body into health without the side effects caused by some synthetic chemicals in modern pharmaceuticals.
3. **Identify and treat the cause.** For healing to take place, practitioners must remove the underlying root causes of disease. These root causes can exist at many levels: physical, mental, emotional, and spiritual. It is the naturopathic doctor's role to identify the root cause, as well as alleviate suffering by treating symptoms.
4. **Treat the whole person.** A core tenet of naturopathy is the belief that health must go beyond treatment of immediate symptoms and instead care for the person's entire well-being. That means treating the whole body, as well as the spirit, soul, and mind.
5. **The physician as teacher.** The naturopath's role also is to educate the patient in naturopathic practices and encourage patients to "take responsibility for their own health." This cooperative relationship between doctor and patient is essential to healing.
6. **Prevention.** The ultimate goal of the naturopathic physician is prevention. The emphasis is on building health, not fighting illness. NDs do this by fostering healthy lifestyles, healthy beliefs, and healthy relationships.

What Conditions Does the Naturopathic Doctor (ND) Treat?

A review of practitioners' Web sites and naturopathic medical schools provides information about the types of conditions that NDs commonly treat. According to the Association of Accredited Naturopathic Medical Colleges (*www.aanmc.org*), the top 10 conditions that NDs treat are:[14]

1. Fatigue
2. Menstruation/hormonal issues
3. Allergies
4. Depression/insomnia
5. Thyroid disorders
6. Weight/appetite problems
7. High Cholesterol
8. Headaches/migraines
9. High blood pressure
10. Fibromyalgia (pain of the connective tissues and muscles)

Naturopathic Medical Schools

Currently, there are six accredited naturopathic medical schools, four in the United States and two in Canada. They are:

- Bastyr University (Washington)
- Boucher Institute of Naturopathic Medicine (British Columbia)
- Canadian College of Naturopathic Medicine (Toronto)
- National College of Natural Medicine (Oregon)
- Southwest College of Naturopathic Medicine & Health Sciences (Arizona)
- University of Bridgeport College of Naturopathic Medicine (Connecticut)

ND Coursework

Figures 14.1–14.4 highlight the ND's four-year curriculum compared with the courses and topics in traditional medical schools. Because the definition of CAM is constantly changing, and mainstream medicine increasingly incorporates more CAM treatments there are fewer topics solely in the CAM list.

Figure 14. 1 ND Courses: Year 1

Courses in Both Naturopathic and Mainstream Medical Schools	Courses Specific to Naturopathic Medical Schools
Biochemistry 1 and 2	Naturopathic Clinical Theory
Human Anatomy 1, 2, and3	Principles of Chinese Medicine
Human Physiology 1, 2, and 3	Massage
Histology	Hydrotherapy
Embryology	Physiotherapy
Research Methods and Design	Fundamentals of Ayurvedic Medicine
Determinants of Health	Botanical Medicine 1
	Vis Medicatrix Naturae
	Hydrotherapy/Physiotherapy Lab
	Physician Heal Thyself

The number of required and elective courses in mainstream medical schools is much greater than those listed above. Most mainstream schools vary course titles, making it impossible to create one representative listing. Mainstream medical school students take at least the same numbers of hours of classroom training as naturopathic doctors. In addition, to become licensed physicians after graduation from medical school, MDs and DOs must complete a minimum of three years of full time residency practice. You can find information about MD training in chapter 12. As of the writing of this book, no national standards for residency requirements exist for NDs after graduation from naturopathic medical school.

Figure 14.2 ND Courses: Year 2

Courses in Both Naturopathic and Mainstream Medical Schools	Courses Specific to Naturopathic Medical Schools
Human Pathology 1, 2, and 3	Botanical Medicine 2 and 3
Immunology	Homeopathy 2 and 3
Clinical Lab Diagnosis 1 and 2	Naturopathic Counseling 1 and 2
Physical and Clinical Diagnosis	Foods, Dietary Systems and
Lecture and Lab	Assessment
Infectious Diseases	Macronutrients and Micronutrients
Pharmacology	Preceptorship
Clinic Practice	Naturopathic Manipulation

Figure 14.3 ND Courses: Year 3

Courses in Both Naturopathic and Mainstream Medical Schools	Courses Specific to Naturopathic Medical Schools
Normal Maternity	Botanical Medicine 4
Environmental Medicine	Naturopathic Manipulation 3
Public Health	Nutrient Therapy
Gastroenterology	Botanical Medicine Dispensary Lab
Eye, Ear, Nose, and Throat	Clinical Ecology
Sports Medicine	Naturopathic Case Management
Addictions and Psychiatric Disorders	
Clinical Practice	
Practice Management 1	
Neurology	
Pediatrics	
Family Medicine	
The Health Systems	
Cardiology	
Minor Surgery	
Medical Procedures	

Figure 14.4 ND Courses: Year 4

Courses in Both Naturopathic and Mainstream Medical Schools	Courses Specific to Naturopathic Medical Schools
Geriatrics	Naturopathic Case Analysis and Management
Urology	Advanced Naturopathic Therapeutics
Practice Management 2	Preceptorship
Radiographic Interpretation 1, 2, & 3	Jurisprudence
Pulmonary Medicine	
Clinical Practice	
Endocrinology	

Licensing of NDs

In states where NDs can diagnose and provide medical treatment, they must also pass a state examination. For the states that license NDs, the applicant is required to have a four-year undergraduate degree and a four-year ND degree from an accredited naturopathic medical school. In 2007, the 14 states that license NDs to practice medicine are: Alaska, Arizona, California, Connecticut, Hawaii, Idaho, Kansas, Maine, Montana, New Hampshire, Oregon, Utah, Vermont, and Washington.

EVOLUTION OF ACCEPTANCE

Any concept, like CAM, that is new or different from the traditional, endures a process to be accepted into conventional practice. In healthcare, this process includes government regulation, accreditation by professional associations, and even plaintiff lawsuits. Government regulation is necessary to ensure consistency and set minimum acceptable standards. It includes licensing the individual practitioners, educational institutions, and locations where care is provided. Both federal and state governments are involved in healthcare regulation. Self-policing agencies, such as associations and regulatory bodies, are also important. In traditional healthcare, respected non-governmental regulatory bodies, such as the Joint Commission on Accreditation of Healthcare Organizations and the National Committee for Quality

Assurance, set accreditation criteria for healthcare groups to ensure continuous, high-quality care. Other examples of self-policing agencies in conventional medicine include the Liaison Committee on Medical Education for medical schools and the Accreditation Council for Graduate Medical Education for residency programs.

Another self-regulating mechanism, sometimes used overzealously, is the medical malpractice lawsuit. Unfortunately, the pursuit of some medical malpractice cases without merit has caused many traditional (or allopathic) physicians to practice medicine defensively. However, when used legitimately, one of the benefits of medical malpractice actions is that they weed out incompetence in the profession. The primary objective of a legitimate medical malpractice suit is to prove that the healthcare practitioner's negligence harmed the patient. Generally, lawyers prove negligence by showing that the practitioner's treatment was below standards accepted in the profession. Therefore, to find a lawyer willing to represent you on a medical malpractice claim, well-published and well-practiced standards of care must exist in the profession.

There is not nearly the same level of published and accepted standards in naturopathic medicine as there is in mainstream medicine. The harm to the public from the lack of standards is that we are robbed of one of our abilities to eliminate incompetence in the profession. One way to increase the standard of care data is to increase the amount of data on successes and failures in the profession. There are two ways to do this. The first is by providing care to increasing numbers of patients. The second is to fund and conduct many studies on the treatments and their outcomes. We should be conducting studies first, and then, using the results of the studies to treat patients. While there are some published CAM studies, much more research is necessary. Most allopathic physicians, who support CAM but refuse to use it in their practices, cite the lack of sufficient research as the primary reason.

Because there is an increasing demand for CAM, it appears that patient treatment may continue to be the primary way of increasing data on CAM standards of care. If you have an interest in

CAM, do your own research of the industry. Use only licensed practitioners who have graduated from accredited schools. And use only practitioners who rigorously articulate the components of informed consent. (See chapter 8 for more details on informed consent.) You may also proactively use self-policing mechanisms to help weed out incompetence in the profession.

Healthcare Organizations with CAM Integration

Many academic medical centers and larger hospitals today have integrated CAM into their practices, usually through an Integrative Medicine Program. The program at the University of Arizona that Andrew Weil, MD, directs is a good example. These programs focus on fusing the best of Western allopathic medicine (drugs and surgery) with alternative approaches to health and healing. AANMC, which supports the academic efforts of accredited schools of naturopathic medicine, discusses many of the recent trends in CAM on its Web site, including the following:

- More than 80 million Americans use CAM every year
- Sixty-eight percent of adults have used at least one kind of CAM therapy
- At least one-third of cancer patients turn to a CAM therapy, used in combination with mainstream treatment
- Sixty-seven percent of HMOs offer at least one form of alternative care
- Eighty-five percent of HMOs think traditional and alternative medical care will grow closer in the future
- From 1998 to 2000, the number of hospitals offering alternative therapies nearly doubled

The Federal Government's Acceptance of CAM

The federal government has only recently begun to accept CAM as a legitimate treatment for some conditions. A big step for CAM came in March 2002. The White House Commission on Complementary and

Alternative Medicine Policy presented to President George W. Bush its recommended blueprint for increasing public access to safe and effective CAM healthcare services. While not approved as of 2007, full implementation of the report's recommendations would fundamentally change CAM legislation and expedite the integration of CAM into U.S. mainstream medicine.

According to the AANMC, the White House Commission on CAM Policy report contains 104 action steps and 29 recommendations, including:[15]

- Improve public access to CAM providers by removing inappropriate barriers to insurance coverage
- Incorporate CAM concepts and practices into federal and corporate health promotion
- Increase financial support for CAM research
- Provide education on CAM practices and professions to conventional practitioners
- Make available CAM education grants, including curriculum and faculty development
- Offer assistance to states to develop consistent regulatory standards

Alternative to Mainstream: The Story of Osteopathic Medicine

Twenty-seven accredited osteopathic medical schools exist in the United States compared to the 125 accredited mainstream medical schools. DOs participate in the same residency programs as MDs, though this was not always the case. The story of osteopathic medicine is included in this chapter as an example of an alternative form of medical treatment that eventually became part of mainstream American medicine. Looking at this process may help to understand CAM's evolution better.

Dissatisfied with mainstream medical care, Andrew Taylor Still, MD, founded osteopathy in 1876. Two osteopathic medical schools still carry his name. He believed that mainstream physicians of his time over-prescribed harsh and often toxic medications. His vision was that someday "rational medical therapy" would include manipulation of the musculoskeletal system and surgery, and sparingly use drugs. He believed that a disordered musculoskeletal system caused disease and dysfunction. He further held that by diagnosing and treating the musculoskeletal system, doctors could spare patients the negative side effects of drugs.

By the early 1900s, providers incorporated proven osteopathic medicine into mainstream medical practices, resulting in DOs and MDs practicing together. The complete integration process for osteopathic medicine into mainstream medicine took about 70 years. During that time, many heated debates and disagreements about the legitimate role of the osteopathic medical doctor occurred.

One of the key turning points in osteopathic medical history was a 1967 decision of the California Medical Association to convert physicians with a DO degree to an MD designation instead. The California Supreme Court reversed the decision in 1974. Had the court upheld the 1967 decision, it would have essentially eliminated the DO designation, at least in California.

Also in the late 1960s, the U.S. Army made a controversial decision to allow DOs to enter the military as physicians. Over time, a study of the conflict and conflict-resolution activities around osteopathic medicine may provide a benchmark for what to expect with CAM.

Side-by-Side with Mainstream: Podiatric Medicine

Podiatric medicine focuses on diagnosing and treating foot, ankle, and lower extremity disorders. Although orthopedic surgeons treat musculoskeletal disorders, in the early 1900s there was no medical profession dedicated to foot and ankle care and treatment. Dr. Scholl, the owner of the name on Dr. Scholl's footwear and foot care products, is the father of podiatric medicine. He started his career in a shoe store and then became so concerned with customers' painful foot conditions that he enrolled in medical school. He earned his MD degree at Illinois

Medical College and made it his life-long mission to improve the health, comfort, and well-being of people through their feet.

In 1912, he founded the second college of podiatric medicine in the United States. Today, podiatrists must attend four years of medical school through one of the eight podiatric medical schools in the United Stated to receive a Doctor of Podiatric Medicine (DPM) degree. Then, they must complete a two- or three-year residency program and meet state licensing requirements.

While podiatric medicine is not an alternative or complementary healthcare approach, it is a good example of filling an unmet need in the medical community. Both Dr. Scholl and Dr. Still began their careers in mainstream medicine, identified deficiencies or gaps in healthcare, and created solutions that eventually took hold in mainstream medicine. Both men are good examples of medical entrepreneurs.

Another Alternative: Chiropractic Medicine

A complementary and alternative healthcare profession, chiropractic medicine focuses on diagnosing and treating mechanical disorders of the spine and musculoskeletal system. The treatments are designed to affect the nervous system and improve overall health. Doctors of Chiropractic medicine (DCs or chiropractors) practice a drug-free, hands-on approach to healthcare that includes physical examination, diagnosis, and treatment. Chiropractors have broad diagnostic skills with training to recommend therapeutic and rehabilitative exercises, as well as to provide nutritional, dietary, and lifestyle counseling.

In the early 1900s, chiropractors' philosophy of the supremacy of the "nerve" differentiated chiropractic medicine from osteopathic medicine (with its supremacy of the "artery" philosophy). Today, there are 19 chiropractic medical schools in the United States, all four-year programs, each requiring a minimum of 90 undergraduate credit hours (about three years). As chiropractic medicine moved into the mid-1900s with licensing in all states, the profession made sure that MDs and DOs did not regulate them. Chiropractors feared they might lose their identity, and be absorbed like osteopathic medicine was into mainstream medicine. (For more information, visit the American Chiropractic Association's Web site at *www. amerchiro.org.*)

FIVE MAJOR TYPES OF COMPLEMENTARY AND ALTERNATIVE MEDICINE

NCCAM describes the following five types of CAM:

1. **Whole Medical Systems** are built upon complete systems of theory and practice. Often, these systems have evolved apart from and earlier than the conventional U.S. medical approach. Examples of whole medical systems that have developed in Western cultures include homeopathic medicine and naturopathic medicine. Examples of systems that have developed in non-Western cultures include traditional Chinese medicine and Ayurveda.
2. **Mind-Body Medicine** uses a variety of techniques to enhance the mind's capacity to affect bodily functions and symptoms. Some techniques previously considered CAM are now mainstream treatments (for example, patient support groups and cognitive-behavioral therapy). Other mind-body techniques still considered CAM include meditation, prayer, mental healing, and therapies that use creative outlets such as art, music, or dance.
3. **Biologically-Based Practices** use substances found in nature, such as herbs, foods, and vitamins. These practices include dietary supplements, herbal products, and other so-called *natural* but scientifically unproven therapies (for example, using shark cartilage to treat cancer).
4. **Manipulative and Body-Based Practices** use manipulation and movement of one or more parts of the body. Some examples include chiropractic or osteopathic manipulation, and massage.
5. **Energy Medicine** involves the use of energy fields. There are two types. Providers use biofield therapies to affect energy fields that purportedly surround and penetrate the human body. Scientists have yet to prove such fields exist. Some forms of energy therapy manipulate biofields by applying pressure to and manipulating the

body by placing the hands in or through these fields. Examples include Qigong, Reiki, and therapeutic touch. Bioelectromagnetic-based therapies involve the unconventional use of electromagnetic fields, such as pulsed fields, magnetic fields, or alternating-current or direct-current fields.

Is CAM for You?

The NIH-sponsored CAM Web site (*www.nccam.hih.gov*) provides good suggestions for determining how to find a qualified naturopathic doctor or other CAM practitioner. These suggestions are summarized as follows:[16]

1. Speak with your primary healthcare providers regarding the therapy you are interested in. Ask if they have a recommendation.
2. Make a list of CAM practitioners and gather information about each before making your first appointment. Ask basic questions about their credentials and practice: Where did you receive your training? What licenses or certifications do you have? How much will the treatment cost?
3. Check with your insurer to see if they will cover the cost of therapy.
4. After you select a practitioner, make a list of questions to ask at your first visit. You may want to bring a friend or family member who can help you ask questions and note answers.
5. Come to the first visit prepared to answer questions about your health history, including injuries, surgeries, and major illnesses, as well as prescription medicines, vitamins, and other supplements you may take.
6. Assess your first visit and decide if the practitioner is right for you. Did you feel comfortable with the practitioner? Could the practitioner answer your questions? Did he respond to you satisfactorily? Does the treatment plan seem reasonable and acceptable to you?

Key Highlights

CAM is a diverse group of medical systems, practices, and products that conventional medicine does not consider to be standard treatment. Complementary medicine is used *along with* conventional medicine. And, alternative medicine is used *in place of* conventional medicine. Over time, many CAM practices (like acupuncture for headaches) have become part of traditional, mainstream practices. A licensed ND or an MD with CAM training is most qualified to practice CAM. Through the Center for Complementary and Alternative Medicine (CAM), the federal government supports and researches CAM practices. Government regulation, accreditation by professional associations, and increased development of CAM standards of care must be expanded so that quality in CAM care can be assured.

Key Actions

- Read some of the books written by MDs mentioned in this chapter to get a better idea of CAM.
- Ask your primary care provider if some type of CAM might be a good option for you.
- Research CAM at AANMC's Web site at www.aanmc.org.

Key Take-Away

It is important to educate yourself objectively about all available healthcare options to help you make the best possible decisions for your healthcare.

Endnotes

---

[1] Rose, Natalia. Raw Food: Life Force Energy. HarperCollins, 2007 and The Raw Food Detox Diet, HarperCollins, 2005.
[2] National Center for Complementary and Alternative Medicine, *www.nccam.nih.gov.*
[3] Hoffman, Ronald L., MD. *Intelligent Medicine: A Guide to Optimizing Health and Preventing Illness for the Baby-Boomer Generation.* Fireside, 1997.

[4] Hoffman, Ronald L., MD. *How to Talk with Your Doctor: A Guide for Patients and Their Physicians Who Want to Reconcile and Use the Best of Conventional and Alternative Medicine.* Basic Health Publications, 2006.
[5] Ibid.
[6] Oz, Mehmet C., MD. *Healing from the Heart: A Leading Surgeon Combines Eastern and Western Traditions to Create the Medicine of the Future.* Plume, 1999.
[7] Oz, Mehmet C., MD; and Roizen, Michael, MD. *YOU: The Owners Manual: An Insider's Guide to the Body that Will Make You Healthier and Younger.* Collins, 2005. (See information on other *You* books in the bibliography in the back of this book.)
[8] Weil, Andrew, MD. *Spontaneous Healing: How to Discover and Embrace Your Body's Natural Ability to Maintain and Heal Itself.* The Ballantine Publishing Group, 1995. (For more Dr. Weil products, go to *www.drweil.com.*)
[9] For information about all of Christiane Northrup's books and other products, go to *www.drnorthrup.com.*
[10] Roizen, Michael F., MD. *Real Age: Are You as Young as You Can Be?* Cliff Street Books, 1999.
[11] Devinsky,Orrin, MD; Schachter, Steven C., MD; and Pacia, Steven, MD. *Complementary and Alternative Therapies for Epilepsy.* Demos Medical Publishing, 2005.
[12] Fuhrman, Joel, MD. *Fasting and Eating for Health: A Medical Doctor's Program for Conquering Disease.* St. Martin's Press, 1995.
[13] Fuhrman, Joel, MD. *Eat to Live: The Revolutionary Formula for Fast and Sustained Weight Loss.* Little, Brown and Company, 2005.
[14] Association of Accredited Naturopathic Medical Colleges (*www.aanmc.org*).
[15] The White House Commission on Complementary and Alternative Medicine Policy report is available at *whccamp.hhs.gov.*
[16] The NIH-sponsored CAM Web site *www.nccam.hih.gov.*

STEP

6

KNOW THE PLACES

CHAPTER

15

Serving as the Common Thread in a Fragmented System of Healthcare

That which is static and repetitive is boring. That which is dynamic and random is confusing. In between lies art. —John A. Locke

In the summer of 2006, I ran the New York borough half-marathons, five half-marathons in all. I finished the last one of the summer, the Bronx half-marathon, and beat my own personal record by 8 seconds. I finished with an average 7 minute 26 second mile. What I did not realize at the time was that the heavy training miles combined with the long-distance racing efforts were destroying my body, the result of which was a complete stress fracture of my pelvis.

An orthopedic surgeon diagnosed my fracture initially, based primarily upon my symptoms. A radiologist performed an MRI at a nearby diagnostic center to confirm the diagnosis. But when the radiologist was not able to give a definitive diagnosis, I decided to seek input from a sports medicine physician. During my third outing to have the condition assessed, the sports medicine physician definitively diagnosed the stress fracture. She designed a comprehensive treatment plan. She gave me a list of *do's* and *don'ts.* Then, she sent me to a lab for blood tests to rule out a thyroid disorder and for a bone density scan to rule out osteoporosis. She also prescribed 12 weeks of physical therapy and recommended a physical therapy group in yet a different location.

For the next four months, as my fracture healed, I bounced back and forth among providers at six different locations. With the exception of the fact that the MRI physician faxed the MRI results to my orthopedic physician, none of these healthcare providers interacted directly with each other. Instead, they all used copies of the MRI or medical records I brought with me to each visit.

No one asked me to cart around the information. No one told me it was my responsibility. I knew if I did not have the original information, there was a good chance the providers would make assumptions that might lead to less-than-the-best diagnosis and treatment. In all, I received diagnostic and therapeutic care for my fracture in the following locations:

- Orthopedic surgeon's office
- MRI facility
- Sports medicine physician's office
- Laboratory
- DEXA (bone density) scan office
- Physical therapy office

I was the only common thread among all of these locations. If I had arrived at the sports medicine physician's office without my MRI films, the doctor would have ordered additional, unnecessary testing for me, and the healthcare system would have incurred additional costs. And, if I had not taken the results of my DEXA scan to the physical therapy office, the therapy program designed for me might not have been aggressive enough and my healing time may have increased. So you see, the information that you bring from place to place helps the healthcare provider in each location to give you the best possible care.

THE EVOLUTION OF WHERE YOU RECEIVE CARE—ONE TO MANY LOCATIONS

Three generations ago, healthcare was provided in the hospital or the physician's office. Care provided in the hospital was often charitable because all hospitals were nonprofit and affiliated with a religious organization or government entity. In the 1940s, U.S. employers began to use private health insurance for the first time as a benefit to attract and retain employees.[1] From 1950 to 1970, the size of the healthcare industry increased from $1.2 million to $3 million employees and healthcare expenditures increased from $12.7 billion to $71.6 billion.[2] Today, U.S. healthcare expenditures are about $2 trillion. In addition to rising costs over the past several decades, the U.S. healthcare system has become a much more complex web of delivery mechanisms. Five main factors contribute to the increasing complexity of the healthcare system:[3]

- Advanced technologies used to diagnose and treat patients
- Higher frequency of use of medical and surgical specialists
- Growing costs of healthcare
- Increased use of testing
- Growing number of medical malpractice claims

A decade or more ago, a physician would have only ordered an x-ray of my fractured pelvis for my post-running pain. Even with a negative x-ray report, given my symptoms and the physician's expertise, the diagnosis and treatment would have been the same—stress fracture with crutches initially and no impact exercise for four months. Although my MRI may not have actually been necessary, it did provide the confirmation I needed.

You may need to go to more than one location to treat one condition. From your perspective, you can easily see all of your different visits as being part of the same overall treatment for one problem. However, each provider in each location views your condition somewhat differently. Like looking through a telescope, they see only the part of your care that they are involved in. Everything outside of that view gets cut out of the picture. Information from every provider at every location who previously treated you for the same condition can widen the view and give each of your providers a better perspective on your care.

As an example of the fragmentation within the healthcare system, figure 15.1 shows the number of different healthcare locations the average patient who has a hip fracture and requires a hip replacement is likely to encounter. Each location creates a unique medical record for this patient. The typical patient may or may not need to receive care in all of these locations.

Figure 15.1 Typical Treatment Locations for a Patient with a Hip Fracture in Need of a Hip Replacement

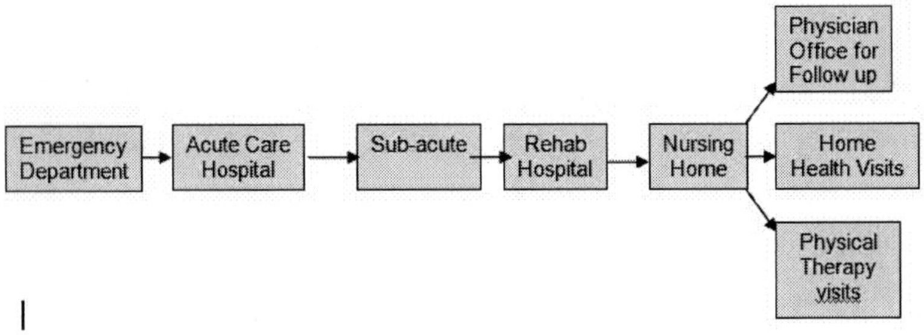

Each location is designed to deliver the best quality and decreased cost of healthcare for that level of care. And, each location creates another medical record for the care you receive there. Consequently, when multiple providers in multiple locations are involved, your medical records, all addressing the same condition or illness, are extensive, fragmented and poorly coordinated.

Even as fragmented as it is, most people consider healthcare in the United States to be the best in the world. But, unless you are the catalyst to ensure all your information gets to each provider at every treatment location, you may have less than the best outcomes. For example, besides having unnecessary testing, you may end up taking medications that do not interact well.

Many healthcare teams recognize the importance of coordinating your health information. If you request, they will assist in sending your records to providers in other locations. When providers forward copies of your records don't assume the records get to the right place. Providers at some locations are better than others at integrating records from another location. You or your medical mentor should take responsibility to ensure continuity by following up with each location where you received care.

Are the Contents and Format of All Records the Same?

Every provider creates his own version of your story. While ideally the basic content of medical records should be the same or similar, there are differences due to approach, clinician training, time, and regulations. As you review your own medical records you will see different approaches used to document information in various locations. An example of a difference in format is when one provider allows physicians to document your history and physical "freehand," while other providers may use a specific form to document specific information. If your physician uses a detailed form, your record may contain more particulars about your care.

The amount of training provided to physicians, residents, and other clinicians also impacts the content of your medical record. More intensive training may result in more attention to detail in medical record documentation. Some locations assign a higher priority to training than others. For example, acute care hospitals usually provide more training about documentation practices than nursing homes or physician offices.

The amount of time available to a physician to document can impact your record. In emergency rooms, a fast-paced environment, providers write their progress notes very quickly. In acute care, also a fast-paced environment, providers make up for some of the time limitations in part, by using additional resources, like residents and mid-level practitioners. Time limitations are not as great in rehabilitation or skilled nursing locations. Regulations also set minimum standards regarding the amount of documentation. For example, in the acute care hospital, physicians are required to document at least one progress note per day in your record. In other settings, like some nursing homes, the attending physician must only document once per week or less.

WHERE CAN I RECEIVE CARE?

The numbers and types of locations where you can receive healthcare in this country are extensive and continue to grow. One contributing factor is the increasing number of physician entrepreneurs who have created their versions of services provided in hospitals. These service locations include urgi-care centers, diagnostic-testing facilities, ambulatory surgery centers, and specialty hospitals often dedicated to heart surgery.

A summary of most types of healthcare provider settings categorized using location and length-of-stay criteria follows. I also include a description of common types of services provided or conditions treated at each location. This is not a complete list of healthcare locations. And keep in mind that your choices, particularly of outpatient locations, continue to grow. Through all of your visits, you remain the one common thread.

Outpatient Locations

You will not spend more than 23 hours in an outpatient location. In most cases, you will be there for a much shorter time. In some locations, such as the physician office, you will need to schedule an appointment. In others, like the ER, an appointment is not required. If you know that you need care in one or more locations, it will be helpful to determine what your local options are. Find out details, such as the size, ownership, and any affiliations with hospitals or other centers. You can find JCAHO quality and accreditation information on their Quality Check Web site at *www.qualitycheck.org.*

Physician Office

The most common location for a physician-patient encounter in the United States is the physician office. You visit your physician either because you have a specific health complaint or for a physical examination. If you are an established patient, the Department of Health and Human Services estimates that your physician will spend an average of 16 minutes with you, more if you are a new patient. In

2005, 963.9 million visits were made to physician offices, or an average of three visits per person. This accounts for 27 percent of all spending in healthcare.[4]

Is the size of the physician practice important to you? Are you more comfortable seeing a solo practitioner or a physician who is part of a small or large group? Your VVMS from chapter 1 will help you answer these questions. According to the AMA, about one-third of physicians are in solo practice. About 25 percent are in groups of two to four physicians, 15 percent are in groups of five to nine physicians, 17 percent are in groups of 10 to 49, and 5 percent are in groups with more than 50 physicians.[5] These statistics give you some idea of physicians available by practice size.

The most frequent conditions seen in physician offices in 2005 were hypertension, arthritis, hyperlipidemia (high levels of lipids or fatty molecules), diabetes preventive care, immunizations, and annual exams. Physician office appointments include visits to primary care, specialists, and surgeons. In 2005, 52 percent of all physician office visits were to primary care physicians. The number of visits increases each year.[6]

Clinics: Non-Academic Medical Centers

Most clinics provide services similar to those in a physician's office. They are usually sponsored and managed by a government entity, community, or religious organization. Clinics typically focus on primary care, but may also provide obstetrical and gynecological, dental, mental health and substance abuse services.

The federal government provides nationwide free-clinic care through the Health Resources and Services Administration (HRSA). You can find clinic locations on the HRSA Web site (*ask.hrsa.gov/pc*). Most of these clinics provide primary medical, obstetrical and gynecological, dental, mental health, and substance abuse services. The federal government's definition of a clinic requires that the facility meet the following test of physician participation: three or more physicians practicing medicine together provide the clinic's medical services, and at least one physician is present during all clinic hours to perform medical services. Residents often provide a lot of the services at clinics.

The most common services clinics provide are immunizations, prenatal and post-natal care, and contraception. The most common conditions clinics treat are allergic reactions, asthma (mild to moderate wheezing), broken bones, burns (minor), cuts (minor), dehydration, diarrhea, earaches and infections, low fevers, rashes and bumps, sprains, and sore throats.

Clinics: Academic Medical Centers (AMCs)

The depth and breadth of care academic medical centers (AMCs) provide is significantly different from other types of clinics. For most AMCs, *clinic* is simply a term to describe services offered in one specialty or subspecialty area, in one location, by a group of physicians employed by or affiliated with an AMC. In some ways, AMC clinics are large, multi-specialty, physician office practices. Physicians in these clinics are either employed by or affiliated with the AMC.

Stanford Hospital Clinics is a group of about 70 different specialty clinics. Many of the clinics are highly specialized, like the pigmented lesion clinic, the sleep disorder clinic, the women's health clinic, or the obesity clinic. Specialized AMC clinics do not have specific financial need criteria to see a physician. In fact, if you have a specific problem and are not sure how to find the best specialist, a specialty clinic at the AMC nearest you may be a good first step. You can obtain the complete listing of AMCs from the Association of Academic Medical Center's Web site at *www.aamc.org*.

Ambulatory Surgery Center (ASC)

An ambulatory surgery center (ASC) provides outpatient surgery to patients. ASCs are freestanding or based within a hospital. The plan for these patients is to admit and discharge them on the same day. However, some ASC patients who experience complications may require admission to a hospital. Because complications may arise from any surgical procedure, you should consider the ASC's affiliation with a hospital. If it does not have one, determine how far away the ASC is from a hospital in case providers need to transfer you.

Physicians or physician-run corporations own most freestanding ASCs. The attraction of a freestanding ASC is usually convenience, personalized attention, and posh accommodations. If you need a hysterectomy, you might want to ask how many surgeons at your ASC perform hysterectomies and how many are performed each year. The more, the better in both cases.

In some instances, it may be helpful to have your surgery performed in an ASC that specializes in your type of surgery. For example, Harvey, a colleague of mine, is a PhD nurse. He had bariatric surgery performed for obesity. Being in the healthcare business, he was aware of the high complication rates often associated with bariatric surgery. As a result, he scheduled his surgery at one of the Bariatric Surgery Centers of America. These centers only perform bariatric surgery and, at least at the time of his surgery, had the lowest postoperative complication rates for the procedure. In addition to specializing in one type of surgery, their high success rate is also due to the amount of education and structure that the centers provide to patients before and after their procedures. Harvey's surgery was successful and he had no complications.

The most common procedures performed at an ASC are: hernia repair; skin repair or excision; ear tube insertion or removal; eye surgery, such as cataract removal or retina repair; plastic or cosmetic surgery; repair of muscles tendons, ligaments, and joints; carpal tunnel release; tonsillectomy; cardiac catheterization; colonoscopy; other gastric endoscopies; gallbladder removal; and hysterectomies. The types of outpatient surgeries continue to grow.

You can find data on ASCs on the CMS Web site at *www.cms.hhs.gov*. You can find general information on ASCs at the American Association of Ambulatory Surgery Centers at *www.aaasc.org*. And, you can search facilities accredited and quality rated by the Joint Commission on Accreditation of Healthcare Organizations (JCAHO) on their Quality Check Web site at *www.qualitycheck.org*.

Outpatient Rehabilitation Center (ORC)

The outpatient rehabilitation center (ORC) provides an integrated, multidisciplinary program. It brings together specialized rehabilitation personnel to upgrade the physical functions of disabled individuals. The center's staff must include a physician and provide services of physical therapists, occupational therapists, and speech therapists. Generally, patients receive physical therapy care in an outpatient setting for a minor injury or following discharge from an inpatient rehabilitation hospital.

ORCs usually treat patients following injury, fractures, heart attack, or stroke. Some ORCs also offer addiction and substance abuse treatment. The Commission on Accreditation of Rehabilitation Facilities (CARF) accredits ORCs. CARF accredits the following types of ORCs: alcohol and substance abuse treatment, blind rehabilitation services, opioid and methadone treatment, physical rehabilitation, and stroke specialty. You can find an accredited ORC on the CARF Web site at *www.carf.org/consumer.*

Emergency Room (ER)

The ER provides expert, immediate care for serious illnesses and traumatic injuries. Care is available 24 hours a day, which physicians provide regardless of ability to pay, at least until you are stabilized. Emergency rooms are attached to acute care hospitals so that if patients are in need of acute care, they can be easily transferred to a hospital room for that care.

Another important consideration is whether the facility has a trauma unit. Trauma units are highly specialized emergency units that can make the difference in life and death situations. Many ERs use a triage system to determine the immediacy of patient medical needs. In a triage system, a nurse assesses the level of severity of the patient's condition and determines the order in which the ER physicians see patients.

ERs treat conditions such as heart attack, stroke, acute chest pain, poisoning, asthma attack, difficulty breathing, uncontrolled bleeding, medication overdose, fractured or broken bones, head injuries, burns, and trauma.

Urgent Care Center (Urgi-care)

Generally, when your primary doctor's office is closed, or you are unable to get a timely appointment you may want to seek care at an urgi-care center. Urgi-care centers also offer some services that usually are not available in a doctor's office, such as x-ray and wound management.

Common conditions treated at urgi-care centers include allergic reactions, asthma (mild to moderate wheezing), broken bones, burns (minor), cuts (minor), dehydration, diarrhea, ear aches and infections, low fevers, rashes and bumps, sprains, and sore throats.

Hospital Outpatient Department (OPD)

The Hospital OPD provides services to diagnose or treat an injury or a problem. Diagnostic services include tests provided in the lab, radiology, cardiology, neurology, or nuclear medicine departments, where patients receive treatment, including physical, occupational, or speech therapy. All hospitals have an OPD on the hospital campus. However, to better serve their patients, most hospitals today have established OPDs throughout their communities.

Common services provided and conditions treated in the OPD include diagnostic lab or radiology tests for common symptoms like chest pain, dizziness, fever, cough, shortness of breath, weakness, lethargy, or pain.

Inpatient Locations

Inpatient locations are overnight-stay facilities. Levels of care are acute, sub-acute, rehabilitation, and skilled nursing. Some patients may only need care in the acute care setting. Others may need care in every setting from acute care to a skilled nursing facility (nursing home). The phrase *level of care* describes the intensity of treatment a patient needs. As the level of care that a patient needs changes, the treatment location changes as well.

The concept of providing different levels of care for different conditions has evolved over time for both quality and cost-savings purposes. First, from a quality perspective, staff is trained to provide a specific level of care. In addition, the facility is equipped with tools and resources most appropriate for patients needing a particular level of care. From a cost perspective, care is the most expensive at acute care hospitals. The equipment there is also the most expensive and the ratio of staff to patients is the lowest.

Separating out levels of care is cost effective for insurance companies, providers, and patients. Your condition and your doctor's order determine your level of care. You have a choice where you receive care. Based on your VVMS decide where you want to receive care. Unless otherwise noted under the location description, you can find JCAHO quality and accreditation information on their Quality Check Web site at *www.qualitycheck.org* for each location.

Acute Care Hospital

An acute care hospital is a short-term hospital that has facilities, medical staff, and all necessary clinical personnel to provide diagnosis, care, and treatment of a wide range of acute conditions, including injuries.[7] The average length of time in the hospital is five days. There are 3,767 acute care hospitals in the U.S. Hospitals are usually classified by location (urban versus rural), ownership (nonprofit versus for-profit), and teaching status (residents versus no residents). About 70 percent of U.S. hospitals are nonprofit entities.[8] You will read additional details on hospitals in chapter 16.

While some hospitals employ a limited number of physicians, most physicians working in a hospital are not employees. Instead, the hospital grants them privileges to admit patients to the hospital. This status provides physicians with considerable influence over hospital processes, as they are one of two primary means by which patients flow into hospitals. The other primary conduit for patient admissions into the hospital is the ER.

Common conditions treated in the acute care hospital include heart failure, heart attacks, pneumonia, urinary tract infections, sepsis, seizures, strokes, respiratory failure, acute asthma, infectious gastroenteritis, dehydration, uncontrolled diabetes or diabetic complications, head injuries, trauma, and poisonings.

Since acute care hospitals are probably the most complex of all healthcare facilities, it is helpful to understand how they are organized. Generally, administrators organize acute care hospitals by floor, and within each floor, by nursing unit or clinical service. For example, the second floor of a hospital may be comprised of all obstetrics patients. The third floor may be general surgery and orthopedic surgery. Most hospitals, depending on their size, have two to four nursing units on a floor.

The reason for separating patients by service is twofold. First, it is more efficient for physicians to visit patients if they are all in the same location. If orthopedic surgeons only have to go to the third floor to visit patients, they likely will be able to spend more time with each one. Second, nurses who staff the units become experts in providing care specific to the service. Chances of higher quality care and improved outcomes generally increase on service-specific units.

The severity of illness and level of care also separates patients, such as the intensive care unit, or ICU. Most hospitals have a general ICU for patients who need constant monitoring while attached to complex machinery, including ventilators. Typically, the nurse-to-patient ratio is two to one. Many hospitals have service-specific ICUs as well like the surgical ICU (SICU), newborn or neonatal ICU (NICU), and cardiac ICU (CCU). Patients in the progressive care unit (PCU) need more monitoring than acute care, but less than in the ICU. Some hospitals also call the PCU the *step-down unit.*

Most patients are discharged from the acute care floor in the hospital to home or another facility. However, some hospitals have a transitional care unit (TCU) for patients who no longer require acute care, but need nursing care. Usually, these patients need some type of rehabilitation. As a patient progresses from ICU levels to transitional care, it generally means the patient is improving. It also means that the resources and cost to care for the patient are less.

Sub-Acute Care Hospital

A sub-acute care hospital is a facility that provides 24-hour nursing care, skilled nursing care, and short-term rehabilitation. Care is more intensive than a nursing home and less intensive than acute care. Coordinated services of physicians, nurses, and therapists are necessary for sub-acute care. Some sub-acute care hospitals are in the same building, but in a separately designated area, as an acute care hospital. This close proximity makes it easier to transfer patients, if necessary.

Common conditions treated in sub-acute care hospitals include Alzheimer's, cancer, neurologic disease, stroke, and brain injury.

Rehabilitation Hospital

Rehabilitation hospitals use a combination of medical, social, educational, and vocational services to enable patients disabled by illness or accidental injury to achieve the highest possible function. An organized staff of physicians provides or supervises services. A registered nurse provides continuous nursing services, and physical, occupational, and speech therapists may be involved in the care of the patient. Often, outpatient and inpatient rehabilitation hospitals offer similar services. The primary difference is the intensity or frequency of the therapy.

Common conditions treated in rehabilitation hospitals include stroke recovery, spinal cord injury, amputation, major multiple trauma, brain injury, neurological disorders (for example, multiple sclerosis, Guillain-Barré syndrome, Parkinson's disease), congenital deformity, hip fracture, burns, severe osteoarthritis, and joint replacement recovery.

Rehabilitation hospitals are accredited by CARF. You can find a listing of all CARF accredited facilities in your area on the CARF Web site at *www.carf.org/consumer.*

Skilled Nursing Facility (SNF) and Nursing Home

Skilled nursing facilities are one category of nursing homes. Nursing homes in general encompass a wide variety of levels of care. Some include personal care facilities that offer a more independent living arrangement.

Generally, the only level of nursing home care that Medicare or other insurers pay for is skilled nursing. Skilled nursing care means that the patient requires care that only a registered nurse can provide. Usually, the patient has a tube in her stomach to help with feeding (gastronomy tube) or other device, or physician orders for other care that a registered nurse needs to manage. If licensed practical nurses (LPNs) or other non-registered nursing staff can manage a patient's care in a nursing facility, then the patient's stay in a SNF may not be covered by insurance. Common conditions treated in nursing care facilities include dementia, Alzheimer's disease, and Parkinson's disease.

Psychiatric Hospital

Psychiatric facilities meet the general hospital requirement for acute care hospitals. However, providers at psychiatric facilities primarily diagnose and treat (under the supervision of a physician), individuals with mental health conditions. Some psychiatric facilities are located on the same campus as an acute care hospital, though less frequently in the same building. There are also many freestanding psychiatric hospitals.

Common conditions psychiatric hospitals treat include schizophrenia, bi-polar disorder, suicide attempts, and major depression. JHCAO also accredits psychiatric hospitals.

Hospice

A hospice provides care to terminally ill individuals at a patient's home or at a hospice location. Hospice is an approach to caring for terminally ill individuals that stresses palliative care (relief of pain and uncomfortable symptoms), as opposed to curative care. In addition to meeting the patient's medical needs, hospice care addresses the patient's physical, psychosocial, and spiritual needs—as well as the psychosocial needs of the patient's family or caregiver.

Common conditions hospices address include cancer, amyotrophic lateral sclerosis, and other terminal illnesses.

Homecare

Other than hospice, home care is the only healthcare service that comes to you. Usually, a registered nurse provides these services. Depending on the situation, though, other healthcare professionals may provide services as well. Home care services for individuals and families in their place of residence focus on promoting, maintaining, restoring health, or minimizing the effects of disability and illness, including terminal illness.

In the Medicare Current Beneficiary Survey and Medicare claims and enrollment data, home healthcare refers to home visits by professionals including nurses, doctors, social workers, therapists, and home health aides.[9] A home health agency is an organization that provides skilled nursing services and other therapeutic services.

Common conditions home healthcare addresses include post-hospitalization management of stroke, heart attack, pneumonia, trauma, and major surgery.

Figure 15.2 Summary of Healthcare Locations

Healthcare Provider	< 24 Hours	> 24 Hours	Comments
Physician Office	X		Need an appointment
Clinic	X		Usually need an appointment
Same-Day Surgery or Ambulatory Surgery	X		Need to schedule and prepare ahead of time
Outpatient Rehabilitation Center	X		Need an appointment; may see a physician or a therapist
Emergency Room or Emergency Department	X		Walk-in emergency conditions
Urgent Care Center or Urgi-Center	X		Walk-in non-emergency conditions
Hospital Outpatient Department	X		Walk-in for most tests
Acute Care Hospital		X	Very sick; average five-day stay

Healthcare Provider	< 24 Hours	> 24 Hours	Comments
Sub-Acute Care Hospital		X	Step down from acute care; average 30-day stay
Rehabilitation Hospital		X	Same level of care as sub-acute hospital but may have more specialized services and resources
Skilled Nursing Facility		X	Insurance may cover depending on level of care needed
Psychiatric Hospital		X	Specialized care
Hospice	X	X	End-of-life care
Home Healthcare	X		They come to you

Key Highlights

You will likely need to see providers in multiple locations for medical and/or surgical treatment. Providers at each location only see their view of you and your condition. Especially when you receive care for one condition in multiple locations, it is your responsibility to ensure your information gets from one provider site to the next. In many cases, your best solution may be to bring copies of your records with you from one location to the next.

Key Actions

- Obtain copies of your records at each provider location to share with all the providers you see.
- Gain an understanding of the various types of healthcare facilities where you may receive care.
- Familiarize yourself with facilities in your area.
- Bring copies of your records with you from one location to another, when possible.
- Ask your physicians to refer you to facilities that best meet your criteria.

Key Take-Away

You are the common thread ensuring that information and communication flows back and forth to the various locations where you receive care.

Endnotes

[1] Starr, Paul. *The Social Transformation of American Medicine.* Basic Books, 1984.
[2] Ibid.
[3] Newhouse, J. "Central findings and policy implications," Chapter 11 in *Free for All? Lessons from the RAND Health Insurance Experiment* (pp. 338 – 371). Harvard Press, 1993.
[4] Cherry, D.K.; Woodwell, D.A.; and Rechtsteiner, E.A. "National Ambulatory Medical Care Survey: 2005 Summary," *Advance data from vital and health statistics*, no 387. Hyattsville, MD: National Center for Health Statistics, June 29, 2007.
[5] Kane, Carol. "Practice Arrangements of Patient Care Physicians," *Physician Market Report.* American Medical Association, 2001.
[6] Middleton, K.R. and Hing, E. "National Hospital Ambulatory Medical Care Survey: 2003 Outpatient Department Summary." *Advance data from vital and health statistics,* no 366. Hyattsville, MD: National Center for Health Statistics, Dec. 14,2005.
[7] Connecticut State Department of Public Health Regulations, 10-13-D1.
[8] Health Forum. *AHA Hospital Statistics 2005.* American Hospital Association, 2004.
[9] Federal Interagency on Aging-Related Statistics. *Older Americans: 2000 Key Indicators of Well Being,* Diane Publishing Co., 2000.

CHAPTER

16

Choosing a Hospital: Teaching Versus Non-Teaching—Important Criteria to Consider

By learning you will teach; by teaching you will learn. —Latin Proverb

In December 2006, Emmalea spent three days in the NYU Medical Center inpatient epilepsy unit. She was there for 24-hour video and EEG monitoring, meaning that she had 30 electrodes glued to her head to read her brain waves as she was monitored and filmed 24 hours a day. A group of physicians and nurses sat in the monitoring room watching the EEG strips for any abnormalities. NYU physicians use this intense process to collect base-line data on every patient with epilepsy to determine the best treatment plan for each patient. Eight days before Christmas, patients of all ages from all over the world filled the unit's 16 beds.

We had a beautiful view of the east side of New York City from the ninth floor of the hospital, plenty of DVDs to watch, dinners delivered from any restaurant within a five-block radius, and visitors on a rolling basis. This type of hospital stay is probably one of the rare occasions when patients spend time in a hospital without being sick. For us, it was a visit of anticipation. What would the data show? Would we learn anything new? How would Emmalea's treatment regimen change after this visit? And, most important, would the treatment control the seizures?

The morning after her first full night of EEG monitoring, 12 healthcare professionals, all decked out in scrubs and white coats filed into Emmalea's room. They lined up, backs against the wall, facing the foot of her bed, except for Dr. Vazquez. She walked over and wedged herself between the bed and the convertible chair-bed that I had slept in the night before. Dr. Vazquez was the attending neurologist who was managing the epilepsy unit during the entire month of December. That meant that she saw every patient in the unit at least once a day and she worked with each patient's primary neurologist to design a plan based on all of the data collected.

Neither Emmalea nor I had met Dr. Vazquez previously, but we knew right away that she was the attending physician in the group, not just because of the way she separated herself from the rest of the pack, but also because she was the only one who spoke to us. The myriad of other individuals standing against the wall were medical school students, interns, residents, fellows, and nurse practitioners. The key evidence anyone can use to identify rank in a hospital is to check the length of the white lab coat. Medical students wear the shortest coats. Other lengths are based upon status in the following order: interns, residents, fellows, and finally, attending physicians who wear the longest lab coats.

You may wonder if Emmalea needed all of these people to manage her care. No, she did not. But, she was in a *teaching* hospital. We chose NYU for treatment because of its reputation in epilepsy management. When we made this choice, we knew that it was a major teaching hospital affiliated with the NYU Medical School. We expected that Emmalea would receive the best possible care. However, we also knew that her case would be used as a learning experience for residents.

THE PURPOSE OF A TEACHING HOSPITAL

At teaching hospitals, also called *academic medical centers* (AMCs), a quid pro quo exists between patients and the clinicians who treat them. AMCs use residents (physicians in training) to provide some patient care. You agree, as a patient, to allow an entire team of clinicians to participate in your care. As a result, you generally must spend more time being examined by and answering questions from, different members of the team. In return, the hospital provides you with the combined expertise of brilliant minds and progressive medical advances for your diagnosis and treatment, all of which can add up to critical advantages in your healthcare.

Your treatment team in an AMC will likely include students, interns, residents, nurses, mid-level practitioners, and of course, attending physicians. You allow the team to observe your care so they can learn. Our country depends on this process to produce well-prepared new generations of physicians. At the same time, the team in the teaching hospital is also there to serve as a check and balance and to provide continuity on all of the care they observe. For the patient this means that, with all of these eyes watching you, nothing should be missed. Since more clinicians are involved in your treatment in an academic medical center, the chances of someone familiar with your case responding to an emergency generally is greater than in non-academic medical centers.

So the unspoken quid pro quo between the patient and the AMC is, "As the patient, I give up some privacy and time, so you can learn. In return, I get peace of mind, an intense level of care, and nothing should slip through the cracks." AMC treatment teams provide an additional safety net that you would not have in a hospital without residents. At the end of our three days in the NYU epilepsy unit that December, Emmalea's healthcare team provided her with a new plan and gave us new hope. The best Christmas present ever.

The Definition of *Resident*

A resident is a physician in her first three to four years of post-medical school training. In the United States, every graduate of an approved medical school must complete a minimum of three to four years of residency training in his specialty before he can practice as an independent, licensed physician. Hospitals employ residents. Licensed physicians, more experienced residents and fellows, supervise these residents.

First-year residents are sometimes referred to as interns. Fellows are technically still residents, in a training mode. They are training in a certain medical or surgical specialty. Hospitals often hire fellows to serve in a senior residency role, conduct special research, and sometimes even manage residents. (You can find additional details on specialties and fellowship requirements in chapter 13.)

The number of residents in a hospital is usually proportionate to the number of patients treated, and the number of beds in a hospital determines the number of patients treated. For example, a small hospital with 100 beds will treat about 3,500 patients per year, on average. Whereas, a large teaching hospitals may have about 1,000 beds and treat approximately 35,000 patients per year. The 100-bed hospital may employ 10 residents, while the larger hospital may employ 150 to 200 residents.

Different AMCs, Different Cultures

The type of hospital, resources available, and depth and breadth of expertise are all crucial aspects when deciding where to receive care. Ultimately, deciding where you want to receive care depends on your definition of quality of care. Referring back to your VVMS from Chapter 1 will help you to decide what type of hospital environment will match your values. Ask yourself: “How do I, as the patient, define quality?” Location, size, infringement on your time, access to research studies, and new technologies—all of these may be considerations for you. Consider all of your values in terms of where you want to receive care, whether it is preventive maintenance or care for a more acute condition.

Physicians often affiliate with a healthcare facility that reflects and exemplifies their professional philosophy. In visiting three academic medical centers (AMCs) with Emmalea, I found this to be true. With each of these encounters, we were able to evaluate the hospitals by communicating with their representative physicians. Because I want to focus on the cultural differences and not criticisms of individual physicians and AMCs, I have omitted the names of the AMCs and changed the names of the physicians.

AMC 1 was located in an urban inner city location. The first thing Emmalea and I noticed was that there was one overworked receptionist in the dingy, messy office, and the chairs were very uncomfortable. Dr.White invited us into his office, and he spent about 30 minutes with us. I found this physician on the Internet, and I learned that he was noted for his book on epilepsy, which I read. We made the appointment the day before, and although no one requested that we bring any medical records or test results, Emmalea and I brought them along. Dr. White used a computer that was wedged between us. The computer blocked the doctor's face, and we were unable to make eye contact. He asked closed-ended questions, and Dr. White seemed to listen intermittently during the half hour we spent with him. He took the "wait and see" approach in devising an action plan. Emmalea's primary neurologist later received a copy of Dr. White's assessment, but we did not.

AMC 2 was nestled in the middle of another urban city. The office was spacious, clean and well furnished. The friendly staff made us feel relaxed as we waited in the peaceful surroundings. We had just gotten situated in the comfortable chairs near an aquarium when we were invited by a nurse to follow her to the examining room. My sister-in-law, Linda, referred us to this group. Her co-worker had been very pleased with the attention and treatment he received with Dr. Jordan. (Fortunately, it only took only one day to get an appointment). Dr. Jordan has written several books on epilepsy, and he directs the

Epilepsy Institute. Again, we brought Emmalea's prior test results and her records with us. Dr. Jordan did not use his computer during our visit although it was in arm's reach. He asked several questions but they were limited mostly to his goal of finding a drug to control seizures. During the half hour visit, a variety of clinicians were in and out of the consultation room. Dr. Jordan immediately started planning an intensive regimen.

Our visit to AMC 3 involved going to one of the hospital's suburban satellite offices. The office, although small and modesty furnished, was immaculate. It had taken five months to get the appointment with Dr. Sheridan. He has published studies that link seizures with hormones, and I found these articles on the Intranet. The receptionist immediately greeted us, and in a very short time, we were introduced to Dr. Sheridan. Dr. Sheridan led us to his office. Dr. Sheridan listened intently to very word we said during the hour he spent with us. He provided several choices for treatment, and Dr. Sheridan asked Emmalea to help make the decisions. The follow up care was carefully planned, and Emmalea concurred with the treatment program. Several days after the visit, we received a phone call from Dr. Sheridan and a detailed e-mail with helpful information. A copy of the consultation report was immediately sent to us and to Emmalea's PCP.

In the informal analysis, you can see that there was a consistent culture of personalized patient focus in the third academic medical center, AMC 3. Whereas, AMC 1 lacked a personalized, patient-focused culture. And, AMC 2 was somewhere in the middle. Use this example to help you determine how to assess whether your hospitals' and physicians' values are congruent with your own.

THE TEACHING HOSPITAL VERSUS THE NON-TEACHING HOSPITAL

The primary difference between a teaching hospital and a non-teaching hospital is the presence of residents in the hospital. A teaching hospital employs residents to assist in patient care. A non-teaching hospital (often a community hospital) does not employ residents to assist in patient care.

Within teaching hospitals, there is a further distinction based on whether the hospital has a relationship with a medical school. Teaching hospitals, (like the NYU Medical Center), that are part of a system that includes a medical school are AMCs (academic medical centers). Other teaching hospitals may or may not be affiliated with a specific medical school.

Figure 16.1 Snapshot of U.S. Hospitals 2007[1]

Acute Care Hospitals in the United States	**Number of Hospitals**
All hospitals	3,767
Hospitals with residents	1,134
Hospitals with residents *and* affiliated with a medical school	284
Hospitals with residents *and* affiliated with a medical school in the Northeast	101

The Hybrid Option in Hospital Care

Some patients want small-town hospital attention with major teaching hospital capabilities. Many teaching hospitals have built networks to funnel their expertise into the community through smaller, sometimes more personalized hospitals. You can generally tell from the Web site if a teaching hospital owns or affiliates with a smaller hospital. Usually, the Web site will say something like "an affiliate of ABC University Medical Center".

When an academic medical center owns a hospital, it has more control over the hospital's management than when it only affiliates with the hospital. Many AMCs and larger hospitals purchase or merge with other hospitals. When a large academic medical center buys a hospital, it may be because the community hospital is in financial trouble or because it makes sense to absorb the hospital into the larger organization.

A merger is a major change that may present some challenges. People inside and outside of the organization naturally resist change. We go through a series of steps in accepting change, much like the five stages Elizabeth Kubler-Ross discusses in her book *On Death and Dying.* [2] The first stage is denial, followed by anger, bargaining, depression and acceptance. It may take a while to reach acceptance. The stress of a merger may weaken overall effectiveness of the organization. For this reason, it is important to know whether your hospital has recently been part of a merger. If it has been at least three years since a merger, chances are you will find some significant benefits from the small hospital being absorbed into the teaching hospital's system.

A good example of a renowned academic medical center merging or affiliating with regional hospitals is the Cleveland Clinic. The Cleveland Clinic has organizations in Ohio, Florida, and Canada. I address here only the system in Cleveland, Ohio. The relationships between Cleveland Clinic and the community hospitals have existed for more than a decade in most cases. The Cleveland Clinic Health System Web site at *www.clevelandclinic.org,* details the names and locations of every hospital in the Cleveland area that is in its system. As a patient of any of the Cleveland Clinic's community hospitals, you also have access to the experts in the main hospital.[3] There are 11 community hospitals in Cleveland Clinic's Ohio network.

OTHER WAYS TO CATEGORIZE HOSPITALS

Ownership

The primary difference in hospital ownership is whether the hospital is a for-profit or nonprofit organization. Government entities, educational organizations, and religious organizations own nonprofit hospitals. Nonprofit hospitals can also be community-based organizations. A few examples of nonprofit hospitals are Johns Hopkins Hospital in Baltimore, Maryland; Mount Sinai Hospital in New York City; and Baylor University Medical Center in Dallas, Texas.

A nonprofit organization is established for charitable, humanitarian, or educational purposes. Individuals do not own nonprofit organizations. Therefore, unlike for-profit organizations, individuals cannot profit or lose based on the financial performance of the nonprofit organization. You may have seen the terms nonprofit and not-for-profit used interchangeably. However, there is a difference between the two. Nonprofit organizations are generally corporations or other legally organized groups. Whereas, not-for-profits are generally groups of individuals without any formal legal action, like a club or small association. Nonprofits, like hospitals, are exempt from some taxes. In return, nonprofit hospitals have certain obligations to give money back to the community and to patients. Although it may seem oxymoronic, nonprofit hospitals can generate profits. If they do, they need to invest the profits to benefit the communities they serve.

For-profit hospitals are private or public. One or more individuals or a private corporation owns private, for-profit hospitals. Public, for-profit hospitals are publicly traded and are owned by the corporations' stockholders. Examples of for-profit hospitals are Tenet Healthcare and Hospital Corporation of America. In 1968, Hospital Corporation of America (HCA) became the first for-profit hospital corporation. Both HCA and Tenet are based in Nashville and own hospitals throughout the country.

Today, HCA generates approximately $25 billion in income annually. According to annual filings, the corporation made a profit of $1 billion in 2006.[4] By contrast, New York- Presbyterian Hospital in New York City, the single largest hospital, with more than 2,000 beds generates approximately $2.4 billion in income annually. According to annual filings, the hospital made a profit of $69 million in 2005. The dollar amounts are proportionate to the size of the organizations. In addition, the percentage of profitability is not disparate with HCA bringing in a 4 percent profit and New York-Presbyterian Medical Center bringing in a 3 percent profit. For a for-profit hospital to generate a profit of 4 percent, it must be an after-tax profit. Since the average corporate tax rate is 20 percent, Columbia/HCA had to make significantly more money than New York Presbyterian to generate a 4 percent on the bottom-line profit.

Approximately 30 percent of hospitals are for-profit and 70 percent nonprofit. Of the nonprofit hospitals, the government owns one-third and religious groups own two-thirds. These issues may not be significant to you operationally or philosophically. To determine your hospital's status, see the American Hospital Directory Web site at *www.ahd.com.* The site provides facts about hospitals in addition to ownership status.

Location

Generally, hospitals are categorized within their geographic region as urban, suburban, or rural. Based on where you live, you may have limitations regarding where you can receive care. Also, location of a hospital does not automatically determine whether you will receive high-quality care. I have visited hospitals in the biggest, most expensive cities, which are on Medicare's bottom 10 percent list for quality indicators. Yet I have also visited remote hospitals that have taken me two plane flights and a three-hour car ride to find, which are on the top 10 percent list.

Range of Services

Most hospitals consider themselves to be "all things to all people," so they can treat anyone who walks in the door. In the future, it is less likely that most hospitals, especially smaller ones, will be able to function in this manner. Michael Porter, in his book *Redefining Healthcare* discusses the need for hospitals to specialize to ensure the highest quality of care.[5] Some hospitals already specialize to an extent. For a list of top specialty hospitals, see the *U.S. News and World Report Best Hospitals* list published each July or visit *health.usnews.com/sections/health/best-hospitals.*

Size

The number of beds a hospital has defines hospital size. The smallest hospitals may have as few as 8 beds, though most of the smallest have at least 25. Generally, these hospitals are located in remote rural areas of the country, and usually designated as "critical access hospitals." They receive certain government benefits to ensure they stay in business since their services are critical in the area. Size alone should not determine your decision making. Be sure to combine this comparison criterion with your other quality ratings.

Values, Vision, and Mission Statements at Top Hospitals

If your values and your hospital's values are aligned, you are more likely to be satisfied with your care. You can usually find a hospital's VVMS in the "about us" tab on their Web site.

Figure 16.2 contains a list of the top 10 values, compiled from a random sampling of hospitals. I list the values in order, from those most frequently mentioned to those least frequently mentioned.

Figure 16.2 Top 10 Values for Sample Hospitals (in Order by Most Common)

1. Quality of care
2. Compassion and respect for the patient
3. Cost effectiveness
4. Community service and community health
5. Caring for those who cannot afford care or are uninsured
6. Customer service
7. Stewardship
8. Ethical actions
9. Accountability and responsibility
10. Teamwork and collaboration

A Compassionate Culture: Can Hospitals Turn Away Poor or Uninsured Patients?

Until about 10 years ago, hospitals could turn away patients, even if they were acutely ill. Additionally, particularly among for-profit hospitals, many outrageous stories of patients having heart attacks on a hospital's lawn after it denied care in the emergency room made front-page news. In 1999, along with several other healthcare reforms, the federal government passed the Emergency Medical Treatment and Active Labor Act (EMTALA). This law requires all hospitals to ensure access to emergency services to all patients, regardless of their ability to pay. At a minimum, hospitals must provide stabilizing treatment for patients who have an emergency medical condition. This means that, while the law does not require hospitals to treat patients without an emergent condition, it does provide some basic protections.

The hospitals in the previous VVMS analysis state their fifth highest value is to provide care to patients regardless of their ability to pay. It is highly likely that hospitals with this value hold themselves to this standard and probably provide more care to the uninsured and disenfranchised than the minimum required by law. These hospitals, which value care to *all* patients, regardless of ability to pay, also are some of the most profitable hospitals nationally. You can see whether your preferred hospital is one that values providing care to patients regardless of ability to pay. (For more information about paying for care if you are not insured, see chapter 3.)

Customer Satisfaction: A Unique Promise by a Hospital

Rush-Copley takes an innovative approach in customer service. For example, its policy is to give movie passes or grocery store gift certificates to patients who are not completely satisfied. (See the full promise below.)

Whether this same type of customer service benefits hospitals and patient quality of care or not is yet to be determined. Certainly, the list of promises the hospital makes shows the high value they place on healthcare consumers. With these high standards and commitment to patient satisfaction, at minimum, hospitals are moving in a good direction.

Rush-Copley Medical Center's Promise to Patients, As Posted on Its Web site:[6]

Our Promise

At Rush-Copley Medical Center, we pride ourselves on providing everyone with extraordinary service. In fact, we're so confident that you'll love our service, we're offering you this guarantee—the first of its kind in Illinois and among the first in the country. If you feel we haven't lived up to our Promise for any reason, we will give you two movie ticket passes or a grocery store gift certificate. Just tell a caregiver or any hospital representative.

Promise to our patients, families, and guests:

1. Warm, friendly greetings in every interaction
2. The offer of a personal escort to your destination
3. To do everything possible to ensure your comfort, safety, and to please you
4. Comprehensive and timely information
5. To give you every opportunity to participate in your care
6. To answer call lights immediately
7. To respect your privacy
8. A sparkling, clean environment
9. Healthy, tastefully prepared food

Hospital Revenue, Profits and Losses

Although 70 percent of hospitals are nonprofit organizations, it is still important for them to generate enough revenue to cover their expenses. Financial losses may cause the hospital to close or be sold. Economic instability has a negative impact on both the hospital and the patients they serve. As you research your hospital choices, find out about the hospital's financial status. You can find profit and loss statements for every hospital at *www.ahd.com.* Financial status should not be your sole or primary criteria. But, all other things being equal, you may be able to use it as a tie-breaker for your choice in hospital care.

The table below contains a random sample of financial information for six hospitals for 2006. Only one hospital, Immanuel Medical Center, made a profit on hospital operations. For University of Missouri, you can see that although they generated $298 million in patient related revenue, it cost them $325 million to run the hospital. So, they lost $27 million operating the hospital. Hospitals have other sources of income including investments and fund raising. The column on the right, net income, shows that, even with additional "non-patient" income, three of the hospitals lost money. For the two hospitals with the largest net income, Tampa General and University of Missouri, both received governmental appropriations in excess of $10 million.

Figure 16.3 Revenue, Profits and Losses for a Random Sample of Hospitals

Hospital	City, State	Net Patient Revenue	Total Operating Expenses	Operating Income	Net Income
Desert View	Pahrump, NV	18,422,741	18,650,297	(227,556)	(207,989)
Immanuel	Omaha, NE	222,033,683	221,746,807	286,876	11,049,403
Memorial Hospital	Gardena, CA	66,390,849	75,037,223	(8,646,374)	(2,454,770)
Renaissance Hospital	Groves, TX	25,720,225	32,494,925	(6,774,799)	(6,642,693)
Tampa General	Tampa, FL	697,349,967	715,971,834	(18,621,867)	45,022,560
University of Missouri	Columbia, MO	298,623,639	325,776,669	(27,153,030)	42,202,802

Key Highlights

Hospitals are classified in many ways, using criteria such as whether the hospital is a teaching or non-teaching hospital, and its for-profit or nonprofit status and ownership. These hospital characteristics affect how a hospital does business. As a result, they drive the hospital's values and the quality of care you receive.

Key Actions

- Seek treatment in hospitals that manifest your values.
- Understand differences in treatment at a teaching versus a non-teaching hospital.
- Know the difference in treatment based upon hospital ownership and profit status.
- Visit the lobby to see if a hospital is a place where you will feel comfortable.
- Check out annual rankings on the *Top 100 Hospitals* to see how your hospital compares to other hospitals.
- Visit the American Hospital Directory Web site (*www.ahd.com*) to view hospital financial information.

Key Take-Away

Evaluate the culture and teaching designation of a hospital to choose one that shares your values.

Endnotes

[1] American Hospital Directory, *www.ahd.com.*
[2] Kubler-Ross, Elizabeth. *On Death and Dying.* Scribner, 1997.
[3] Cleveland Clinic Web site, *www.clevelandclinic.org.*
[4] American Hospital Director, *www.ahd.com.*
[5] Porter, Michael E., and Olmstead Teisberg, Elizabeth. *Redefining Health Care: Creating Value-Based Competition on Results.* Harvard Business School Publishing, 2006.
[6] Rush-Copley Medical Center Web site, *www.rushcopley.com/consumer/discover/promise.aspx.*

STEP

7

LEARN THE LANGUAGE

CHAPTER

17

Learning the Language of Medicine

Language is the source of misunderstandings. —Antoine de Saint-Exupery

Last Christmas, my family and I went to Paris. I had not been to Paris since my college years, when I lived in Nantes for a semester and attended the university there. Back then, I was quite at home with the language. I had to be. I was proficient and used this knowledge to my advantage. Later, as a mother, when Emmalea and John were young, I would speak to them in simple French phrases. But when I stepped off the plane some 25 years after college, I found that phrases like "brush your teeth, please" and "give me your foot" (for putting on socks) did not come in very handy. I wished I had brushed up on my French before taking the trip. Shortly after we arrived, Emmalea and I left the hotel to find a local bistro off the beaten path. When we got there, I realized this was not at all the type of place tourists frequented. Suddenly, I broke out in a sweat as I realized that I was not sure how to order a drink or understand what the waiter said to us. When you do not understand the spoken language, you are on the periphery, the outside. You miss something, but you are not sure what.

If you are fine with just being a tourist, that's okay. You may want more. You may want the experience of understanding what it is like to be French, Italian, or Polish—your experience is less than complete without some understanding of the language of the land you are visiting. Returning home, we decided as a family that before returning to France (or visiting any other non-English speaking country) in the future, we would take a crash course in the language to fully immerse ourselves in the culture of the country we planned to visit.

When you are in the land of medicine, you may feel the same way as we did in France. Only in healthcare, you have more at stake than feeling as if you missed a unique experience during vacation. Knowing the language of medicine allows you to feel more confident in your healthcare communications. You can take the approach like we did in France and rely on the English-speaking French citizens to help you. But, if you rely solely on your healthcare providers, you may always wonder, *am I missing something*?

The language of medicine or medical terminology is, in many respects, a foreign language. It has its own vocabulary and methods for combining words in an understandable format. With any language, the more immersed you are in it, the more fluent you become.

Physicians and other healthcare professionals spend the great majority of their lives immersed in medical terminology—the language flows as smoothly for them as baseball jargon does for a New York Yankee or ballet terms for a prima ballerina. They live it, know it, and visualize every word easily. Baseball jargon like *dish, balk, or "K"* may be as difficult for the ballerina to understand as ballet terms like *cabriole*, *rond de jambe*, or *ballon* may be for the baseball player to comprehend. It's the same in the field of medicine. Just like my next trip to France, it may take some homework and good communication skills on your part.

ELIMINATING BARRIERS IN THE LANGUAGE OF MEDICINE

In this chapter, I describe a systematic approach that can make the process easier and may even be fun. Learning the basic rules that guide the combination of root words, prefixes, and suffixes in medical terminology helps decode words. Looking up definitions, asking physicians for clarification, and verbalizing your understanding also helps develop your comprehension, and hence, better communication and decision-making skills about your healthcare.

When my father-in-law was in the hospital for a pericardial effusion (fluid around the heart) last year, Joe called me to tell me my father-in-law was going to have a *thoracentesis*. Joe could not pronounce the word, let alone understand what it was. He spelled it out for me. A thoracentesis is a procedure in which a surgeon inserts a needle into the chest to remove the excess fluid that has built up, in this case, around the heart. Although the surgeon had explained the procedure to him, my father-in-law had no idea what procedure he had given permission for. Clearly, here was a difference between *hearing* an explanation and *understanding* it.

The second time Emmalea was in the ER after a seizure, no neurologists were available. Only an ER physician could see her, but I insisted we needed at least a phone consultation with a neurologist. When I talked to the neurologist, he was not familiar with Emmalea's case. I explained that she had juvenile myoclonic epilepsy, diagnosed three months ago, and that there was a family history. I described her current medication regimen and explained that she was neither sleep-deprived nor drinking alcohol (two possible triggers for seizures).

I spoke fast but confidently, choosing my words carefully, to give him the best possible description of Emmalea's situation. Once I finished, there was silence on the line for a moment and then he asked, "Are you a nurse?" I found it extremely odd but telling that he would assume I must be a nurse because I could articulate some medical terms.

Many clinicians assume patients do not know medical terminology. Yet if more healthcare consumers had a better grasp of it, communication between patients and healthcare providers would likely be better. Lack of understanding terminology is just one more thing that can separate patients from caregivers.

You are disadvantaged when you cannot communicate effectively with your healthcare providers. It is not in your best interest to wait until you are suddenly entrenched in the world of healthcare to try to understand the language of medicine.

Check Your VVMS

Check your values, vision, and mission statement (VVMS) to determine where knowing medical terminology falls in your priorities. Do you have the interest and time to dedicate, or would you rather just ask your doctor to translate? Are you a person who simply enjoys words? How about Scrabble? Word games? Do you diligently complete the daily crossword puzzle? You may enjoy intellectual exercises as a means of keeping the brain stimulated. Learning medical terminology can be akin to these activities.

In his book *Healthy Aging*, Dr. Andrew Weil discusses two activities that have a proven protective effect against dementia and Alzheimer's disease.[1] The first is learning a new computer operating system and the second is learning a foreign language. When individuals learn these new concepts, they are less likely to develop either condition. In both cases, Dr. Weil explains, learning these specific concepts creates new neural pathways in the brain. Although no one understands the exact mechanism for the protection, the activity that creates the new neural pathways appears to produce the protective effect. Dr. Weil does not specifically classify medical terminology as a foreign language. But if the learning concepts are the same, perhaps learning medical terminology not only benefits your healthcare, but your health as well.

Depending on your VVMS, you can skim this chapter, or you can plunge into it. If you have an even greater interest, there are many books and online courses available, some of which I have included in an appendix to this book. You can choose one or a combination of options in terms of your knowledge of medical terminology:

1. Rely solely on your healthcare providers
2. Learn the basics (this chapter will provide that for you)
3. Find a mentor who can translate for you

If you educate yourself on the basics, you will likely feel more confident in your healthcare discussions and decisions. But, if you are more of a numbers person than a linguistics person (you prefer Sudoku to Scrabble) you can still take an important step. Choose a medical mentor who already knows medical language or is adept at deciphering medical vocabulary. When we visited the Louvre and the Musée d'Orsay, we hired a French tour guide to explain everything to us. We didn't want to miss anything. It is the same with healthcare—you want to identify someone who understands the language to be your tour guide if you don't know the language.

Do It Now!

It is important to apply your values, vision, and mission statements (VVMS) from chapter 1 to using medical terminology in your healthcare experiences. Write your plan for addressing the language of medicine in the space provided below. Regardless of the approach you choose, the important part is to have a plan that works best for you.

How I Will Address My Need to Understand Medical Terminology?

____

____

____

MEDICAL TERMINOLOGY: IS IT A PURPOSEFUL BARRIER IN HEALTHCARE COMMUNICATIONS?

You may feel healthcare providers use medical terminology to put a barrier between you and them. Healthcare providers use medical terminology to be more efficient. Saving 30 seconds by using medical shorthand might make a difference between life and death in an emergency. A good example is the term *bacterial gastroenteritis*. This term means "inflammation of the stomach and the intestines due to a bacterial infection." Using two words versus 12 words is significant.

String several terms together and you could save a minute or more. In the ER a physician could save a life in this amount of time.

Dissecting a Discharge Summary

The following paragraph is excerpted from a discharge summary, a document the physician dictates when a patient leaves the hospital. Definitions for medical terms are included in parentheses.

Figure 17.1 Sample Hospital Discharge Summary

The patient is a 93-year-old who noted increasing dyspnea *(difficult breathing),* pedal edema *(swollen feet),* palpitations *(irregular heart beat),* hoarseness, and nonproductive *(not spitting up any material from the respiratory system)* cough over a three-week period. Patient is afebrile *(without a fever).* No history of prior myocardial infarction *(heart attack)* or CHF *(congestive heart failure; heart is not pumping correctly)* or cyanosis *(bluing of the skin).* In the emergency room the patient was noted to be in pulmonary edema *(swelling in and around the lungs)* and was treated with IV *(intravenous)* Lasix *(drug to treat congestive heart failure)* and diuresed *(administered medicine that increases urine excretion to decrease fluid pressure on the heart).* He was given oxygen. Rhythm *(heart beat)* appeared to be sinus *(normal heart rhythm originating in the sinoatrial node of the heart)* with frequent atrial *(top chamber of the heart)* ectopic *(arising from abnormal site or tissue)* beats and then was noted to be in and out of atrial *(top chamber of the heart)* fibrillation *(abnormal heart rate marked by rapid, randomized contractions of the atrial chamber of the heart)* and some tachycardia *(fast heart beat).*

Reading this report, the efficiencies in using medical terminology become startlingly clear. If this report did not use medical terminology to explain the clinical issues, it would contain almost 70 additional words. Using medical terminology in this report resulted in using about 50 percent less words. This percentage, translated to everyday care, might indicate that clinicians are twice as productive when they use medical terminology.

Breaking Down Words for Understanding: -otomy, -algia, and -itis

The first thing I learned as a student in medical terminology is that the suffix *otomy* means "incision." With that one piece of information, I felt empowered. Knowing that any term with the suffix *otomy* meant that the body part would have an incision made into it gave me instant understanding of a plethora of medical terms. For example, a *gastrotomy* means "incision into the stomach (or gastric region)."

The more I learned, the more empowered I felt. That same day, I also learned two other suffixes: *algia*, which means "pain," and *itis*, which means "inflammation of." I now knew that the term *neuralgia* means "pain from the nerves or caused by a nerve." And I now knew that *arthritis* means "inflammation of the joint" (*arth* being a prefix meaning "joint"). I became so interested in the language that I spent nearly every waking moment learning it. Once you learn the basic rules of the language, root words, prefixes, and suffixes, the process of learning a language is much easier.

BASICS OF LEARNING MEDICAL TERMINOLOGY

There are three basic parts to medical terms: a prefix (which is at the beginning and usually identifies some part of the central meaning), a root word (the middle of the word and its central meaning), and a suffix (which is at the end and modifies the central meaning as to what or who is interacting with it or what is happening to it).

Medical terminology uses a root word, generally a body part, with various prefixes and suffixes. For example, the prefix *peri* (around) and the suffix *itis* (inflammation), combined with various root words, form several medical terms, like the following:

- Pericarditis, inflammation around the heart (*card* means heart)
- Periadenitis, inflammation around the glands (*aden* means gland)

- Periaoritis, inflammation around the aorta (*aort* means aorta, the largest artery in the body)

Keep in mind that most medical terms will have either a suffix or a prefix but not both.

You can mix and match most of the common root words, prefixes, and suffixes in medical terminology to learn about 75 to 100 of the most common medical terms. The next three brief sections highlight short cuts to learning some basics. The remaining sections highlight words associated with body parts and systems.

Common Prefixes

A prefix is a word element put at the beginning of a word to form another word. The prefix generally has the same meaning in every derivative word. Some examples of common prefixes used in medical terminology appear in figure 17.2.

Figure 17.2 Common Prefixes in Medical Terminology

Prefix	Meaning	Example	Definition
A, An	Not, without	Afebrile	Without fever
Cyano	Blue	Cyanosis	Bluing of the skin
Brady	Slow	Bradycardia	Slow heart beat
Dys	Difficult	Dyspnea	Difficult breathing
Exo	Outside of	Extracranial	Outside the skull
Hyper	Excessive, too much	Hypertension	High blood pressure
Hypo	Low, too little	Hypotension	Low blood pressure
Intra	Within	Intramuscular	Within the muscle
Leuko	White	Leukocytes	White blood cells
Peri	Around	Pericardium	Around the heart
Onco	Tumor	Oncology	Study of tumors
Retro	Behind	Retrosternum	Behind the sternum
Tachy	Fast	Tachycardia	Fast heart beat

Common Suffixes

A suffix is a word element put at the end of a word to create another word. The suffix generally has the same meaning in every derivative word. Some examples of common suffixes used in medical terminology appear in figure 17.3.

Figure 17.3 Common Suffixes in Medical Terminology

Suffix	Meaning	Example	Definition
Algia	Painful condition	Arthralgia	Joint pain
Asthenia	Weakness	Myasthenia	Muscle weakness
Cele	Tumor, hernia, swelling	Cystocele	Herniated bladder
Centesis	To puncture	Pneumocentesis	Puncture of the lung
Cyte	Cell	Leukocyte	White blood cell
Dynia	Pain	Otodynia	Ear pain
Ectomy	Excision	Colectomy	Removal of the colon
Itis	Inflammation	Colitis	Inflammation of the colon
Lithiasis	Stone	Nephrolithiasis	Kidney stone
Oma	Tumor	Hepatoma	Liver tumor
Otomy	Incision into	Gastrotomy	Incision into stomach
Pathy	Disease	Cardiomyopathy	Disease of the heart muscles
Penia	Shortage of	Leukopenia	Shortage of white blood cells
Plasty	Repair	Angioplasty	Blood vessel repair
Ptysis	Spitting	Hemoptysis	Spitting of blood
Rrhage	Excessive flow	Hemorrhage	Excessive blood flow
Rrhaphy	Suture	Herniorraphy	Suture of hernia
Rhea	Flow or discharge	Rhinorhea	Discharge from the nose
Tripsy	To crush	Lithotripsy	Crushing of stone

Common Root Words

A root word is a word combined with a prefix or a suffix to form a derivative word. The root word generally has the same meaning in every derivative word. Some examples of common root terms combined with suffixes used in medical terminology appear in figure 17.4.

Figure 17.4 Common Root Words in Medical Terminology

Root Word	Meaning	Example	Definition
Aden	Gland	Adenoma	Tumor of a gland
Angi	Blood vessel	Angioplasty	Repair of blood vessel
Arthr	Joint	Arthritis	Inflammation of joints
Broncho	Airway in the lung	Bronchitis	Inflammation of the airways
Ceph	Head	Cephalgia	Headache
Chole	Gall, bile	Cholelithiasis	Gallstones
Cost	Rib	Costoplasty	Repair of the ribs
Cyst	Bladder	Cystitis	Inflammation of bladder
Enceph	Brain	Encephalopathy	Disease of the brain
Gastr	Stomach	Gastritis	Inflammation of the stomach
Hem	Blood	Hematuria	Blood in the urine
Hepat	Liver	Hepatitis	Inflammation of the liver
Nephro	Kidney	Nephrolithiasis	Kidney stone
Phleb	Vein	Phlebitis	Inflammed vein
Pneumo	Lung	Pneumonitis	Inflammed lung
Rhino	Nose	Rhinoplasty	Repair of the nose

Do It Now!

Here is an opportunity to exercise your linguistic abilities. Use the figures in this chapter as your starting point. Start with the definitions that interest you the most. Spend just 10 minutes to make a list of them, and say the definitions to yourself or to a friend who wants to learn along with you. Check your learning as you go.

I provide a word match as a practice for you in figure 17.5. When you are ready, try it out. See how you do. Use the medical terminology charts if you want to help you find the meaning of the words. You'll likely be surprised to discover it is easier than you thought. (You can find the answers at the end of this chapter.)

Figure 17.5 Medical Terminology Word Match

Word Match (Draw a line from the word to its definition.)

1. Tachycardia	A. Disease of the heart muscle
2. Afebrile	B. Difficult breathing
3. Cyanosis	C. Inflammation of the bronchus
4. Hematuria	D. Low white blood cell count
5. Leukopenia	E. Disease of the brain cells
6. Myalgia	F. Muscle pain
7. Dyspnea	G. Bluing of the skin
8. Encephalopathy	H. Blood in the urine
9. Bronchitis	I. No fever
10. Cardiomyopathy	J. Fast heart beat

Reading Versus Pronouncing Medical Terminology

Seeing a word and saying the word are two different things. Often, the best way to learn to pronounce medical terms is to hear someone say them and repeat them. I have recorded the correct pronunciation of every medical term in this chapter's figures at *www.7stepshealth.com.* Please listen at your convenience.

Common Medical Abbreviations and Acronyms

Abbreviations can complicate learning medical terminology. If you do not understand a term, how can you understand its abbreviation? Figure 17.6 provides a list of some of the more common medical abbreviations.

Figure 17.6 Abbreviations for Medical Terminology and Acronyms

Abbreviation	Meaning
b.i.d.	Two times a day
Bx	Biopsy
C	With
CA	Cancer
CHF	Congestive heart failure
COPD	Chronic obstructive pulmonary disease
CVA	Cerebrovascular accident (Stroke)
CXR	Chest x-ray
Fx	Fracture
H & P	History and Physical
I & O	Intake and output
I.M.	Intramuscular
I.V.	Intravenous
M.I.	Myocardial infarction (heart attack)
n.p.o.	Nothing by mouth
p.c.	After meals
PERRLA	Pupils equal, round, and reactive to light and accommodation
p.o.	By mouth
p.r.n.	As necessary, as needed
q.i.d	Four times a day
t.i.d.	Three times a day
S	Without
SOB	Shortness of breath
TIA	Transient ischemic attack
UA	Urinalysis
UTI	Urinary tract infection

MEDICAL TERMS BY BODY SYSTEM

For learning, it is easier to organize medical terminology by body system. Examples of terms in the most common body systems are provided below.

Nervous System

The nervous system is composed of the brain, the spinal cord, and all the nerves of the body. A physician who treats disorders of the nervous system is a neurologist. These disorders include strokes (blood flow has been cut off to a portion of the brain), transient ischemic attacks (may be a precursor to a stroke), seizure disorders, and multiple sclerosis. Surgeons trained in neurology are neurosurgeons and generally perform surgery related to the brain.

Figure 17.7 Common Medical Terms for the Nervous System

Term	Meaning
Aphasia	Inability to speak (may occur with stroke patients)
Ataxia	Unstable gait (may occur with stroke patients)
CNS	Central nervous system
Craniotomy	Incision into the cranium (skull)
CSF	Cerebrospinal fluid
CVA	Cerebrovascular Accident (stroke)
Encephalitis	Inflammation of the brain
Encephalomalacia	Softening of the brain tissue
Hydrocephalus	Excess water in the head
LP	Lumbar puncture (spinal tap)
Myelocele	Herniation of the spinal chord
Myelodysplasia	Abnormal formation of the spinal cord

Eyes, Ears, and Respiratory System

While the eyes, the ears, and the respiratory system are complex in nature (and not necessarily interrelated), their medical terminology is fairly simple and therefore, easy to explain in one section. Physicians who treat the eyes (medically and surgically) are ophthalmologists.

Physicians who treat disorders of the ear (usually in conjunction with the nose and the throat) may be primary care physicians (for sinus or ear infections). However, when patients need specialized treatment or surgery, they go to an otolaryngologist (formerly known as an ENT or ear, nose, and throat physician).

Otolaryngologists perform complex surgeries on the ears, nose, throat, and related structures.

Medical physicians who treat the respiratory system also may be primary care physicians (for bronchitis, mild asthma, or pneumonia). However, patients who have severe asthma or respiratory failure see pulmonologists, who specialize in treating respiratory disorders. And general surgeons or thoracic surgeons may treat patients who need respiratory surgery, depending on the complexity of the procedure.

Figure 17.8 Common Medical Terms for the Eyes, Ears, and Respiratory System

Term	Meaning
Apnea	Temporary cessation of breathing
Blepharoptosis	Drooping of the eyelid
Bronchitis	Inflammation of the bronchus
COPD	Chronic obstructive pulmonary disease
Diplopia	Double vision
Dyspnea	Painful breathing
Emphysema	Difficulty breathing from over distention of the lungs
HEENT	Head, eyes, ears, nose, throat
Laryngitis	Inflammation of the larynx (voice box)
Otalgia	Pain in the ear
Pleurisy	Inflammation of the pleura (lining around the lung)
Pneumothorax	A collection of air in the chest cavity where it does not belong
Retinopathy	Disease of the retina
Rhinoplasty	Repair of the nose, plastic surgery of the nose
Tachypnea	Rapid breathing
Tympanotomy	Incision into the eardrum
URI	Upper respiratory infection

Circulatory System

The circulatory system includes the heart, blood vessels, and the spleen. Some of the most common disorders in this system, commonly known as the cardiac system, involve the heart. Physicians trained in this area are cardiologists.

Surgeons trained in this area are thoracic surgeons, sometimes also referred to as cardiothoracic surgeons. They perform the most extensive open-heart surgeries, such as heart valve replacements and cardiac bypass surgery. General surgeons, however, also perform other types of surgery on the circulatory system, such as on the blood vessels.

Some physicians perform heart and blood vessel surgeries using radiology procedures. These physicians are interventional radiologists. They also may surgically treat patients who have circulatory problems.

Figure 17.9 Common Medical Terms for the Circulatory System

Term	Meaning
Aneurysm	Weakening in an artery wall
Arrhythmia	Abnormal heart rhythm
Cardiovascular	System of heart, arteries, veins, and capillaries
Cardiothoracic	Related to the heart and the chest (lungs)
Iscehmia	Death of tissue caused by lack of blood flow to tissue
Lymphoma	Lymphatic tissue tumor
Phlebitis	Inflammation of the veins
Thrombocyte	Platelet cell in blood (used for clotting)
Thrombophlebitis	Inflammation of a vein (phleb) with a clot (thrombo) formation
TIA	Transient ischemic attack

Gastrointestinal System

The gastrointestinal or digestive system includes all parts of the body involved in digestion, from the mouth to the anus. More than 20 organs or specific subcomponents of organs are involved in digestion. For example, the large intestine consists of the ascending, transverse, descending, and sigmoid colon, which each have slightly different functions in the process of digestion.

Also included in the digestive system are the liver, pancreas, and gallbladder. Physicians who treat patients with digestive disorders are primary care physicians or gastroenterologists. Two of the most common conditions gastroenterologists treat are gastroenteritis (inflammation of the stomach and intestines) and GERD (gastroesophageal reflux disease).

Figure 17.10 Common Medical Terms for the Gastrointestinal System

Term	Meaning
Cholelithiasis	Stones in the gallbladder
Colitis	Inflammation of the colon (large intestine)
Diverticulosis	Pouches that develop in the colon wall
Dyspepsia	Painful digestion
EGD	Esophagogastroduodenoscopy (examination of the esophagus, stomach, and duodenum with a scope)
Enteric	Related to the small intestine
Gastritis	Inflammation of the stomach
GERD	Gastroesophageal Reflux Disease
GI	Gastrointestinal
Glossitis	Inflammation of the tongue
Hepatomegaly	Enlargement of the liver
Rectocele	Hernia of the rectum
Sublingual	Under the tongue

Musculoskeletal System

The musculoskeletal system provides support for the body and protects internal organs. Physicians who treat musculoskeletal disorders are orthopedic surgeons. Orthopedic surgeons generally perform surgery on two types of patients: those who have suffered trauma or injury or those who have "worn out" joints. The most common types of surgery performed on patients with trauma include repairs of fractured bones, torn muscles, ligaments, or tendons. The most common types of surgery performed on patients with "worn out" joints are replacement of hip or knee joints and excision or repair of herniated vertebral discs.

Patients who have non-surgical musculoskeletal disorders, such as arthritis, fibromyalgia, or pain, typically see primary care physicians, sports medicine physicians, rheumatologists, and even neurologists (for pain management).

Figure 17.11 Common Medical Terms for the Musculoskeletal System

Term	Meaning
Arthritis	Inflammation of the joint
Costectomy	Excision of a rib
Discectomy	Excision of a herniated disc
Laminectomy	Excision of the posterior arch of the vertebrae (performed for a herniated, or "slipped" disc)
Kyphosis	Posterior curvature of the spine
L1, L2, . . . L5	Lumbar vertebrae, first, second . . .fifth
OA	Osteoarthritis
ORIF	Open reduction and internal fixation (for fracture repair)
Osteochondritis	Inflammation of the bone and cartilage
Metacarpals	Bones of the hand
Metatarsals	Bones of the foot
Osteomalacia	Softening of the bones
RA	Rheumatoid Arthritis
Scoliosis	S-shaped curvature of the spine
Thoracolumbar	Pertaining to the chest and lower back

Endocrinology, Infectious Disease, and Immunology

The endocrine system involves organs, such as the pancreas and the pituitary gland, which secrete hormones into the blood. Physicians who specialize in this area of medicine are endocrinologists. The most common disorders endocrinologists treat are diabetes and obesity.

Physicians who treat infectious diseases may be primary care physicians. However, for particular infections, like HIV/AIDs, or severe pneumonias, patients would receive care from physicians specializing in infectious disease.

Immunology is the study and treatment of the human immune system, or the body's ability to resist disease. Patients who have chronic infections, certain cancers, or transplanted organs may develop immune disorders. Immunologists treat patients with these types of disorders.

Figure 17.12 Common Medical Terms for the Endocrine and Immune Systems

Term	Meaning
AIDS	Acquired immunodeficiency syndrome
Hypoglycemia	Low blood sugar
Hyperglycemia	High blood sugar
IDDM	Insulin-dependent diabetes mellitus
IgG, IgM, IgE	Immunoglobulins (antibiodies made by your immune system to protect you from disease)
Immunodeficiency	A disease characterized by the inability to fight off disease
NIDDM	Non-insulin-dependent diabetes mellitus
Onychomycosis	Fungal infection of the nails
Pyothorax	Accumulation of pus in the chest
Sx	Symptoms
T3, T4	Thyroid hormones
TSH	Thyroid stimulating hormone

Genitourinary System

The genitourinary system includes the male and female reproductive systems and the urinary system. Physicians who treat the urinary system are urologists. When a patient has a specific kidney disorder that requires continuous treatment (for example, kidney failure), a nephrologist generally provides treatment.

A gynecologist treats disorders of the female genital system. Many gynecologists also practice obstetrics, delivering babies. However, because of technological developments in reproductive medicine as well as increased medical malpractice cases in obstetric medicine over the past two decades, many physicians trained in obstetrics and gynecology choose to specialize in only one of these two areas.

Figure 17.13 Common Medical Terms for the Genitourinary and Female Genital Systems

Term	Meaning
ARF/CRF	Acute renal failure/chronic renal failure
Cystorrhaphy	Suture of the bladder
D&C	Dilation and curettage (of the uterus)
Ectopic pregnancy	Pregnancy that occurs outside of the uterus
Endometritis	Inflammation of the inner uterine lining
ESRD	End-stage renal disease
Hysterectomy	Removal of the uterus
Menorrhagia	Excessive menstruation occurring at irregular intervals
Multigravida	A woman who has experienced two or more pregnancies
Neonatology	Study of newborns
Nephritis	Inflammation of the kidney
Nocturia	Urination at night
Puerperium	The time period just after giving birth
Polyuria	Frequent urination
Primigravida	Woman who is experiencing her first pregnancy
Prostatitis	Inflammation of the prostate
Salpingo-oophorectomy	Removal of the fallopian tubes and ovaries
TAH	Total abdominal hysterectomy
TURP	Transurethral resection of the prostate

Mental Disorders

The U.S. Substance Abuse and Mental Health Services Administration (SAMHSA) defines mental health as:[2]

How a person thinks, feels, and acts when faced with life's situations. It is how people look at themselves, their lives, and the other people in their lives; evaluate their challenges and problems; and explore choices. This includes handling stress, relating to other people, and making decisions.

Mental disorders can be divided into neuroses and psychoses. Psychoses are mental disorders that involve a loss of a sense of reality. Neuroses are mental disorders that do not involve a loss of a sense of reality. Physicians who treat mental disorders are psychiatrists.

Primary care physicians also may treat some mental disorders, especially neuroses. In fact, according to statistics the National Center for Health Statistics publishes annually, the most common drug primary care physicians prescribe is antidepressant medication.[3] Other clinicians who treat individuals with mental health disorders include psychologists, licensed social workers (LSWs), and, depending on the state where you live, other licensed mental health therapists or counselors.

Figure 17.14 Common Medical Terms for Mental Disorders

Term	Meaning
Bipolar disorder	Fluctuation between mania and depression
DSM-IV	*Diagnostic and Statistical Manual of Mental Disorders*, 4th edition
ECT	Electroconvulsive therapy, uses low-voltage electrical stimulation of the brain to treat some forms of major depression, acute mania, and some forms of schizophrenia.
Group therapy	Groups of 4 to 12 people who have similar problems and meet together regularly with a therapist. The therapist uses the emotional interactions of the group's members to help them get relief from distress and possibly modify their behavior.
Hallucinations	Experiences or sensations that have no source, such as hearing nonexistent voices, seeing nonexistent things, and experiencing burning or pain.
OCD	Obsessive compulsive disorder, recurrent and unwanted thoughts or rituals, and an obsessive need to perform those rituals.
Psychoanalysis	Long-term, intensive individual therapy with a psychoanalyst three to five times a week, using "free association" to explore unconscious motivations; focuses on past conflicts as the underpinnings to current emotional and behavioral problems.
SAD	A form of depression that appears related to fluctuations in the exposure to natural light. It usually strikes during autumn and often continues through the winter when there is less natural light.
Schizophrenia	Literally, "condition of a split mind"

See How Far You Have Come

Below is the discharge summary information presented earlier, but without the definitions of the medical terms. Read the paragraph to see if you feel more confident about the meaning of some of the words. Do not expect to master the entire paragraph, but defining a few terms after this short read gives you an idea of how far you can go in learning medical terminology, the language of medicine.

The patient is a 93-year-old who noted increasing dyspnea, pedal edema, palpitations, hoarseness, and nonproductive cough over a three-week period. Patient is afebrile. No history of prior myocardial infarction or CHF or cyanosis. In the emergency room the patient was noted to be in pulmonary edema and was treated with IV Lasix and diuresed. He was given oxygen. Rhythm appeared to be sinus with frequent atrial ectopic beats and then was noted to be in and out of atrial fibrillation with some tachycardia.

Key Highlights

The language of medicine is a foreign language, but if medical terminology is new to you, it is possible, with effort, for you to acquire at least a basic understanding. Medical terminology allows clinicians to be more efficient when caring for patients. Depending on your VVMS, it may be a priority to have a good grasp of medical terminology, the language of medicine.

Key Actions

- Refer to your VVMS to decide how much time you want to spend learning the language of medicine.
- Choose a strategy to manage medical terminology: rely on your healthcare providers to explain everything to you, learn the basics, or find a mentor who can translate for you.
- Remember that most medical terms consist of a root word with a prefix or suffix, used in various combinations.

- Read the common terms and definitions in this chapter, as well as listening to the pronunciation of the words at *www.7stepshealth.com.*

Key Take-Away

The more you are able to understand the language of medicine, the more empowered you become as a healthcare consumer, and the more you increase your ability to get the best possible healthcare.

Answers to figure 17.5

1. Tachycardia	J. Fast heart beat
2. Afebrile	I. No fever
3. Cyanosis	G. Bluing of the skin
4. Hematuria	H. Blood in the urine
5. Leukopenia	D. Low white blood cell count
6. Myalgia	F. Muscle pain
7. Dyspnea	B. Painful breathing
8. Encephalopathy	E. Disease of the brain
9. Bronchitis	C. Inflammation of the bronchus
10. Cardiomyopathy	A. Disease of the heart muscle

Endnotes

[1] Weil, Andrew, MD. *Healthy Aging: A Lifelong Guide to Your Well-Being.* Anchor, 2007.

[2] U.S. Substance Abuse and Mental Health Services Administration, *www.samhsa.gov.*

[3] National Center for Health Statistics. Health, United States, 2006, with Chartbook on Trends in the Health of Americans (Table 92, page 332). Hyattsville, MD:2006. (*www.cdc.gov/nchs/hus.htm*).

CHAPTER

18

Coding: Another Medical Language You Should Know About

A different language is a different vision of life. —Federico Fellini

In 2006, after 12 years of making the same New Year's resolution, Phoebe finally had a routine medical checkup at the age of 47. She made the first resolution the year she turned 35, right after her second child was born. Two of Phoebe's friends highly recommended Dr. Grujanac, a local family practice physician.

Dr. Grujanac was a burly man of Serbian descent. He asked Phoebe questions and conducted the exam in a very structured way, completing many forms as he moved through the process. "Everything looks good so far, but I would like to run several tests on you," Dr. Grujanac explained as he wrote a few last notes on the pages in front of him. He divided the pages into two stacks. One stack, he kept in Phoebe's record. The other stack, he gave to Phoebe. Phoebe looked down at the myriad of small papers in her hands. Dr. Grujanac had written an order for a different test on each paper: an EKG, a DEXA scan, a urinalysis, a mammogram, and several orders for blood tests. "Once I get the results of all of the tests, we can schedule a follow up visit to discuss them. But so far, everything looks fine to me," he said.

As she reviewed the orders, Phoebe noticed that Dr. Grujanac had written the numbers 401.9 and 250.00 on the orders. What Dr. Grujanac didn't know was that Phoebe was a health information management (HIM) professional, trained as a coder. While the typical patient would not know the meaning of these numbers, Phoebe knew immediately. The code 401.9 is for hypertension and code 250.00 is for diabetes. These numbers on her record meant that she had these conditions.

Surprised, because she had neither of these conditions, Phoebe asked Dr. Grujanac why he wrote the numbers on the orders for the tests. "Well," he said, "that's pretty much the way I always write the orders. Over the years, I have found that when I use these numbers, insurance companies will usually pay for the tests. It's really helping *you* out." He further explained that he uses certain numbers based on what he sees during the exam with the patient. Phoebe's blood pressure was slightly high, he said, and the slight dizziness she described upon rising from a seated position could be due to abnormal blood sugar levels. If that was the case, left untreated, she *could* develop diabetes.

Then it was Phoebe's turn. She had spent most of her professional life educating physicians how to code and bill correctly. She explained to Dr. Grujanac how using these codes on her order would be documenting something about her that was not true. Furthermore, she said, "My diagnoses are sent to my insurance company. While I know it won't affect my current insurance, in the future it could be a reason for increasing my rates, especially if I ever need to purchase insurance individually."

In fact, Phoebe had been contemplating starting her own consulting firm. If she did, she would be shopping for health insurance. Phoebe refused to have the tests performed unless Dr. Grujanac wrote new orders that were accurate. Dr. Grujanac thanked Phoebe for explaining the problems with using inaccurate codes. He had never heard this explanation before and appreciated Phoebe enlightening him.

Phoebe smiled politely. She thought about all the other physicians she had worked with over the years. They had all responded the same way as Dr. Grujanac. The coding of diagnoses was not only important to her as a coder, it was also important to insurance companies, hospitals, departments of health, and medical researchers.

However, with patients and doctors, she thought, it is just different. Doctors often don't realize the impact the codes make on the patient and on the healthcare system. Patients usually are not aware of the codes at all.

Dr. Grujanac asked for Phoebe's help in writing out the orders for her tests. Given her training, Phoebe knew it was important for the information to come directly from the physician, ordering the tests. But she could ask him questions that would help him to clarify how he could document these orders. "Why *exactly* are you ordering these tests for me?" she asked him. "Are you ordering them because I have a symptom or a problem that you are investigating? Or, are you just ordering them because you believe I am healthy, and you just want baseline test results for my record?"

Dr. Grujanac thought for a minute and then replied that generally he was looking for baseline information. However, the slight dizziness upon rising that Phoebe described, combined with her slightly elevated blood pressure, did cause him to order additional tests. For example, he ordered the baseline EKG when he ordinarily would not have ordered it for a new patient unless she was at least 50. He ordered additional blood tests based upon the symptoms she described.

"Okay," Phoebe said, thinking that Dr. Grujanac should be paying her for her services or at least call this visit a wash. "You have described my dizziness and elevated blood pressure as the reason for additional testing. So, you can use the code 780.4 for dizziness and 796.2 for elevated blood pressure on my orders." Dr. Grujanac was already scribbling the numbers as Phoebe was reciting them.

"One last thing," she said as he was making his way toward the door, "documenting my symptoms, the dizziness and elevated blood pressure that you described in my record is important. It will support the fact that you used these codes. I am also happier because now my test orders accurately represent me." "Got it," Dr. Grujanac said as he exited the door. Seconds later, he popped his head back in the room. "The visit's on me, he said. It's the least I can do." Phoebe smiled. This was a first for her.

WHAT IS MEDICAL CODING AND WHY SHOULD I CARE?

Medical coding involves assigning a number, from an established coding system, to each of the diagnoses and procedures your physician documents in your medical record. The two principle systems for coding used in the United States are ICD-9-CM and CPT.

ICD-9-CM is the *International Classification of Diseases, 9th Edition*, used since 1927 to assign a code to every patient's diagnoses and procedures. The World Health Organization (WHO) originally created the ICD coding system. The United States, under the direction of the Centers for Disease Control (CDC) adopted its own version of the system. The initials "CM" stand for the United State's own "clinical modifications" to the international classification. Because of government regulatory requirements relating mainly to reimbursement, the United States is the only country in the world still using the 9th revision. All other countries use the 10th revision, which is more detailed.

CPT is the Current Procedural Terminology classification system, which the American Medical Association (AMA) developed in 1974. It is used to assign codes to physician office visits, diagnostic tests and procedures. Physician payments are determined based upon the level of visit (1 to 5) they provide to a patient. The higher the level, the higher the physician's bill will be.

Coding is important for a few reasons. First, like Phoebe's codes, the codes assigned to your medical record could have potential negative ramifications for your health insurance. Second, your insurance could reject your bill based upon the code or codes assigned. If the information causing the rejection is incorrect, you will want to resolve this issue.

Third, researchers throughout the country use data from healthcare visits. If the data is not correct, then the research will be flawed and not helpful to anyone. You can ensure accurate data in your records by checking the explanation of benefits (EOB) for each visit statements and by explaining your symptoms to your physician as accurately, detailed, and completely as possible. As you can see, your attention to your own medical record coding has many advantages, not just for you, but for everyone.

How Are Codes Assigned to My Health Information and Me?

Professional medical coders assign codes to diagnoses and procedures that your doctor has documented in your medical record. Coders, especially those who work on inpatient and surgical records, must successfully complete years of training and pass national certification exams to be proficient at the process.

As a patient, you do not need to have the same level of understanding of coding as professional medical record coders. A basic understanding of coding, along with a list of references is sufficient to be an empowered healthcare consumer—one who verifies the diagnostic codes in your medical record and on health insurance statements.

Detailed Example of Coding for a Heart Attack

The following list includes all the different codes available for patients admitted to the hospital with a heart attack. There are additional codes for patients who have had the heart attack prior to hospital admission, or when the physician has not documented exactly when the heart attack occurred.

You can see how each code designates very specific information. The digits to the left of the decimal represent the main condition [Heart attack]. The digits to the right represent the specific location and timing of the patient's heart attack.

410.01	[Heart attack] of the anteriolateral wall
410.11	[Heart attack] of other anterior wall (for example, anterioapical or anteroseptal wall)
410.21	[Heart attack] of the inferolateral wall
410.31	[Heart attack] of the interoposterior wall

410.41	[Heart attack] of other inferior wall (for example, diaphragmatic wall)
410.51	[Heart attack] of other lateral wall (for example, basal-lateral, high lateral)
410.61	[Heart attack] of the true posterior wall
410.71	[Heart attack] of the subendocardium (also nonstransmural infarct)
410.81	[Heart attack] of other specified sites (for example, atrium, papillary muscle)
410.91	[Heart attack] of unspecified site of heart

The details used in codes in the ICD-9-CM coding book are generally to facilitate medical research. For example, certain areas of the heart affected by heart attacks may respond better to certain drugs or interventions than others. However, if coders grouped all patients' heart attacks together under one general code, there would be no effective way of comparing large databases of patients with heart attacks as researchers do today.

Insurance companies and Medicare also use the detailed ICD-9-CM coding to determine if the information is sufficient for them to pay the bill. Certain insurance companies and Medicare may reject codes that are "unspecified." For example, the heart attack code 410.90 represents "heart attack of unspecified site of the heart, unspecified as to episode of care." If this code is submitted on a patient's bill, it could be a red flag for an insurance company, and the bill could be rejected unless more detailed codes are submitted by the provider. The insurance company's perspective is that if the hospital staff treated the patient for a heart attack, they should know if it was a current, acute attack (a fifth digit of "1" instead of "0"), and they should probably know where in the heart muscle the blood flow was stopped.

It Doesn't Take an Expert to Catch a Coding Mistake. As Jay's medical mentor and his wife, one of Christine's self-imposed responsibilities is reviewing the bills sent to his insurance company. Since he was 12, Jay has needed daily insulin injections for type 1 diabetes. Although Jay, now 39, has developed some common complications associated with diabetes, he has had a lot of success with the insulin pump for the past several years. This new technology now keeps his diabetes under control most of the time.

In his late 20s, Jay developed diabetic retinopathy. When his endocrinologist told him that he could lose his sight, Jay and Christine searched the eastern seaboard for the right treatment team. Eventually, they found that team at Wills Eye Hospital in Philadelphia. The team there used new technology, and performed hundreds of the laser treatments instead of the dozen his original physician had recommended. Treatment at the Wills Eye Hospital was successful. Jay retained his eyesight, and the team continues to manage his diabetic retinopathy.

Recently, Jay had a follow-up laser surgery for his diabetic retinopathy. For reasons unknown to him or Christine, the insurance company refused to pay for this surgery, although they had paid for all of the prior laser surgeries. Christine checked the insurance benefits, which indicated no limitations on the number of times Jay could receive this type of surgery. The rejection notice that they received simply said, "Diagnosis does not match procedure."

Neither Jay, a sales professional, nor Christine, a human resources director, was ever formally trained in the health insurance process. They learned "on the job." Christine looked at the diagnosis code on the EOB. It was the same code she had seen on Jay's other bills: 250.01, the code for type 1 diabetes. However, Christine didn't stop there.

She then compared the paid bills with the current bill to see if she could find some other difference. She was sure that the insurance company had made a mistake. As she reviewed the old bills, she quickly saw that the first three had the code 250.01, just as she remembered. When she got to the fourth bill, however, she saw a slight difference. On this bill, the number was 250.51, one digit different. This one-digit difference seemed too easy a solution to Christine. She thought this could not possibly be the difference between the insurance company paying an $18,000 bill or not. Still, it was a difference worth checking out. Seeing the designation of "ICD-9-CM code" in the box to the left of the 250.51 on the bill, she decided to Google the term *ICD-9-CM code* and found a Web site that listed every ICD-9-CM code. Next to the number for each code was a diagnosis or a description. As she scrolled down the 200s, right after 250.00, she found 250.01.

Comparing the descriptions of the two codes, she saw that 250.01 said, "Type 1 diabetes without complications" and 250.51 said, "Type 1 diabetes with *retinal complications.*" "So, that explains it!" Christine thought, realizing that the hospital had made the mistake, not the insurance company. Feeling newly schooled in the nuances of coding, Christine made the necessary phone calls to the physician and the hospital to change the number, and the insurance company paid the bill.

WHAT RESPONSIBILITIES DO I HAVE REGARDING HOW MY MEDICAL RECORDS ARE CODED?

As a patient, it is not your responsibility to make sure your physician uses the correct documentation. However, it is your responsibility to provide your physician with detailed, accurate, and complete information about your health status. In addition, checking your bill for accuracy of the diagnoses can help keep the process in check.

At the end of your visit to your physician, you will usually receive a one-page summary from your physician or his office assistant. This summary form, also called a *superbill* lists diagnoses and visit codes. If you do not receive one, ask for a copy before you leave. The physician checks the boxes on the form that represent your diagnoses and the level of your visit. Before you leave the office, review the superbill to make sure, like Phoebe, that your physician is not mistakenly recording a diagnosis on your bill.

Check your explanation of benefits (EOB) that you receive from your insurance company, whether they pay or deny your bill. If they deny the bill, you may be able to find a problem with the coding, as Christine did. Even if the insurance company pays your bill, it still is a good idea to make sure that the bill does not contain erroneous codes and diagnoses. Not only will this type of verification help ensure that your insurance records are accurate, but it will also ensure that the insurance company does not pay for treatment you did not receive. You may wonder why you should go this extra step for an insurance company—well, aside from being honest, it helps prevent unnecessary increases in insurance costs for everyone.

Coding: Another Form of Medical Shorthand

In chapter 18, I discussed how healthcare professionals use medical terminology to be more efficient, saving seconds or minutes, which in some cases can make the difference between life and death. Of course, the use of coding is not a life or death decision. However, it does significantly condense medical record information. For example, a coder can turn a 50-page patient record into 10 to 20 numbers that represent the most relevant patient information.

Coding Examples for Some Common Conditions in the Hospital

In this section, I briefly describe a few examples for coding hospital patients' diagnoses and treatments. Following each patient care summary, I list the appropriate codes. (Keep in mind that some codes may change after publication of this book.) These examples give an idea of the detail used in coding, as well as how coders translate your diagnoses into numbers for easy analysis. A good example was Jay's diagnosis of type 1 diabetes with diabetic retinopathy. The code for this diagnosis translates to 250.51, a more efficient way of stating the diagnosis.

Coding for a Patient Who Has Several Diagnoses

A patient is admitted to the hospital with asthma and develops respiratory failure and pneumonia. The patient's medical history shows that his father died of a heart attack. The doctor gives him medications for diabetes and hypertension, and documents that the patient was noncompliant with taking this medicine prior to entering the hospital. For 56 pages of medication orders, progress notes, consultant reports, and history and physical information, seven codes sum up the patient's clinical condition:

493.90	Asthma
518.81	Respiratory failure
486	Pneumonia
250.00	Diabetes, unspecified
401.9	Hypertension
V15.81	Noncompliance with medications
V17.3	Family history of heart disease

The first column (the one with the numbers) is the part of your coded information that hospitals send to insurance companies, the government, and, once they remove your name, to research organizations and other groups. You may have noticed your own diagnostic codes on your insurance bills.

The second column, to the right of the numbered codes, lists the medical terminology. The difference between coding and medical terminology is that as a patient, you do not have to communicate with your physician using the coding. In fact, most clinicians do not even know coding. They rely on trained coders to translate their documentation into coded data.

Coding for Routine Delivery of a Baby

A 41-year-old female in labor with her first child is admitted to the hospital. Her water broke on the way into the ER. Five hours later, she delivers a healthy baby girl. The baby develops slight jaundice later that evening and she receives phototherapy. The jaundice resolves, and the following morning, the hospital discharges both mom and baby. Mom and baby came into the hospital as one patient, but they leave as two patients, they have separate records, codes, and bills.

Codes on the mom's record:

658.11	Rupture of amniotic sac less than 24 hours prior to delivery
659.51	First pregnancy in a woman who will be 35 years of age or older at expected date of delivery
V27.0	Single live born (the outcome of delivery is coded on every mother's medical record)

Codes on the baby's record:

V30.00	Single live born delivered without mention of caesarean section in the hospital
774.6	Unspecified jaundice of the newborn

Coding for a Stroke Patient

An 82-year-old man is admitted to the hospital with a stroke. Doctors determine his stroke is due to a cerebral bleed that necessitated surgery. The patient was not able to speak, walk, or swallow. He also required an abdominal feeding tube and transfer to the hospital's rehabilitation unit, where he received physical and occupational therapy. Within 40 days, he was able to walk, talk, and feed himself. The rehab unit discharged him to home 45 days after his initial admission to the hospital. The patient's coding:

Codes for diagnoses:

431	Stroke due to cerebral bleeding
784.3	Inability to speak (aphasia)
781.2	Inability to walk alone (ataxia)
787.2	Inability to swallow/painful swallowing (dysphagia)

Codes for procedures:

01.39	Draining cerebral bleed
43.11	Placement of feeding tube through abdomen

Coding Examples for Some Common Conditions in the Physician's Office

In this section, I describe a few examples for coding patients' visits to physician offices. Following each patient care summary, I list the appropriate codes.

Coding for Patient with Fever and Other Conditions

A 42-year-old man schedules a visit to his physician for a fever and sore throat. The physician diagnoses the patient with an upper respiratory infection. He also notes that he has hypertension.

99212	Office visit, level 2
465.9	Upper respiratory infection
401.9	Hypertension

Coding for Patient with High Cholesterol and Other Conditions

A patient sees her physician for high cholesterol. She also has hypertension, cataracts, and is obese.

99215	Office visit, level 5
272.0	High cholesterol
401.9	Hypertension (high blood pressure)
366.9	Cataract
278.00	Obesity

WIKINOMICS AND CODING

For a little less than a decade, millions of individuals, through a loose system of shared intellectual capital, have been collaborating to create concepts like Wikinomics, Web sites like Wikipedia, and open software systems like Linux. Likewise, the healthcare data sets that are available nationally and internationally may be some of the first examples of common intellectual healthcare capital. Each data point represents one encounter with a healthcare professional.

From an individual perspective within this huge data set, the information you provide to healthcare professionals, through both your own verbal communication and the information from your symptoms and test results are translated to create a single record with many diagnoses. How you communicate your own information influences what your data looks like. How your information is translated by the physician and then the coder also influences what your data looks like. While you cannot totally control the coding process, you can, like Phoebe did, self-police the process by looking at your bills and your test orders to validate that the information about you is accurate.

ICD-9-CM RESOURCES

For a general guide, figure 18.1 shows some of the more common diagnoses along with their ICD-9-CM code, for each chapter in the *ICD-9-CM 2007* . It is helpful to understand what is in each chapter to locate codes and other information you may need as you review your medical record and insurance billing statements.

The table does not represent the complexities of the coding system and the many rules that credentialed coders apply to determine the best code for a particular diagnosis. You can purchase a current version of the ICD-9-CM coding book from various publishers. Most are available on *amazon.com*. For more information on coding, see this Web site: *icd9cm.chrisendres.com/200.*

Figure 18.1 *ICD-9-CM 2007* Codes in Order by Body System

Type of Condition	Diagnoses and Codes
Infectious diseases	HIV = 042; Herpes = 054.9; Hepatitis = 070.9; Mononucleosis = 075; Chlamydia = 079.99
Cancer and other tumors	Colon cancer = 153.9; Lung cancer = 162.9; Skin cancer = 173.9; Breast cancer = 174.9; Prostate cancer = 185; Hodgkin's disease = 201.90
Endocrine and nutritional	Type 2 diabetes = 250.00; Type 1 diabetes = 250.01; Obesity = 278.00; Morbid obesity = 278.01; Malnutrition = 263.9; Dehydration = 276.5; Hypercholesterolemia = 272.0
Blood	Anemia = 285.9; Sickle-cell anemia = 282.69; Aplastic anemia = 284.9; Hemophilia = 286.0

Type of Condition	Diagnoses and Codes
Mental health and substance abuse	Schizophrenia = 295.90; Depression = 311; Bipolar disorder = 296.80; Anxiety = 300.00; Alcohol abuse = 305.00; Tobacco abuse = 305.1; Bulimia = 307.51; ADD = 314.00
Nervous system	Alzheimer's disease = 331.0; Parkinson's disease = 332.0; Multiple sclerosis = 340; Epilepsy = 345.90; Migraine = 346.9
Heart and circulatory system	Hypertension = 401.9; Angina = 413.9; Heart attack = 410.91; Arrhythmia = 427.89; Heart failure = 428.00; Stroke = 436
Respiratory system	Pneumonia= 486; COPD = 496; Emphysema = 492.8
Digestive system	Esophageal reflux = 530.81; Hernia = 550.90; Gastroenteritis = 558.9; Gallstones = 574.20; Gastrointestinal bleeding = 578.9
Urinary system and sex organs	Urinary tract infection = 599.0; Kidney failure = 585
Pregnancy	Normal delivery of one child = 650; Twin delivery = 651.01
Skin	Diaper rash = 691.0; Psoriasis = 696.1; Acne = 706.1
Muscles and bones	Rheumatoid arthritis = 714.0; Arthritis = 716.99; Bunion = 727.1
Congenital conditions	Spina bifida = 741.90; Congenital heart defect = 746.9
Newborn	Preterm infant = 765.19; Jaundice of the newborn = 774.6
Symptoms	Fainting = 780.2; Seizures = 780.39; Headache = 784.0; Palpitations = 785.1; Cough = 786.2; Chest pain = 786.50 Nausea and vomiting = 787.01; Abdominal pain = 789.00
Injuries	Fractured ribs = 807.09; Fractured vertebrae = 805.9
Non-sick reasons for visiting a healthcare provider	Personal history of cancer = V10.X; Family history of cardiovascular disease = V17.X; Newborn = V30.0X

Key Highlights

Every time you see a healthcare provider, he documents in your medical record. Coders then translate that documentation into ICD-9-CM and/or CPT codes. Insurance companies, researchers, government agencies, and healthcare planning organizations all use medical codes for different purposes. Understanding what medical coding is, and how the coding process works, enables you to be alert for mistakes that could negatively affect your insurance payments, insurance rates, and, most importantly, your health.

Key Actions

- Understand that coders assign diagnostic and procedural codes using a complex, detail-specific process, so it is possible for mistakes to occur that can affect your bill.
- Ask you provider what the codes on your bill or medical record mean, or look them up in the newest version of the *ICD-9-CM,* or on the Internet.
- Check the codes on the EOB from your insurance company for bill and medical record accuracy.

Key Take-Away

You can use your basic coding knowledge and online resources to make sure your healthcare bills and medical records are correct.

Afterword

Today, Emmalea has been seizure-free for six months, a huge milestone for anyone with epilepsy. We began the six-month countdown so many times during the first year and a half without success, that all of us are almost afraid to mention that we are finally there. So, we celebrate silently, each in our own way. Some are celebrating through prayer and positive thoughts, others simply rejoicing in the knowledge that Em is finally on a clear path towards a seizure-free life. As for me, I am celebrating by writing the conclusion to this book on this day. I have waited purposefully, and may have even delayed the publication date a bit. Call me superstitious, but when I first began writing this book with Emmalea as my primary inspiration, I pictured myself writing the conclusion on this date.

The next seizure-free milestone is one year. So, we begin the next count down. I feel certain that her seizures will still be in control in a year (and beyond) because she is committed to and responsible for her health, has an excellent healthcare team, and a complete record of all of her healthcare interactions. Emmalea may not have a formal written VVMS, but she does have one that she carries in her head that she follows religiously and with a positive spirit. Also, unlike most of us, Emmalea began developing these life skills, out of necessity, at the age of 19. Her strength, focus, and maturity through this difficult period leaves me both awestruck and immensely proud.

In our family's journey with Emmalea, who is now 21, we have learned about her body, her brain, and her dietary needs. We have also seen her willpower and determination to reach the six-month milestone. She was a child who, for the first 18 years of her life could not swallow a pill. The day after her first seizure, along with continuous coaching sessions from her brother and her cousin Valerie, she taught herself to swallow 16 pills a day. That number is now down to six pills a day. Although she has gotten slightly discouraged after each seizure, her attitude has always been, "whatever it takes." With that attitude, her plan and her resources, she has a higher likelihood of staying healthy and in control.

When I gave the unpublished manuscript of this book to Emmalea to read, I feared the worst—that she would be uncomfortable with revealing the details of her epilepsy to you. After all, as I discuss in the book, we all have a high expectation of privacy in our health information. Having your health story printed for the world to read is certainly a violation of privacy unless you agree to it. However, Emmalea is a talented poet and artist. After reading the manuscript, she turned to me and thoughtfully said, "I think it's important for artists to use their own experiences to communicate their message. That's what this book does." She then went on to say that if her story can help even just one other person, revealing some private details would be worth it.

As for the other stories in this book, hopefully they have helped effectively illustrate the *7 Steps* for you. As for Vera, she remains on a positive healthcare path. And, like Emmalea, she also has created a VVMS that she is using to manage her healthcare moving forward. For the 2,000 individuals who shared their positive stories in healthcare with me, it is clear that although healthcare is complex and confusing, there is much good that does come from even some of the worst experiences. If this weren't true, I would not have received 2,000 responses to my request in less than 24 hours. It also tells us that people have a need to share their stories. While sharing may be therapeutic for each of them, we can all learn from the stories of others.

So, here you are, at the end of reading some, or all, of this book. From the beginning of the book where we first created your VVMS together through all of the discussions on healthcare providers, places, and information, hopefully you now realize that even though the healthcare system is indeed complex, you *can* learn to manage it. In fact, you owe it to yourself and to anyone who loves or cares about you to learn to manage the system and the people in it.

Once you boil any complex process down into its component parts, such as understanding how to manage the healthcare system in *7 steps*, it becomes much easier to grasp. If you create your vision, own your story, build your relationships, access quality, understand the people, know the places and learn the language, you, like Emmalea, will have a greater probability of reaching your healthcare goals. And, most important, you will be empowered as you continue moving forward on a positive path to improved healthcare and improved health.

As you do move forward and apply the concepts I have shared with you in this book, I hope you will let me know about your own victories and the victories of your loved ones. Please also let me know about questions you have or issues you would like to know more about. You can submit questions through the *7stepshealth.com* Web site. Once there, you can also share your own positive experiences in healthcare through the Web site as a way for others to learn from your story.

Thank you for joining me in this journey. I hope you will refer back to this book often as you move toward and then continue to maintain your best possible healthcare.

Appendix 1 How to Review Your Medical Record

Your hospital medical record is a complex document. Every piece of your medical record serves a separate purpose. As you learned in chapters 4 and 5, different people use your medical records in different ways. In this appendix we address the different parts of the most multifaceted medical record—the hospital record. It also provides some information about the contents of medical records in other settings. You will find it helpful to refer to your own medical record as you read—particularly if you have a hospital record.

WHY SHOULD I CARE ABOUT THIS?

By now, I'm sure you can see how important it is for you to take responsibility to create, understand, and manage your medical records. For years you have most likely received healthcare without knowing anything about your medical record, what it looked like or why healthcare providers collected certain types of information about you. So you may be asking yourself, why do I need to know now?

First, gaining a greater understanding of your own medical records and health information helps you to take charge of your own healthcare decisions. Second, if you understand the significance of the information you provide to your healthcare team, you are more likely to provide the most accurate, detailed, and complete information. A greater understanding of how your healthcare team relies on that information also enables you to be a participating partner in your healthcare outcome.

Third, as I addressed in chapter 6, federal law gives you the right to review and request corrections to your record. To an extent, having this right makes you accountable for the quality of information in your medical record. If you choose not to exercise this right, then you must take at least partial responsibility for incorrect information in your records. Knowing how to review your records may help you to be more accountable for its contents.

Finally, understanding what is in your medical record may enable you to better appreciate the process used to provide your treatment. The format of your medical record is reflective of medical treatment philosophies. You may not be aware of, or may not recall, the many types of treatment and testing you have received in the past. I will discuss some of the built-in redundancies and checks and balances in the system for documenting your healthcare. Familiarity with the content of your medical record builds confidence in healthcare decision making.

DO I REALLY WANT TO *READ* MY MEDICAL RECORD?

Perhaps the thought of reading the details of your hysterectomy, prostatectomy, or open-heart surgery is not appealing. This is understandable. Here, then, is another opportunity to review your values, vision, and mission statement (VVMS) and define how extensively you want to interact with your records.

Chapter 4 explains the benefits of obtaining and maintaining all of your medical records in one location for continuity of your care. However, *obtaining* your records and *reading* them are two very different things. You can obtain your records and never read them, leaving that to the clinicians. Or you can read every page of every record, line by line. The best approach for most patients is probably somewhere in the middle. Part of the goal of this chapter is to give you a strategy for reading your medical records: which reports are most important to read and what are the key pieces of information in a report.

Remember this caveat: reviewing a medical record for a novice may be daunting. As you review your record, it is important not to jump to conclusions based on discrete pieces of data. If you do have questions or concerns, you need to ask your physician to provide his or her interpretation of *all* the information. Start out your review by using my suggested approach and, as you become more familiar with your records, delve into different parts in more detail.

WHEN SHOULD I READ MY MEDICAL RECORD?

The short answer to this question is that it is best to obtain and review your medical records *after* you have received care. And long enough after so that you are feeling well enough to get value out of anything you may read in your record.

Although you have a responsibility to obtain, maintain, and be familiar with the content of your medical records, your physicians and other healthcare providers have the primary responsibility for creating your record. It is their ultimate responsibility to document information in your record that is correct, accurate, reliable, consistent, legible, and timely. Unless you have some significant, immediate concern, it is best not to question your healthcare team's process at the time they are treating you. You should be entering into a relationship with a physician and other members of your healthcare team that is trusting and positive. They are the experts. It is important for you to trust that they will create your medical records with your best interest in mind.

WHAT CAN I DO IF PARTS OF MY RECORD ARE ILLEGIBLE?

Legibility of physician handwriting is an issue in every hospital. Nearly every medical record I have ever reviewed—more than 100,000 so far in my lifetime—had at least one illegible note. Some were completely illegible. Many accrediting and government agencies have created sanctions or fines for hospitals with illegible medical records. In the meantime, what can you do if you obtain your medical record and cannot read it?

Under the Health Insurance Portability and Accountability Act (HIPAA), you have the right to request a correction in your medical record if you believe the information is incorrect, inaccurate, or incomplete. If you cannot read the information in your record due to illegibility, you can file a request for correction with the hospital. Ask that the physician rewrite the information legibly so you can read it. This is a reasonable request. And, if more patients exercised this right, maybe more physicians would provide legible documentation. The downside to this approach is that it may take several days or weeks for the physician to document the information you are requesting.

If you want more immediate results, you might seek help reading the illegible record from several experienced individuals, including staff in the HIM department, another clinician, or even the physician who created the record. You also may consider sending a letter, along with copies of the illegible information (minus your identification information), to the hospital administrator. Providing this feedback may not only help you, it may help other patients by making the physician more accountable for the legibility of his future documentation.

HOW TO REVIEW YOUR HOSPITAL RECORD'S CONTENTS

The following sections highlight contents of hospital medical records, taken mostly from electronic sources. The information is based on actual patient records, but all patient identifying information has been removed. It's important to note that specific medical record formats and forms vary from hospital to hospital. The forms in your record may look different from these examples, but the content is probably similar. The contents presented in this chapter are in the same order that they are generally created in your record, from the history and physical (first) to the discharge summary (last).

Not all forms will be part of every patient record. For example, if you receive treatment during a stay for pneumonia, you will not have an operative report in your record. For forms that are required for every patient record, I have marked *Required* next to the title of the form or medical record entry. I also have added *Key Report* to those reports that are most important for you to review. In general, if you only have a brief amount of time, review your history and physical, and discharge summary. Together these reports should address most key information in your record. I also have marked *Look For* notes with each report. These notes identify what parts of the form or medical record entry are the most important to read.

History and Physical (*Required, Key Report*)

As you may recall from chapter 4, your history and physical (H&P) is, by far, the most comprehensive document in your medical record. During a hospital stay, your H&P is the first document completed. It contains key information about your condition, including symptoms upon admission, current medications, and any chronic conditions, such as hypertension, diabetes, or asthma. Physicians usually document their initial "impression and plan"—their first instinct regarding the symptoms and the best course of action to pursue—at the end of the H&P.

In the hospital, physicians may handwrite or dictate (for transcription into a typed document) your H&P. Federal and state laws and guidelines drive the contents of the reports, so that the minimum requirements are consistent from hospital to hospital.

In a teaching hospital, your H&P has multiple authors. Interns are most likely the first clinicians to interview you and gather information for your H&P. They record your H&P and then a more senior resident reviews it. Finally, your attending physician reviews the report, signs it, and places it in your medical record for other clinicians' reference.

Look For: the physician's initial assessment or impression about the cause of your symptoms, usually at the end of the document. This assessment usually includes plans for testing and possible treatment. You should not be surprised when you read the initial assessment, as your physician should have talked to you about it while you were in the hospital. If this is not the case, read further in your record to see if the documentation becomes more consistent with your final diagnosis. If it does not, ask your physician to clarify the documentation for you.

Figure A1.1 Sample: H&P Report

Patient name: **Medical record #:** **Date of admission:**

Chief complaint: severe obstruction during sleep

History of present illness: The patient is a 29-year-old female with nothing significant in the past medical history who was here for sleep study arranged by her primary care physician. As per parents, patient started snoring at age 15 and the snoring has worsened in the past few months. It was associated with brief pauses in respiration lasting a few seconds, occasionally waking her up from sleep approximately 2 to 3 times a night. The patient feels very tired during the day. On sleep study she had 50 episodes of apnea and hypercapnea de-saturating to the fifties, needing further management.

Review of systems: The patient's review of systems is remarkable for that mentioned above in the history of present illness. All other systems are negative.

Allergies: Patient is allergic to penicillin and ampicillin and shell fish.

Family history: There is a family history of asthma and eczema.

Social history: The patient lives with her parents. No siblings, no tobacco use at home, alcohol only on special occasions, no HIV risks.

Physical examination: On physical examination, the patient's vital signs are weight of 88 kg, temperature of 97 degrees, blood pressure 118/69 mmHg, respiratory rate is 17 per minute, pulse ox is 100% on room air, pulse 111 beats per minute. The patient is a healthy appearing female in no acute distress. HEENT: Normocephalic, atraumatic. Ears, nose throat examination is within normal limits. Nasopharynx, hypertrophic mucosa. Oropharynx, tonsils enlarged left greater than right, no erythema or exudate. Exraocular movements are intact. No icterus. Neck is supple, no lymphadenopathy. Lungs are clear to auscultation bilaterally. Cardiovascular has a regular rate and rhythm, S1 and S2 are normal. 2+ pulses symmetric. The patient's abdomen is soft and nontender, nondistended. Musculoskeletal, normal gait, no joint swelling or tenderness. Skin has no rash. Neurological, normal.

Initial Assessment and Plan: Patient will be evaluated for possible tonsillectomy and adenoidectomy.

Progress Notes (*Required, Key Report*)

Progress notes are notes that the physician or other clinician documents, usually on blank, lined paper in your record. In hospital records, they are almost always handwritten, often with varying degrees of legibility. The progress note section is like the "town hall" of the patient record. This is where all the clinicians treating a patient document their current observations, plans, and treatments. Assuming they are legible, you may enjoy reading progress notes. There is something about the candid nature of progress notes that cannot be captured in a formal report. Just keep in mind that clinicians usually handwrite progress notes.

At smaller, non-teaching hospitals, one progress note per day generally is the norm. However, at an academic medical center, you could have several progress notes per day. In one academic medical center in New York City, we calculated the mean number of progress notes per day to be nine. On average, patients had two entries from an intern, two from a resident, one from a fellow, one from a medical school student, one from a consulting physician, and one from an attending physician—an example of the "check-and-balance" system of the academic medical center environment.

In some hospitals, progress notes are integrated, which means that all clinicians treating a patient document their notes in the same place. In an integrated progress note environment, on one given day, you might have entries by all of your physicians, the three different nurses who cared for you during each of their shifts, your nutritionist, your physical therapist, and your respiratory therapist. Integrating the notes is generally the best way for the healthcare team to have a good idea about everything that is going on with each patient from day to day. However, in a non-integrated environment, nurses have their own set of "nursing notes," therapists, their own set, and so on. With this system, team members must flip back and forth among different sets of notes to see everything that happened to a patient on a given day.

A Note on SOAP Format for Progress Notes

The SOAP format is a technique of writing progress notes that requires the physician to document the *subjective* aspects of the patient's care, or how the patient is feeling; the *objective* aspects, or what the test results say; the physician's *assessment* of the subjective and objective components; and the physicians *plan* for the patient. The SOAP format used to be quite popular. Today, healthcare providers' use varies in frequency. Although SOAP format is well structured and clearly written, in our technology-driven, fast-paced world, its main drawback is that it requires more time than an unstructured note. As I've mentioned before, in medical situations, time is always critical. The samples in figure A1.2 show both a SOAP note and a progress note in unstructured form. Information in parentheses provides additional definitions, added for explanatory purposes.

Look For: a final diagnosis or diagnoses at the end of the progress note. In the SOAP format, the diagnosis is in the "P" or plan section of the note. In the following progress note, the patient's diagnosis is bradycardia (*slow heart beat).* Keep in mind that the diagnosis may change based on additional test results. So, it is important to look at the diagnosis in *each* progress note throughout a hospital stay to see the evolution of decision-making around your diagnosis.

Figure A1.2 Samples: SOAP Report and Progress Note

Soap Report (by resident)
Patient 1: 1/16/06 7:40 a.m.

Pt is a 64 y.o. AAF with h/o aortic valve replacement and arrhythmia who was admitted for ↑ SOB (*shortness of breath*) and chest tightness.

S: Patient states that she is feeling good. SOB better. Without further episodes of chest tightness. Pt reports that her legs are swollen. They feel heavy.

O: Vitals: Today am: T: 98.2 R: 18: P 52; BP 164/64; I/O: 700/BR privileges; Wt 93.55 kg. PE: HEENT: Normal; CN: RRR with SEM; ABD: soft; EXTR: 1+ pitting edema *(a swelling in the tissue under the skin of the lower legs and feet)*

A: SOB (*shortness of breath*) most likely secondary to bradycardia, which was due to her digoxin medication.

P: D/C digoxin. Echo showed no wall motion abnormalities. Pt has normal heart function. Pt scheduled for stress test today.

Progress Note (by attending)
Patient 2: 2/4/05 3:00 p.m.

Hypertensive urgency better, but still needs additional meds. No angina or CP (chest pain) since admit. Influenza A → resolving pulmonary infection. Supportive care. Continue infusions.

Consultation Report

A consultation report is a detailed report written by a specialist at the request of your primary care physician. You will only have a consultation report in your record if your primary care physician requests a consultation. The consultant must complete a written report following his examination of and consultation with you.

The contents of the consultation are similar to the H&P, only with additional, detailed information about the specialist's opinion regarding diagnosis and recommended treatment. For example: You are admitted to the hospital with shortness of breath. Your primary care physician (PCP) initially believes it is an exacerbation of your asthma to treat as usual, but she orders some tests just to be sure. The test results cause her to suspect you may also have some cardiac issues going on, but she isn't 100 percent positive. Because cardiology is not her area of expertise, she requests a cardiology consult.

The cardiologist examines you, interviews you, and analyzes all of your test results. The cardiologist may: (1) recommend additional tests and continue to treat you along with your PCP, (2) decide that there is no cardiac condition and recommend that the PCP continue to treat you solo, or (3) decide no additional tests are necessary, diagnose you with a cardiac condition based on the information already collected, and continue to follow you with your PCP. The consultant's report goes in your record once transcribed, for the entire treatment team's reference. The consultant usually also sends a copy of the report to the requesting physician for her office files. (For a sample consultation report, see figure A1.3.)

As you review your record, you may see some disagreement between your primary care physician and the consulting specialist. If, for example, one physician documents a stroke and another physician documents a transient ischemic attack (TIA), a much less serious condition, you will want to know which diagnosis is correct. The official "rules" in the hospital setting dictate that the PCP (or attending physician) documentation takes precedence over any of the consulting physicians' documentation. However, I have spoken with many PCPs who believe that the consultants are the experts, and whatever they say is final. If you are in doubt, ask your PCP to clarify for you. You can also go back to chapter 9 and review the section on what to do when doctors disagree.

Look For: the final diagnosis, which usually is at the end of the consultation report just after the impression or plan. Be sure to read the specific recommendations for testing and treatment that the consultant documents. If any of this information is new to you, read the rest of your record to see if the record becomes clearer. If, after reviewing your entire record, the information in the consultation report still does not make sense to you, ask your PCP or the consultant for clarification.

Figure A1.3 Sample: Consultation Report

Patient name:	**Medical record #:**	**Date:**

Consultation service: ENT/Otolaryngology

Reason for consultation: Evaluate patient for tonsillectomy and adenoidectomy for sleep apnea.
This consultation was requested by Dr. X. This is a 29-year-old female admitted post sleep study. The patient has a history of loud snoring, witnessed apnea, daytime drowsiness, and headaches in the morning. Past medical history: the patient has a remote history of asthma. Past social history is noncontributory. Patient is on no medications. Physical exam shows a large amount of adenoid tissue, larynx is normal.

Plan: It is my recommendation that this patient be cleared for tonsillectomy and adenoidectomy surgery.

Thank you for allowing me to follow this patient with you, Dr. Z.

Surgery/Operative Report

Whenever you have a surgical procedure at a hospital, the surgeon performing the operation must dictate a detailed report about the surgery within 24 hours of your operation. Because a lot can happen in that time, the first thing the surgeon does after the procedure, is handwrite a progress note, documenting the basics of the surgical procedure. Generally, the surgeon's immediate postoperative note includes the diagnosis, the surgery performed, a brief explanation of tissue removed, any unexpected events, and the amount of blood loss during the surgery.

It is important for the surgeon to enter this brief note into your record as soon as possible after surgery. This way, the entire clinical team caring for you is aware that you had the surgery. They will also be able to read about the outcome and the postoperative diagnosis. The formal, more detailed operative report, transcribed sometimes days after your procedure, describes all of the steps involved in the surgery. Your record will also contain anesthesia reports regarding your condition before, during, and after you received anesthesia. (For a sample surgery report, see figure A1.4.)

Look For: pre- and postoperative diagnosis and the surgery performed. This information should be at the beginning of the report. If any of the information surprises you, or you do not understand it, ask your surgeon for clarification.

Figure A1.4 Sample: Surgery/Operative Report

Patient name: **Medical record #:** **Date:**

Operative report

Surgeon: Dr. A
First assistant surgeon: Dr. B
Service: ENT/Otolaryngology

Preoperative diagnosis: Obstructive sleep apnea
Postoperative diagnosis: Obstructive sleep apnea
Operative procedure: Tonsillectomy and adenoidectomy
Estimated blood loss: 50cc
Complications: None
Anesthesia: General endotracheal tube
Pathology: Tonsils and adenoids sent for permanent section.
Description of procedure: The patient was brought to the operating room and underwent general endo-tracheal tube anesthesia. The endo-tracheal tube was taped in the midline position. A Crowe-Davis retractor was used to open the oral cavity. A red rubber catheter was inserted through the nose and the oral cavity to elevate the soft palate. The tonsils were found to be roughly 3+ on both sides. Approximately 4 cc of -.25% Marcaine was injected in both tonsillar fossae that pushed both tonsils medially. We palpated the adenoid bed and found a large amount of adenoid tissue. Using an adenoid curette, the vomer was engaged trans-orally and with several sweeps, a large amount of adenoid tissue was removed from the nasopharynx…the tonsillar capsule was found, and dissection was carried superiorly, laterally, and interiorly to dissect free the left tonsil along the tonsillar capsule. There were a few sites of bleeding that were immediately cauterized using the Bovie cautery. We then retracted the right tonsil medially using an Allis clamp, and a mucosal incision along the anterior pillar was made, and dissection was carried superiorly, laterally and interiorly to dissect free the right tonsil. We then removed the tonsil balls from the nasopharynx and examined the nasopharynx. We then tilted the head forward and found no further bleeding, and thus the patient was extubated. The coral cavity and oropharynx was carefully irrigated, and the patient was extubated and transported to the PACU in stable condition.

Pathology Report

Whenever surgeons remove tissue from your body during a procedure, no matter how small it is, they must send it to the pathology department to examine and diagnose. The tissue could be anything, a cancerous tumor, a piece of infected skin, your appendix. Although surgeons or internists often make a preliminary diagnosis based on what they see, your diagnosis is not final until the pathologist determines the specific results. The pathologist who is examining the tissue must dictate a report describing both the gross and microscopic characteristics of the tissue as well as her final diagnosis. This report also goes into your medical record for your clinical team to read (for a sample pathology report, see figure A1.5).

Look For: the microscopic or pathologic diagnosis. This is the final diagnosis for any tissue removed during surgery. This diagnosis should agree with the surgeon's postoperative diagnosis on your operative report, as well as whatever the surgeon has shared with you. If it does not, ask your surgeon for clarification.

Figure A1.5 Sample: Pathology Report

Patient name: **Medical record #:** **Date:**

Surgical pathology report

Clinical diagnosis and history: obstructive sleep apnea
Specimen source: adenoid tissue; right and left tonsil

Pathologic diagnosis:
A. Adenoid, adenoidectomy: lymphoepithelial tissue with follicular hyperplasia [overgrowth]
B. Tonsils, bilateral tonsillectomy: lymphoepithelial tissue with follicular hyperplasia

Gross description:
Specimen A is received in formalin labeled with the patient's name and "adenoid tissue" and consists of multiple fragments of tan, focally congested soft tissue measuring 3.2 x 1.8 x 0.8 cm in aggregate. The specimen is grossly unremarkable.

Summary of sections:
A-1, one piece

Specimen B is received in formalin labeled with the patient's name and "right and left tonsil" and consists of two pink-tan un-oriented, nodular tissue, and three additional fragments of pink-tan soft tissue. The mucosa-covered, nodular soft tissue measures 2.9 x 2.5 x 1.5 cm, and 2.3 x 1.7 x 1.3 cm. The three additional tissue fragments measure 1.7 x 1.2 x 0.4 cm in aggregate. The nodular tissues show homogenous pink-tan parenchyma. Representative sections are submitted.

Summary of sections:
B-1, right and left tonsils, two pieces

Laboratory Report

Laboratory tests are probably the most commonly performed tests. Given that there are more than 200 different components in human blood, the amount of information that a laboratory test report can provide is quite voluminous. Perhaps you have had a nurse or technician draw your blood and watched as numerous vials filled up. This section explores the results of a laboratory test and the report that represents the analysis of your blood.

As with any test, it is important to have your physician act as the buffer between any abnormal result and your diagnosis, if any, that the lab results represent. Every lab test identifies when a result is high (H) or Low (L) for the expected norms (for a person of your gender and your age). However, the H or L value is not necessarily of concern. Your physician interprets the results for you. In addition, normal ranges vary slightly lab to lab, so the ranges on the sample that follows may differ slightly from your own reports. (For sample results of a complete blood count [CBC] and other common blood chemistries, see figure A1.6.) The National Institutes of Health (NIH) provides an excellent resource for information about laboratory tests (and other diagnostic tests) at www.nlm.nih.gov/medlineplus/.

Look For: any H's (high) and L's (low). For each H or L value, note the blood element and how far out of the normal range the level is. Lab test results are often the most confusing for patients. To review details of your lab tests, make a post-hospitalization appointment with your PCP. Since factors such as age, weight, current medications, or chronic conditions may affect lab test results, the criteria for normal ranges may vary and not every H or L value is significant. Only your physician can make this determination.

Figure A1.6 Sample: Laboratory Blood Test Report

Complete Blood Count	Normal Range	Units	Results for Day One	Results for Day Two
Hemoglobin	12.0–16.0	g/dL	L10.9	L11.1
Hematocrit	36–40%	%	L 30.8	L30.9
WBC	4.5–13.0	Th/cmm	6.9	5.2
RBC	4.2–5.4	Mil/cmm	L 4.1	4.61
Platelet count	150–400	Th/cmm	233	230
Glucose	65–99	mg/dL	77	H 102
BUN	10–26	mg/dL	10	L 9
Sodium	135–148	mEq/L	139	139
Potassium	3.5–5.2	mEq/L	4	3.7
Chloride	96–109	mEq/L	107	104
CO2	22–33	mEq/L	23	23
Albumin	3.5–5	g/dL	4	4.6
Calcium	8.2–10.3	Mg/dL	9.8	9.7
Magnesium	1.8–2.4	Mg/dL	2	1.9

Electrocardiogram Report

Electrocardiogram (EKG or ECG) reports are unique because both the technical information (the EKG strip) and the interpretation from the cardiologist are stored in the medical record. With other diagnostic test results, only the interpretation is stored in the medical record while the technical testing medium (for example, the film) is stored elsewhere

The cardiologist usually dictates a few notes that later are transcribed at the top of the EKG strip. (See figure A1.7.) Non-medical professionals are probably not familiar with how to interpret an EKG strip. However, with a medical dictionary, you may be able to interpret the written portion of your EKG. As with any diagnostic report, keep in mind that your physician views your EKG (and any other reports) together with your entire health profile. Therefore, avoid taking the cardiologist's interpretation of your EKG as definitive without the input from your attending physician.

You need your primary care physician—or cardiologist—to be the buffer between you and your information, especially when you are not feeling well. When Joe was admitted to the hospital for chest pain and "premature ventricular contractures" (PVCs), my family and I were quite concerned until the cardiologist told him that 70 percent of the people on any hospital unit have at least one PVC a day. The cardiologist was able to put the test result into perspective for us.

Look For: the impression. On most EKGs, the terms following the word *impression* will be *normal* or *negative*, or list a diagnosis, such as atrial fibrillation or heart block. If the information surprises you, seek clarification from your primary care physician. The significance of the results, as with any diagnostic tests, can vary based on your specific circumstances.

Figure A1.7 Sample: EKG Report

Patient name: **Medical record #:** **Date:**

Test: Routine EKG
Sinus tachycardia with 1st degree AV block. Nonspecific T wave abnormality. Abnormal EKG.
Impression: Negative exam
Electronic signature of cardiologist

Radiology Reports

Radiology reports can be for x-rays of all parts of the body. In addition, radiology reports can include more complex testing like CT scans and MRIs. In every case, a qualified physician, usually a radiologist, reviews and interprets the films or computer images. The radiologist then dictates his impressions based on what he sees on the films or computer screen and on the patient's history. The radiology diagnostic process is a collaborative one. The radiologist's impression is only one component to arriving at a diagnosis. Your PCP and other physicians who treat you also participate in arriving at a final diagnosis.

During one conversation I had with a group of cardiothoracic surgeons, they said they read and interpreted the post-operative chest x-rays themselves for all of their surgical patients. They felt that they were the only ones who really knew exactly what was going on with their patients and had to consider everything that happened during surgery in making a diagnosis.

More than one physician reading your x-rays may actually produce the most accurate results. A teaching hospital in suburban Philadelphia provides a good example of a team approach that is beneficial to every patient. In this hospital, all the radiologists sit in the same room with their computers and films. As they review the test results, they may ask a colleague to take a look at the film if they want another opinion.

Look For: the impression. On most radiology reports, the terms following the word *impression* will be *normal* or *negative* or list a diagnosis, such as pneumonia or heart failure. If the information surprises you, seek clarification from your primary care physician. The significance of the results, as with any diagnostic tests, can vary based on your specific circumstances.

Figure A1.8 Sample: Radiology Reports

Patient name: **Medical record #:** **Date:**

Portable chest x-ray
Final report, interpreted by: Sally Smith, MD
Indication: shortness of breath
AP portable view of the chest reveals the lungs to be clear. The heart is not enlarged. No adenopathy or effusions are seen.
Impression: Lungs clear, normal x-ray of the chest
Electronic signature of radiologist

Patient name: **Medical record #:** **Date:**
Brain CT scan
Final report, interpreted by Sally Smith, MD
Indication: headache, blurring of vision
Findings: The brain is of normal size, configuration. Ventricles are normal in size and position. There is no hemorrhage. There is no hematoma.
Impression: Negative exam
Electronic signature of radiologist

Physician Orders (*Required*)

A physician order is required for every prescription medication, test, therapy, or intravenous therapy (IV) that your doctor wants you to have. Without an order, you will not receive the treatment or the test. Essentially, a physician order is the "go-ahead" from your doctor directing the nursing staff about the action to take in your case.

Over the past decade, hospitals have been transitioning to computerized physician order entry (CPOE). This process allows physicians to create orders electronically from any computer. The orders immediately alert the pharmacy, radiologist, and nurse. This process—which is one of the grading criteria for the quality review firm, The Leapfrog Group—is the most efficient way to process physician orders. In addition, quality reviews have proven that electronic orders are associated with fewer errors than manually written orders.

In hospitals with no CPOE system, physicians must write an order in your medical record, or dictate the order over the phone to a nurse who then must document the order in your record. After documenting the order, the nurse must alert the pharmacy, radiology department, or other department. The potential for error is greater and the manual order diminishes efficiency.

The typical physician order should include: date, what is being ordered, why it is being ordered, if a drug is ordered, the amount and frequency of the drug, and the physician's signature. (See figure A1.9.)

Look For: the medications and tests ordered for you. If you are confused or concerned, you can always ask your PCP during your next visit.

Figure A1.9 Sample: Physician Order

Physician Orders	
1/6/06	Lasix 40 mg, PO, Daily Sammy Smith, MD
1/7/06	Prevacid, 30 mg and ASA, 325 mg, Daily Sammy Smith, MD
1/7/06	Transfuse 2 U (units) of PRBC (packed red blood cells) Sammy Smith, MD

Medication Administration Report (*Required*)

The medication administration report is an important step in the treatment process. This report confirms that you got the medicine you were supposed to get, when you were supposed to get it. It documents what the physician ordered and what actually happened. There should be no discrepancies between the physician's orders and the medication administration report. The sample of a medication administration report in figure A1.10 shows the detail of events based on the physician orders from figure A1.9.

Look For: the medications you received. You will probably not find anything inconsistent with your care and treatment. If you are confused or concerned, you can always ask your PCP during your next visit.

Figure A1.10 Sample: Medication Administration Report

Medication or Fluid	Dose and Amount	Route	Frequency	Date	Time	Nurse signature
Lasix	40 mg	PO	Daily	1/6/06	900	XXX
Prevacid	30 mg	PO	Daily	4/29/05	1948	XXX
ASA	325 mg	PO	Daily	4/29/05	1948	XXX

Nursing Graphic Record (*Required*)

If you have ever been a patient in a hospital, you have likely noticed the nursing staff at your bedside, like clockwork, to take your temperature, blood pressure, and other vital signs. The nursing staff records all this information and graphs it out in a set of forms known as the *nursing graphic record.* These vital signs are generally taken three to four times in a 24-hour period. This process is yet another set of checks and balances built into the clinical care team process to ensure nothing abnormal about a patient occurs without the team's knowledge.

Look For: information that appears to be different from what you recall happened. This rarely happens, so you don't need to review the nursing graphic record in detail. However, if you notice anything unusual while scanning the data–such as a fever you were not aware of—you may want to put this on your list of questions for your next PCP visit.

Discharge Summary (*Required, Key Report*)

Your hospital discharge summary, about one or two pages in length, is the final document completed in your medical record. It summarizes everything that happened during your hospitalization. Although it may be handwritten, most discharge summaries are dictated and transcribed. Because your physician creates the discharge summary *after* your discharge, healthcare providers will refer to it for any future care you may receive in the same hospital. In addition, if you transfer from the hospital to another location, such as a nursing home, the hospital forwards your discharge summary to that facility. Depending on hospital procedures, your discharge summary may not be filed on your medical records until several days after you leave the hospital.

State and federal laws, as well as accrediting agencies such as the Joint Commission on Accreditation of Healthcare Organizations, have minimum requirements for the contents of a discharge summary. The discharge summary in the figure below is an example of the type of information that physicians may include in hospital discharge summaries.

Look For: several pieces of important information. Because this is such a key document it is probably a good idea to read the entire report. However, you can prioritize the information in the following manner. First, look for your final (or discharge) diagnosis, usually near the beginning of the report. Make sure it matches what your doctor told you. Second, review discharge medications for consistency with your current regimen. Third, read the hospital course to confirm what you recall. Rather than an exercise in identifying information that you did not know, you can view this as a way to learn more about what happened while you were a patient. As with any of the information in your record, if you are surprised or concerned, ask your PCP for clarification.

Figure A1.11 Sample: Discharge Summary

Patient name: **Medical record #:**
Sex/Age: Female/94 years
Admission date: 04/20/05
Discharge date: 04/25/05
Attending physician:
Chief complaint: Back pain, disequilibrium and change in mental status
History of present illness: This is a 94-year-old white female resident of an assisted-living facility who apparently fell on 4/17/01. There was no recorded injury. She fell again today on 4/20/01 while showering. She injured her back. Thereafter she was sent to the emergency room, where her temperature was verbally reported as 102 degrees, though no written documentation of this could be found. The patient became confused while there, though she had been given Vicodin in the emergency room. Her daughter was in attendance and also noted a 4-week history of increased shuffling of her gait.

Past medical history:
1. Osteoporosis.
2. Anemia.
3. Atrial fibrillation status post pacemaker.
4. Hypertension.
5. History of DVT and pulmonary embolism requiring chronic anticoagulation.

Discharge diagnoses:
1. CHF (congestive heart failure)
2 Fluid overload

Family history: Noncontributory
Social history: The patient is a widow. She is Catholic and lives in an assisted-living facility. She is a nonsmoker and a nondrinker.
Medications:
Zyprexa 2.5 mg daily.; Colace 100 mg daily. Fosamax 5 mg daily; Coumadin 3 mg daily.; Protonix 40 mg daily.; Ferrous sulfate 325 mg daily.; Calcium 500 mg daily.; Synthroid 0.05 mg daily.

Figure A1.11 Sample: Discharge Summary (Continued)

Physical examination: Admission recorded temperature could not be found. Pulse was 84, respiratory rate 14, blood pressure 136/82. The patient's 0_2 saturation on room air was 95%. On 2 liters by nasal cannula, it was 100%. The patient did appear somewhat pale. She was nontoxic and complained of back pain. Her skin revealed no rashes. There was scattered bruising. The HEENT examination was negative. Neck: Supple. Chest revealed right basilar rales. Heart: Regular rate and rhythm without murmurs. The ankles revealed 1+ nonpitting edema. There was no obvious external trauma to the back, but there was pain of both upper and lower back on palpation and with movement. The patient was alert and oriented X 3. Her neurologic examination showed no focal deficits.

Hospital course: The patient was admitted and treated for fluid overload and back pain. X-rays of her back showed no new fractures, and an MRI was deferred secondary to presence of a pacemaker. The patient's atrial fibrillation remained stable, and there was no exacerbation of her dizziness. A cardiology consult was requested, and no further testing or changes in treatment were recommended. Prednisone dose was increased to 7.5 mg per day while her Tylenol No. 3 was able to be decreased. Eventually she did get a consult from the pain management clinic. Please refer to their note for their specific recommendations.
The patient's history of hypertension was noted, but her blood pressures remained stable. Synthroid was increased due to a somewhat abnormal thyroid-stimulating hormone. Her anticoagulation was easily controlled. Physical therapy was helpful, and on 04/25/01 the patient was transferred for further nursing care to a skilled nursing facility.

Medications on discharge: Discharge medications according to the medication included calcium carbonate 1200 mg daily, amiodarone 200 mg daily, prednisone 7.5 mg daily, digoxin 0.125 mg daily, Synthroid 0.075 mg daily, Metamucil one pack daily, Zebeta 5 mg daily, Fosamax 5 mg.

PREVIOUS HOSPITAL RECORDS

If you were admitted to the hospital, you may be wondering about your medical records from prior admissions and what happened to them. The hospital makes available all your medical records from prior admissions to that hospital to your current healthcare treatment team. You can imagine that this process is much more efficient if records are electronic or at least imaged so they can be stored electronically. Even as recently as 2006, I visited hospitals where only the original, hard copy of the patient's medical records were stored on the same unit as the patient during the current admission. This storage practice often wreaked havoc when a clinician needed to find one report or piece of information that was buried somewhere in the hundreds of pages in patient's record from his last admission. To be sure that all of your past records are available should you ever require hospitalization at the hospital of your choice, call the health information management department (also called the medical record department) or nursing department for confirmation of their process.

EMERGENCY ROOM RECORD

Every hospital has a very specific format for records used in its emergency room (ER). However, for the most part, hospital ERs will contain a brief history and physical, some progress notes, and many test results. In an emergent situation, usually the analysis of many tests is required. The test results become a part of your emergency record in this case.

The ER physician must document your final diagnosis before discharging you from the ER. This diagnosis will be part of your ER record. If your clinician admits you from the ER into the inpatient hospital, your ER record becomes part of your inpatient record. It is important for the physicians treating you as an inpatient, to have access to everything that happened in the ER. Making your ER record a physical part of the inpatient record ensures that your treatment team will have access to all of the information they need to provide you with the best care.

Look For: the diagnosis or impression at the time you were discharged from the ER. The ER record usually lists this information at the bottom of the first page. If the ER physician discharged you from the ER to home and you have any questions about your record, ask your PCP for clarification. It may be difficult to communicate directly with the ER physician on this issue. If you were admitted from the ER into the hospital, don't be surprised if the diagnosis or impression is different from your final diagnosis or impression on your discharge summary. It is quite common for the ER documentation to differ since the ER physician will not have access to test results or additional exams for you over the next few days.

AMBULATORY SURGERY UNIT RECORD

Similar to ER records, ambulatory surgery unit (ASU) records are more compact than inpatient hospital records. You can understand the ASU record by referencing the documents described for the inpatient hospital stay. The ASU record generally includes an H&P (usually created in the physician's office prior to your surgery); progress notes from the surgeon, anesthesiologist, and nurses; a formal surgical report; a pathology report if any tissue is removed; preoperative and postoperative anesthesia forms; physician orders; and a discharge order. Overall, the ASU record is compact and focused, just like the ASU procedure.

Look For: the preoperative and postoperative diagnosis documented on your surgical report. If the surgeon removed any tissue, look at the pathological or microscopic diagnosis. If you have questions, ask your surgeon or PCP for clarification.

MATERNITY AND NEWBORN RECORDS

Maternity and newborn records have their own specific formats. The maternity record is generally divided into three parts: the antepartum (before birth) record, the labor and delivery record, and the postpartum (after birth) record. The antepartum record is an H&P specific to the obstetrics patient. The labor and delivery record documents all activities during labor and delivery. The postpartum record logs the mother's condition after delivering the baby.

Newborn babies have their own medical records, separate from the mother and specific to the newborn. The record includes an initial profile, or detailed physical. In addition, it contains a flow sheet that collects all data from the nursery stay.

The maternity and newborn records are unique from every other patient record in the hospital. For normal deliveries, the mother and the baby are both healthy, not acutely ill. Different types of information are collected on them than patients who are sick. This is a significant part of the reason that mothers and babies need their own, specifically formatted medical records.

WHAT HAPPENS TO THE FILMS AND THE COMPUTER PRINTOUTS FROM MY TESTS?

In the hospital, you may have tests using media that typically are not included in the traditional patient record, such as films, computer readings, and echograms.

In the most technically advanced hospitals, all of your health information is electronic and can all be accessed from one portal. This medical record storage practice is similar to what many banks use. You can look online to see your balances, even scanned copies of checks. Unfortunately, most hospitals have not yet arrived at this level of information processing. In most hospitals, only the radiology department can access the films or computer media electronically. You can determine what level of detail is accessible at your hospital by asking the following questions:

- **Does the hospital have an online system to access my medical record?** As mentioned previously, Beth Israel Deaconess Medical Center in Boston and the Cleveland Clinic have full electronic patient record systems. Medical records are available to patients and all healthcare providers in the system via the Internet. An ideal methodology for accessing your information, this process hopefully will be available in the future for all hospitals. You may be able to obtain copies of your information (including films and computer printouts) on one CD.

- **Will copies of my records be provided to me in hard copy only?** This is the lowest level of operating. Unfortunately, it is still the most common for most hospitals. If you need to obtain your records in hard copy, chances are the information backing up your medical record (like x-ray films) is not integrated into your record. Therefore, you will probably need to make separate requests for each film from each department. Chapter 6 addresses this process in more detail.

Appendix 2 Raw Food and Nutrition Resources

Raw food experts are a small, dedicated group of people. I have compiled a list of the resources I use and have found helpful in the past few years. The number of credible resources appears to be growing. I will update this list on the *www.7stepshealth.com* website as appropriate.

PLACES TO GO

Arnold's Way (www.arnoldsway.com)
Arnold's Way is a raw and organic café owned and managed by Arnold Kauffman in Lansdale, Pennsylvania. In addition to his own menu of raw meals that you can find on his website, Arnold also sells raw food ingredients, cooking supplies, books, DVDs and rebounders. If you don't live in eastern Pennsylvania, you can see Arnold on YouTube. He has recorded over 30 videos on YouTube.com on raw food preparation and juicing. Arnold has also included many stories of individuals who have reversed very serious disorders through a raw food diet.

Awesomefoods (www.awesomefoods.com)
Awesomefoods is a wholesale and internet raw food service. I order freshly prepared raw food meals that are delivered directly to my door a few times a month from Awesomefoods. There is an extra fee for overnite delivery and the insulated container, but the quality and consistency of the food is worth the expense. Bruce & Marsha Weinstein, from the suburbs of Philadelphia, are the creators of Awesome Foods.

They make mostly food that is unsweetened, however, their sweet prepared foods are made with agave nectar as the sweetner. Agave nectar is very low on the glycemic index. This means that it does not cause a strong insulin reaction, unlike dates and honey, which are very high on the glycemic index.

High Vibe (www.highvibe.com)
High Vibe is a raw retail grocery store and an internet site owned and managed by Robert Dagger, a nutritionist in New York City. The store and site have an excellent selection of raw food ingredients and snacks. The store and site also stock a comprehensive supply of raw food books, organic beauty products and other resources. Bob is a nutritional coach and provides one-on-one counseling in the areas of fasting, cleansing, anti-aging, and increasing energy.

Pure Food and Wine (www.purefoodandwine.com)
Pure Food and Wine is a gourmet food restaurant in New York City that can make the transition from a typical American diet to an all raw diet easy for almost anyone. The restaurant is owned and managed by Sarma Melingailis and serves dinner every night of the week. One Lucky Duck (oneluckyduck.com) is the restaurant's take-away and Internet site tucked right around the corner. There, you can enjoy an amazingly indulgent bowl of ice cream (made with coconut meat and agave), chocolate pudding, or a myriad of other desserts, and not feel guilty.

The Ann Wigmore® Foundation (*www.wigmore.org*)
Anne Wigmore (1909 – 1994), was one of the first raw and natural food proponents to share her knowledge and methods with the public through her books, educational programs and the Hippocrates Institute. Today, her work is carried on by her foundation in San Fidel, New Mexico. You can spend a week or two at the foundation and become certified in the Ann Wigmore methods. She was a big proponent of daily wheatgrass, one of the certification areas at the foundation. In addition to educational opportunities at the foundation, you can read Wigmore's books, still in print today. They include: *The Hippocrates Diet and Health Program, The Wheatgrass Book, Recipes for Longer*

Life, The Sprouting Book, and *Be Your Own Doctor: A Positive Guide to Natural Living.*

BOOKS TO READ

Colin T. Campbell, PhD *(www.thechinastudy.com)* Dr. Campbell has studied the effects of nutritional status on long term health. He wrote *The China Study: Startling Implications for Diet, Weight Loss and Long-term Health*, one of the most comprehensive studies of health and nutrition ever conducted. The book discusses the connection between diet and heart disease, obesity, diabetes, common cancers, autoimmune disease.

Gabriel Cousens, MD, MD (H)*(www.gabrielcousens.com)* Dr. Cousens is a licensed M.D., licensed M.D.(H) (homeopathic physician), Diplomate of the American Board of Holistic Medicine, Diplomate in Ayurvedic Medicine, psychiatrist and family therapist, and creator of Whole Person Healing (WHP) 3-day personal holistic health evaluation. His book *Conscious Eating* is a classic 800-page nutritional tome.

Joel Furhman, MD *(www.drfuhrman.com)* Because Dr. Furhman is an MD who takes a holistic approach to treating patients, he is a featured physician in Chapter 14 of this book. He has published many books that contain principles of a raw food diet including: *Eat to Live: The Revolutionary Formula for Fitness and Sustained Weight Loss, Disease-Proof Your Child: Feeding Kids Right,* and *Fasting and Eating for Health: A Medical Doctor's Program for Conquering Disease.*

Natalia Rose *(www.therawfooddetoxdiet.com*) Natalia Rose is a dietician with a private practice in New York City. In her books, she presents a mainstream approach to transitioning to a raw diet. She also provides some good recipes for both raw foodists and main stream healthy eaters. Her books include *Raw Food: Life Force Energy* and

The Raw Food Detox Diet: A Five-Step Plan for Vibrant Health and Maximum Weight Loss.

Joshua Rosenthal *(www.integrativenutrition.com)* Joshua Rosenthal is a nutritional counselor and founder of the Institute for Integrative Nutrition. His book, *Integrative Nutrition: Feed Your Hunger for Health & Happiness* serves as the keystone for a comprehensive training and nutritional certification program held in conjunction with Columbia University. The philosophy of the institute, is that each individual needs a dietary plan developed specifically for them.

Jeremy Saffron *(www.lovingfoods.com)* Jeremy Saffron has written two books, *The Raw Truth* and the *Raw Foods Resource* that are good resources for anyone interested in learning more about raw foods, where to find them, and how to make them.

Dr. N.W. Walker N.D. Walker, along with (but separate from) Anne Wigmore, was one of the first individuals to practice principles of raw food and vegetable juicing for good health. It is unclear how old he was when he died, but most agree he was well over 100. In 1949, he wrote *Become Younger* and in 1972, he wrote *Vibrant Health (*the updated version of *Become Younger),* still sold today. The books describe vegetable juicing and fasting.

David Wolfe *(www.davidwolfe.com)* David Wolfe is thought by many to be an authority on raw chocolate, raw-food nutrition, superfoods, and herbal healing. He wrote *Eating for Beauty, The Sunfood Diet Success System* and *Naked Chocolate.*

Appendix 3 Medical Terminology and Coding Resources

The following are the some of the best Internet-based medical terminology and coding resources available. Some programs provide a brief overview of the topics, while others have a more in depth approach. You can tell by the price and the length of the program how comprehensive the courses are. If you are interested in classroom learning, you can probably find courses at your local community college. In addition, if you are interested in finding out more about a degree (A.S. or B.S) and credential (RHIT or RHIA) in health information, the AHIMA website (*www.ahima.org*) contains a complete listing of all credentialed programs in the U.S.

MEDICAL TERMINOLOGY

Corexel *(www.corexel.com)* Corexcel is an Internet-based training firm that provides accredited programs. Their medical terminology program is comprehensive, priced between $265 and $395, depending on whether you purchase the text book and one-year access to their Internet resource. They claim that students can submit their coursework to colleges for consideration for college-level credits.

Universalclass (*universalclass.com)* Universalclass is an Internet-based training firm that provides focused programs for continuing education in many areas including medical terminology (Medical Terminology 101), Anatomy and Physiology, and Medical Coding and Billing. Courses range $30 to $55.

CODING

American Health Information Management Association *(www.ahima.org)* AHIMA is my number one recommendation for ICD-9-CM coding training. The association provides a myriad of on-line training programs on anatomy and physiology, coding, and other health information related topics. The courses range in price from $175 to $300 and, because of the shorter, focused courses, allow the student a lot of flexibility. You can use the AHIMA courses to try out different topic areas and determine if you have an interest in delving further into the learning process. You can access the course listings from the "Professional Development" tab on the AHIMA homepage.

American Academy of Professional Coders *(www.aapc.org)* AAPC is my number one recommendation for CPT coding training. The association offers an independent study program that ranges from about $1,200 to about $1,800, depending on whether you are a member or chose to train for physician office or hospital-based training. The AAPC does not allow for much flexibility since you must register and pay for the entire program prior to beginning the coursework. You should know before you begin that this is a profession you are committed to.

Meet the Author

Ruthann Russo, PhD, JD, MPH, RHIT, is an expert in health information management and policy. A presenter, teacher, and a self-described "serial entrepreneur," she has more than 20 years of experience working in and advising healthcare organizations. Dr. Russo designed the revolutionary HealthMap™ program, created to empower healthcare consumers. A steadfast believer in improving the quality of healthcare, she has personally instructed over 3,000 physicians across the country including doctors at hospitals affiliated with the University of Pennsylvania, University of Maryland and Johns Hopkins University. She is the author of five books on how physicians should document in their patient's medical records and how to make sure medical bills are correct.

Dr. Russo is a partner in the Bethlehem, Pennsylvania-based law firm of Russo & Russo and serves as a Managing Director with Navigant Consulting. A lifelong learner, passionate about the field of healthcare and about helping others, she is a graduate of Dickinson College, American University's Washington College of Law, Robert Wood Johnson Medical School's program in public health, and Touro University.

Ruthann and her husband, Joe, have been married for 25 years. Together, they have two children, Emmalea and John, and a Chihuahua named Lola. The family splits their time between homes and offices in both Center Valley, Pennsylvania and New York City. For more information visit *www.RuthannRusso.com.*